AṢṬADAḶA YOGAMĀLĀ

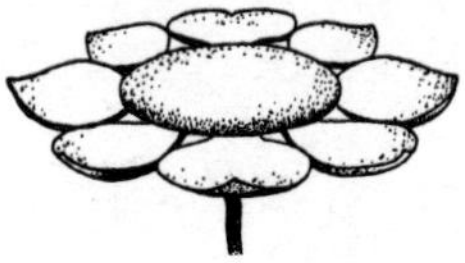

AṢṬADAḶA YOGAMĀLĀ

(COLLECTED WORKS)

B.K.S. IYENGAR

Volume 2

ARTICLES, LECTURES, MESSAGES

ALLIED PUBLISHERS PVT. LIMITED
NEW DELHI MUMBAI KOLKATA CHENNAI NAGPUR
AHMEDABAD BANGALORE HYDERABAD LUCKNOW

ALLIED PUBLISHERS PRIVATE LIMITED

Regd. Off. : 15 J.N. Heredia Marg, Ballard Estate, Mumbai 400001
Prarthna Flats (2nd Floor), Navrangpura, Ahmedabad 380009
3-2-844/6 & 7 Kachiguda Station Road, Hyderabad 500027
16-A Ashok Marg, Patiala House, Lucknow 226001
5th Main Road, Gandhinagar, Bangalore 560009
1/13-14 Asaf Ali Road, New Delhi 110002
17 Chittaranjan Avenue, Kolkata 700072
81 Hill Road, Ramnagar, Nagpur 440010
751 Anna Salai, Chennai 600002

First Published 2001
Reprinted 2004

ISBN : 81-7764-178-6

Cover design : The Author
Artwork : S.M. Waugh

Published by Sunil Sachdev and printed by Ravi Sachdev at Allied Publishers Private Limited, Printing Division, A-104 Mayapuri Phase II, New Delhi 110064

8/2004

Invocatory Prayers

ॐ

Yogena cittasya padena vācāṁ
Malaṁ śarīrasyaca vaidyakena
Yopākarottaṁ pravaraṁ munīnāṁ
Patañjaliṁ prāñjalirānato'smi
Ābāhu puruṣākāraṁ
Śaṅkha cakrāsi dhāriṇaṁ
Sahasra śirasaṁ śvetaṁ
Praṇamāmi Patañjaliṁ

I bow before the noblest of sages Patañjali, who gave yoga for serenity and sanctity of mind, grammar for clarity and purity of speech and medicine for pure, perfect health.

I prostrate before Patañjali who is crowned with a thousand headed cobra, an incarnation of Ādiśeṣa (Anañta) whose upper body has a human form, holding the conch in one arm, disk in the second, a sword of wisdom to vanquish nescience in the third and blessing humanity from the fourth arm, while his lower body is like a coiled snake.

Yastyaktvā rūpamādyaṁ prabhavati jagato'nekadhānugrahāya
Prakṣīṇakleśarāśirviṣamaviṣadharo'nekavaktrāḥ subhogī
Sarvajñānaprasūtirbhujagaparikaraḥ prītaye yasya nityaṁ
Devohīṣaḥ savovyātsitavimalatanuryogado yogayuktaḥ

I prostrate before Lord Ādiśeṣa, who manifested himself on Earth as Patañjali to grace the human race in health and harmony,

I salute Lord Ādiśeṣa of the myriad serpent heads and mouths carrying noxious poisons, discarding which he came to Earth as a single headed Patañjali in order to eradicate ignorance and vanquish sorrow.

I pay my obeisance to him, repository of all knowledge, amidst his attendant retinue.

I pray to the Lord whose primordial form shines with peace and white effulgence, pristine in body, a master of yoga, who bestows on all his yogic light to enable mankind to rest in the house of the immortal Soul.

BY THE AUTHOR

This volume of *Aṣṭadaḷa Yogamālā* published by Allied Publishers, Delhi, is the second volume of the first part of the "Collected Works" of Yogācārya B.K.S. Iyengar. Each part comprises several volumes which are arranged according to the following scheme:

Articles
Interviews
Question and Answer Sessions
Techniques of *Āsanas, Prāṇāyāma, Dhyāna* and *Śavāsana*
Therapeutic Applications of Yoga
Garland of Aphorisms and Thoughts
General Index and Analytical Dictionary
Addendum

Also by the Same Author

Light on Yoga
Light on Prāṇāyāma
Concise Light on Yoga
Art of Yoga
Tree of Yoga
Light on the Yoga Sūtras of Patañjali
The Illustrated Light on Yoga
Yoga Ek Kalpataru (Marathi)
Arogyayoga (Marathi)
Light on Aṣṭāṇga Yoga
Aṣṭadaḷa Yogamālā (Vol 1)
Yoga The Path To Holistic Health

Also on *Iyengar Yoga*

Body the Shrine, Yoga Thy Light
70 Glorious Years
Iyengar His Life and Work
Yogapushpanjali
Yogadhārā

CONTENTS

SECTION III – MY VISION OF YOGA

LIST OF TABLES

LIST OF PLATES

Acknowledgements

The author wishes to extend his grateful thanks to the following people for their assistance, enthusiasm and time which they willingly gave to the publication of this volume.

Smt. Geeta S. Iyengar – For her valuable assistance in researching, checking and overseeing the editing of the works.
Faeq Biria – For editing, as well as overseeing the project.
Patxi Lizardi – Edtorial work, project co-ordination.
John Evans – Editing Guruji's work with understanding into cohesive English.
Stephanie Quirk – Editing assistance, Book design and layout
Raya Dhavale – Layout of the tables and work on preparing the plates
S.M. Wagh – Line drawings and illustrations
Ashok Tamhankar – Illustrations of Indian deities
Devki Desai – Calligraphy
Soni Studios – for reproduction of photos
Mr. Kokate – back cover artwork
Surojit Banerjee – Final editing work.
Allied Publishers (New Delhi).

DEDICATION

RAMAA – THE LIGHT ON MY YOGA*

This volume will remain as an unfinished volume, if I fail to speak of my wife Ramaa to whom I am ever grateful as the source of my devotion to yoga. First of all I am grateful to my mother who gave me birth and my father who nurtured me till I was eight and a half years old and then to my *Gurujī*, who planted the seed of yoga. But it was my wife alone who saw that I continue my *sādhanā* uninterrupted, maintaining the same zeal to this day. Hence my life's journey is incomplete without reference and reverence to my wife Ramaamaṇi.

My wife, Ramaa was born on November 2nd, 1927, at Anekal, 20km away from Bangalore. She was the ninth child of her parents as I am the eleventh of my parents. Like my father, her father was a schoolteacher at a primary school. Though I am told that she was a brilliant student in her school, she could not study beyond the fourth standard.

Our marriage took place on July 9th, 1943, when Ramaa was sixteen and I was twenty-four. After four months of marriage we started our life in Pune in November 1943, when I got a contract to teach yoga in Perugate, at Bhave School for girls for a period of six months. When she arrived in Pune she had only her *mangalsūtra*, the wedding necklace tied by me at the time of our marriage and nothing else. I had nothing in my possession to make her live with ease or comfort. When her date of arrival was fixed I borrowed an aluminium vessel and two plates from Motee (the proprietor and printer of Motee press), from where Maharashtra Herald is Published now, who was my student. The first fire at my home, which then became our home, was lit in a stove that was also borrowed from him and his family members.

With contentment Ramaa shared equally in my hard struggle to maintain ourselves. We continued our life each day with what little we could get and remained unperturbed by our unsolved economic problems, which remained for several years.

Each day I used to get up very early in the morning for my yoga practices. Ramaa too was up at the same time to prepare coffee, which was the only nourishment for both of us.

---

* Courtesy Timeless Publishers, U.S.A.

Though the word "yoga" was unknown to her she used to observe my practices with interest and without any interference. As she was too young she did not know what yoga stood for, and she never ventured to ask what I learned or what yoga teaching was meant for. However, as time went by, she evinced keen interest in practising the art with me. I started teaching her daily while practising myself and she became not only my pupil, but a partner in my profession. As she made progress in her practices, I taught her how to assist me, for me to improve my methods. This in turn helped me to excavate the potentials of the art hidden deep in my heart. My instructions and guidance to her to help me during practice made her to become a good teacher. This enabled her to independently teach the lady students from my group. As our family responsibilities increased and her attention towards the welfare of the children took much of her time, she could not take to teaching on a regular basis, but continued whenever the time was available.

Whenever she found time, she not only practised yoga for herself, but she helped me too. She was always ready to assist and adjust in different *āsana* so that I could master them. Besides all this, she would utilise any available time for her students.

As I had already mentioned earlier[1], we both had dreams the same night in 1946. The dreams came true which indicated bright days ahead. People started enquiring for lessons. With the blessing of God fortune favoured us, our domestic life became secure and our suffering decreased, and by His grace our wants were fulfilled. We had not imagined that our life at home as well as in the field of yoga would make such good and great progress. As time passed we slowly understood each other, and lived happily, mentally and spiritually. We adored each other.

With a strong feeling of togetherness we discussed with each other and worked out that her interest in life must be to take care of our children, and mine to pursue my practices and teaching without any hindrance so that life may move in smoothness. I was everything to her and she was everything to me. We shared the love of the divine through each other. Ramaa was the personification of patience and magnanimity. She was simple, generous and unostentatious. She was kind to one and all. She had great forbearance even towards people who did not wish her well. She was quiet, serene, peaceful and remained unruffled in adverse circumstances. She took everything in her stride coolly. With love, joy and devotion she looked after those who came to her for help or advice. She served all with friendliness and compassion, extending to them both her hands.

---

1 Volume 1, page 19.

I remember how the late Dr. N.B. Parulekar, proprietor and editor of *Sakal*, Pune, compared her to Sharadadevi, wife of Shri Ramakrishna Paramahamsa. How true his words were, as I realise more and more recollecting her majesty in looks and nobility of expression.

Hospitality, kindness and self-sacrifice were very much in her blood. She treated her maidservants and sweepers of the street as if they were members of her family. During festival days, she used to reserve their share of food, lest they should be overlooked. Her feelings and thoughts were virtuous and she never wished ill of anyone. Such was her disposition. Her love was unique, she had a heart full of compassion and people called her *Ammā*, which means "mother". Her physique was big, her mind great and her soul noble.

She was philosophical in her thoughts and philanthropic in her dealings and never brooded over her past discomforts. She betrayed no sorrow in times of distress nor felt jubilant at her affluence.

Ramaa was an accomplished vocalist and while cooking or combing the children's hair, would sing quite a large number of songs composed by Purandaradasa and Thyagaraja. She had a great liking for both Karnataka as well as that of Hindustani classical music. This created in her children a love and interest in music. She was an excellent cook. She was able to prepare a number of dainty dishes at home even for large parties as well as on occasions like festivals and gatherings. These housewifely skills created a unique combination of oneness in the family and children.

I do not recollect any occasion of misunderstanding between us. My impatient nature – speed, quick decisions and impulsiveness – was counterbalanced by her soft voice and the dignified but quiet expression in her eyes. We lived without conflicts as if our two souls were one. She was never harsh to the children; yet she commanded high respect and moulded them proficiently cultivating right discipline in them.

Ramaa suddenly became weak after performing the *Bhūmi Pūjā* on land purchased by us for our proposed new house on January 25th, 1973.

On Friday January 26th, 1973, I had her admitted to a nursing home so that she might rest and recover from fatigue. I was with her for a few hours. As she showed the signs of recovery, I came home, since I had to go to Bombay the next day.

I had left for Mumbai to conduct yoga classes as usual. On the Sunday, January 28th, 1973, at four o'clock in the morning, my pupils, Shri Madhu Tijoriwala and Shri Barzo Taraporewala came to the hotel where I was staying. I had been restless the whole night and I was already up when they knocked at the door. They asked me to proceed to Pune, saying that they had a message from my son that my wife was in a serious condition. As I had seen her the previous day, I did not assess the gravity of the situation and told them that I would finish the Sunday class and then proceed to Pune. My pupils insisted upon my returning forthwith, accompanied by them. I understood the situation although I could not express my fears about the survival of my wife. They hesitated to put the fact to me, with a view to giving me the shocking news as late as possible. On the way, Smt. Freny Motivala, a third pupil, joined us to go to Pune. However I was thoughtful and prepared for any eventuality.

When we were about to reach Pune, my pupils asked me whether we should go home or proceed to the nursing home. I replied that if she was alive, she would be in the nursing home, or otherwise at our residence. Then they broke the news that she was no more. Then I said that my children must have brought her body home and so I advised them to drive straight to the house, which we reached at 6:30 a.m. As I entered the premises, I saw many of my pupils and people and knew that everything was over. With coolness, I comforted my weeping children, telling them not to weep for their mother, who was a pious soul. From then on I was both their mother and father.

As the news spread that Ramaa embraced mother earth, people from all walks of life, known and unknown, thronged the house, as if it were a temple, to pay their homage to the departed soul. Pupils who had come from South Africa for lessons witnessed her body being laid to rest. Messages poured in from all parts of the world, expressing their grief and sorrow. She embraced death with the same graceful serenity with which she had lived – with patience and forbearance.

What a noble lady my wife was! She knew her death was approaching. That night my two daughters, Sunita and Suchita, had a sitar recital. She did not want to disturb them nor had she stopped me from going to Bombay. Noticing the time when the concert would be over, she asked the doctors at the nursing home to phone Dr. Pabalkar, our neighbour, who had a telephone. It was three o'clock in the morning when my son, Prashant and daughter, Geeta, went to see her. She asked them to go home immediately and to light up the lamps to our deity and to come back soon with the other children. All the children could not go, as no transport was available at that odd hour. She just asked them why they did not bring the other children. She said to Prashant and Geeta that her duties and responsibilities were coming to an end and she would be departing in a few moments. She did not want to die on the bed of the nursing home. She wanted to be closer to mother earth and lie on a carpet on the floor but the doctors did not permit it. So she sat reclining. Placing the children's palms in hers, she blessed them and told them to bear the future responsibilities on their own. She breathed her last like a great tapasvini who knew of her death beforehand. Her soul merged with the Universal Divine Soul.

The *Bhūmi Pūjā* foundation which Ramaa had laid, later became the famous Ramaamaṇi Iyengar Memorial Yoga Institute. It was built in her memory by raising donations from friends, pupils and admirers as a token of their love and affection.

As long as she was alive, I lived a carefree life as she managed the house, the children and myself. She left me completely free to devote my time to the practice and teaching of yoga. Since her passing away I have become a householder and now my children are substantially bearing the burden of the house. While she was alive I was married to Ramaa and yoga and now yoga alone remained in my life. I am never separated from her for she is always in my heart.

Today being the twenty-eighth anniversary of her death, I pray the Lord to grace her wherever she exists, to grace this Institute, so that her soul sees its growth as the centre of nourishment to millions of students of yoga throughout the world.

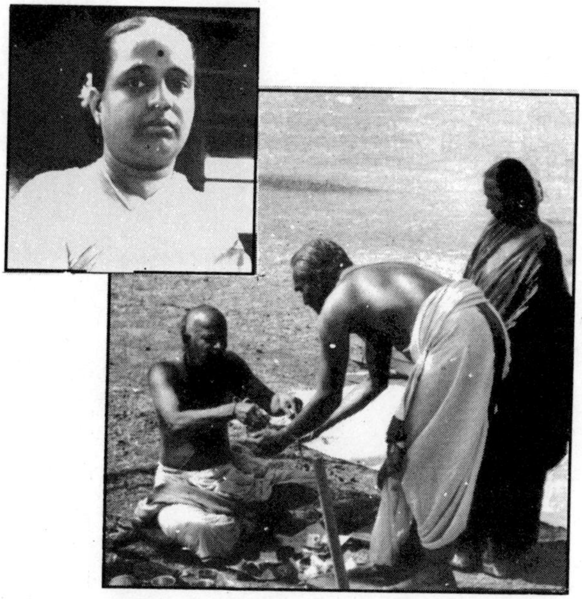

Plate n. 1 – Gurujī and Ramaa Performing the *Bhūmi Pūjā*

PREFACE

All mankind lives unwittingly within the truth of yoga. Yoga is one. Yet we find ourselves in the position of having to portion it up, to compartmentalise it, to search to grasp its mechanisms. Why? It is because we all misapprehend reality *(avidyā)*. Not just partially, but totally. Only the supreme *bhaktan* is capable, with one peerless gesture of surrender, of turning the Universe inside out. We simply cannot. We are like that man who has put on his shirt inside out and back to front. The only way he can rectify his error is to take it off, work out how it should be and start again. Through yoga, we take off the shirt of our ignorance, study it and put it back on correctly, as a shirt of knowledge. To do this (like the man turning out the body and each sleeve of his shirt separately), we examine each petal of yoga as if it were separate. Just as our man knows that there is only one shirt, we should not forget that there is only one yoga.

Though it is now some time since my own practice reached its maturity, the flow of my ideas on how best to present and communicate this subject so dear to my heart, never ceases to evolve. For this reason, although the following chapters remain substantially the same as when they were first delivered as talks around the world, I have nevertheless amended, amplified or cut as I deem necessary in order to transmit my teaching as clearly and precisely as I am currently able. Some slips of the tongue have been removed, as have some repetitions, but I have allowed some of the latter to remain so that each chapter should stand alone, comprehensible within itself without endless cross-referencing.

Because so much of this book concerns *āsana* and *prāṇāyāma,* the two aspects of yoga with which my name is especially associated, I am naturally trepidatious lest this volume should fail to do justice to a subject which is at the core of my life's work. I am perhaps equally anxious lest the emphasis that my teaching has placed on *āsana* and *prāṇāyāma* be interpreted by some as intending to exclude or minimise other limbs of the great body of yoga. On the contrary, the very heart of my teaching has been an attempt to demonstrate in the most practical and useful way how any perfected part of yoga contains the essence of every other aspect, the macrocosm inside the microcosm or the universal couched within the particular, like the genetic code which lies in the DNA of each of our cells.

It was the circumstances of my life that pitched me headlong into the practice of *āsana*, and a tumultuous time I had of it. For me, peace has only been achieved out of life's turmoil. Initially I had no special aptitude for *āsana*. It was by no means love at first sight. But I did persevere, and love of this subject was granted me. So it was that over the years I discovered that in the bubbling cauldron of *āsana*, its practice, perfection, presentation and its teaching, is to be found the entirety of yoga.

Others may enter yoga by different portals. Through the inspired perfection of two aspects of *yama, satya* and *ahiṁsā*, Gandhiji realised the whole of yoga, and in doing so changed the world. The narrow door through which Sri Aurobindo passed was a burning desire for flawless, exalted knowledge. How many of us can, unaided, emulate such giants as these? Trying and failing we are forced either to abandon the attempt, or to act out a life of hypocritical pretence, paying lip service to ideals we cannot match.

The gateway of *āsana* is broad and all may pass through it. Its benefits are immediate, tangible and visible. Though hard, it is accessible, sustainable, motivational and real. The juxtaposition of apparent diversity and underlying oneness, the conundrum at the core of the universe, is most acutely experienced in *āsana*, and as Patañjali so clearly says (II.48), the beauty of *āsana* is its ability to place us beyond the harm of dualities.

Even by his standards, Patañjali's words on *āsana* are concise, in fact lapidary. And, like stones, they form the plinth on which yoga practice is founded. A plinth must above all be firm and stable *(sthira)* and this is the very first word he uses to describe *āsana*. From this base begin the techniques of yogic absorption. At their culmination, he says, when there is joy, effortless effort and all dualities are reconciled, then *yama* and *niyama, prāṇāyāma, pratyāhāra, dhāraṇā* and *dhyāna*, inevitably, must be present.

For most students the grandeur of this statement, however logical, is difficult to grasp and far more so to bring to realisation.

Let me illustrate from my own practice. Look at the two photographs of *Parivṛttaikapāda Śīrṣāsana* and *Pārśva Śīrṣāsana*, some were taken when my physical prowess was at its height, the second when my yogic practice was mature. It is axiomatic that the shape of the self *(svarūpa)* is identical to the shape of the body. Keep in mind that yoga is composed of practice *(abhyāsa)* and renunciation or detachment *(vairāgya)*. Think of *abhyāsa* as a centrifugal force, like a flower opening or a merry-go-round, and *vairāgya* as a centripetal one, like a flower closing or the root of a tree spiralling down to penetrate the hard earth. Now, although these two words, centrifugal and centripetal describe a relationship which exists in duality, it is not a duality of conflicting or antagonistic opposites, but a complementary relationship of polarity. In other words, if you had to draw a line to join them up, it would not be by a straight line but by a circle. If they were antagonistic, Patañjali would not have been able to write *sūtra* II.47 on effortless effort, *sūtra* II.48 on an end to duality or the last word to his final *sūtra* IV.34 – *iti* – "that is all", meaning that there is an end, that a resolution beyond all temporary compromise can be attained.

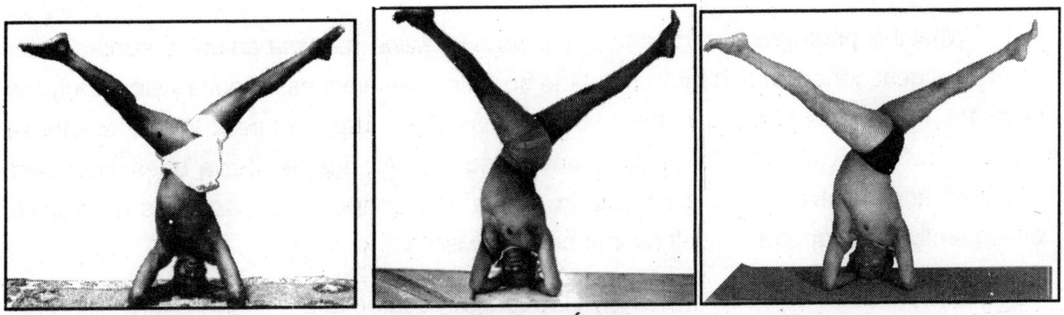

Parivṛttaikapāda Śīrṣāsana

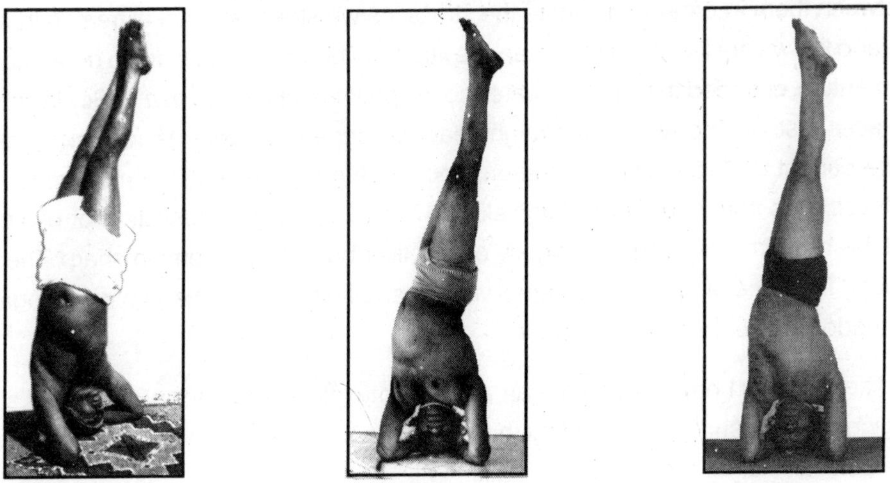

Pārśva Śīrṣāsana

Plate n. 2 – Examples of: *Parivṛttaikapāda Śīrṣāsana* and *Pārśva Śīrṣāsana*

Look back at the first photograph of *Parivṛttaikapāda Śīrṣāsana*. Can you now see that, in spite of all my skill, one leg is more dynamic *(abhyāsa,* centrifugal), the other more passive *(vairāgya,* centripetal)? The list of their relative duality continues: one is exhibitive, the other inhibitive, one is proud, showing off, the other humble and shy. In *Sālamba Śīrṣāsana* there is a spindle of centripetal energy running vertically through the body. Centrifugal energy is expressed by the lift of the arms, the opening of the chest and the spread of the soles of the feet. When we teach, we say, "This is in, this is out, this is up, that is down." These words are shorthand for all the above dualities, including universality and particularity. In the first photo of *Pārśva Śīrṣāsana* the legs are obviously thrown back, here the centrifugal energy is physically and dynamically expressed. Evolving nature has a centrifugal bias which tends towards the creation of multiplicity and therefore particularity. A centripetal movement leads towards integrity or oneness, hence universality.

What this photograph undoubtedly shows is *dhāraṇā* in *āsana,* an uninterrupted linear flow of intelligent concentration throughout the body. Intense alertness is quite visible. Only the *ahaṁkāra,* 'I' shape, is short of perfection. But what of the later pictures? Where are those dualities now? Look at my legs. Is there any inequality? All dualities have been absorbed, reconciled and resolved. This is *dhyāna* in *āsana.* The shape of the *āsana* is meditative. Consequently the shape of the self cannot be otherwise.

There is a tale in Greek mythology of two mighty searocks, Scylla and Charybdis, either one of whose contact would destroy a vessel. The problem was for the ship's helmsman to steer between them in order to navigate the straits. As we steer between extremes in our own practice and life, we are like that helmsman. Inevitably as beginners we want to generate energy and momentum, or speed through the water, so we pull nearer to *abhyāsa,* or Scylla, where the current races fast. Seeing where that might lead we edge over towards *vairāgya,* Charybdis, where the current is slacker but treacherous rocks are concealed, so we must redouble our watchfulness. This corresponds to Patañjali's II.47, exalted effort is cessation of effort. At this moment the helmsman's hand rests lightly on the tiller but his eyes remain sharp. There is an expression, "The price of freedom is eternal vigilance." Likewise must we, aiming in yoga for the goal of freedom, never relax our vigilance.

These words I have written are an attempt to explain, and I hope, to help all students from beginners on, in such a manner that they may reap the benefits of yoga along the way, and one day taste its final and incomparable fruit.

B.K.S Iyengar

B K S IYENGAR

SECTION I

AṢṬĀṄGA YOGA

*YOGA DṚṢṬI**

(With yogic eyes)

Dear lovers of yoga,

Though I am completing seventy years of life, and more than five decades in the field of yoga, I am yet a child in yoga. Yoga is a vast, as well as a life-absorbing subject, and to mature in it is a Herculean task.

The term yoga comes from the root *yuj*, meaning to yoke, to join, to bind, to associate with, and so forth. Actually, yoga means union, the union of the individual soul with the Universal Soul. Yoga is a discipline that removes all dualities and divisions. It integrates body with breath, breath with mind, mind with intelligence and intelligence with the soul. Yoga makes one penetrate from the outer skin towards the core of being and conversely links the core of being to the periphery. Yoga is both an evolutionary path (outward journey) and involutionary path (inward journey), in the quest of the soul.

I have no right to brand my method of practice and teaching as "Iyengar Yoga". It is my pupils that call it "Iyengar Yoga" to distinguish it from the teachings of others. Though I am rational, I am also a man of sentiment and tradition-bound. I trust the statements of others, follow their lines of explanation and experiment with them to gain experience. If my experience tallies with their expressions, I accept their statements. Otherwise I discard them, live by my own experiments and experiences, and make my pupils feel the same as I felt in my experiments. If many agree, then I take it as a proven fact and impart it to others. By the grace of yoga, not only have I imbibed a special awareness of intelligence to penetrate microscopically my inner body, but I also think and act simultaneously. This two-edged quality of intelligence has made me watch distinctly, part by part and as a whole, my body, mind and self kindling with flashes of new thought and ideas in order to act instantly and aptly, and at the same time guide my students to learn better.

---

* Recorded as a cassette, this message was sent to various centres in the world to be played during *Gurujī's* seventieth birthday celebrations on the 14th December 1988.

The only thing I am doing is to bring out the in-depth, hidden qualities of yoga to the awareness of you all. This has made you to call my way of practice and teaching, "Iyengar Yoga". This label has caught on and become widely known, but what I do is nevertheless purely authentic traditional yoga. It is wrong to differentiate traditional yoga from Iyengar Yoga. Likewise it is unfair to market yoga as *rāja yoga, haṭha yoga, laya yoga, mantra yoga, tantra yoga, kuṇḍalinī yoga, tāraka yoga* and so on. In fact, there is no distinction between one yoga and another; they all have the same root and the same purpose.

Yoga, like God, is one. But people call Him by different names. Mother Earth is one. Though the Earth is one single orb, we divide it into hemispheres, into East, West, North and South. These manmade divisions interlace our various cultures. Yet at the same time throughout civilisation there is an essence of life that is the same. What is that essence? That essence is self-progression, self-realisation and integration of one's self to the Divine. It is the same with yoga. Many make a division and say that *haṭha yoga* is physical and *rāja yoga* mental. Can one say where the body ends, and the mind begins? Or where the mind ends, and the self begins? Only armchair yogis or lazy ones can possibly invent such unwarranted distinctions.

Patañjali speaks of *cittavṛtti nirodha,* the restraint of the fluctuations of consciousness *(citta),* commonly termed as mind. Remember that the restraint of the fluctuations of consciousness is the beginning of yoga and not the end. Restraint of mind is a means towards integration.

For example, engineers first build a dam on a turbulent river to regulate its flow. Then the collected water is channelled through canals to various parts of the land for irrigation. Similarly, Patañjali advises the *sādhaka* first to restrain the disorderly behaviour of consciousness, so that he directs it correctly by investigation, study, examination and proper judgement *(vitarka* and *vicāra);* by distinguishing mundane pleasure from that of pure bliss *(ānanda),* and by differentiating between ego and *sāttvic* self *(asmitā).* From here, the *sādhaka* is guided to experience the end of yoga, in the form of *dharmamegha samādhi* or *nirbīja*[1] *samādhi* (a state in which the ego or 'I'-ness is not only absent but has been expunged for ever). Here all imprints *(saṁskāra)* and afflictions are washed away for ever; the consciousness is freed from all flaws so that the stream of wisdom and virtue flows clean and clear like torrential rain.

Svātmārāma in the *Haṭhayoga Pradīpikā* speaks of *prāṇavṛtti nirodha,* restraint of the fluctuations of *prāṇa* or breath. *Prāṇa* means breath, air, wind, vital air, life, vitality, strength, power and aspiration. *Prāṇāyāma* is the restrained control of the breath through the delicate manipulation of the fingers on the nostrils, to harmonise the inflow, control, and release of breath so that consciousness gains calmness and functions positively towards self-realisation.

---

[1] See vol. I, pages 233 and 263.

The *Yoga Sūtra* starts with *Samādhi Pāda*, whereas *Haṭhayoga Pradīpikā* ends with *samādhi*. Patañjali distinguishes between *puruṣa* and *citta* – one eternal and independent, the other transient and dependent. Svātmārāma uses a compound word formed of two syllables, *ha* and *ṭha*. The *ha* stands for *puruṣa*, and *ṭha* for *citta*, which has no light of its own, but borrows from *puruṣa* or the Self.

All yoga students must know that yoga demands a cultivation of the codes of conduct for progression to occur at physical, mental, intellectual and spiritual levels. For this, yoga requires tremendous effort, perseverance and patience.

The yoga I teach is purely *aṣṭāṅga yoga*, known as the eight-limbed yoga, expounded by Patañjali in his 196 terse *sūtra*, each of which reflects profound experiential knowledge. These are supplemented with *haṭha yoga* texts, the *Bhagavad Gītā* and others. Patañjali's *Yoga Sūtra* have attracted considerable attention and there are many commentaries on them. Most commentators have seen the subject of yoga objectively or from an academic angle. On the other hand, I have responded to it subjectively. Through my uninterrupted practice and its refinement I have compared my experiences and feelings with the original text.

According to Patañjali, yoga is the restraint of the fluctuations of the mind. When the fluctuations cease, the soul is uncovered. The fluctuations are summarised in five categories as *vṛtti*. These are real knowledge, unreal or contrary knowledge, imagination, sleep and memory. Naturally, the question of why do fluctuations and modifications in the *citta* arise and how are they to be restrained has to be answered. Fluctuations and modifications arise because of afflictions *(kleśa)*. The afflictions too are summarised in five categories. These are lack of spiritual wisdom, egoism, attraction towards attachment, aversion to pain and clinging passionately to life. Latent subliminal impressions are at the root of the fluctuations and afflictions in the consciousness. When these afflictions become subtle, they become *vṛtti*. These afflictions, fluctuations, modifications and modulations are partly inherited and partly acquired.

Patañjali explains the nine obstacles on the path of self-progression and realisation. These obstacles are easily cognisable. He begins first with physical disabilities, and then the mental and intellectual obstacles which block spiritual growth. He defines the physical obstacles as disease and torpor, the mental obstacles as doubt, carelessness, idleness and sense gratification, and the intellectual impediments as living in the world of illusion, lack of perseverance and inability to maintain the progress achieved. Besides these obstacles, he goes further and says that laboured breathing disturbs the organic body; tremor of the body shakes the cellular body; despair makes the mind weak and fickle, and sorrow affects the intellectual calibre. Thus, all these distractions scatter the consciousness, which is already in a disturbed and shaky state due to fluctuations and disturbed movements from its very existence in the world.

The afflictions and obstacles are nothing but imperfection in the health of the body and in the state of the mind. Hence, the science of yoga begins with the understanding of sorrow, aims at the purification of body and mind and ends with emancipation. Patañjali sums up the effect of yoga in one *sūtra*. He says, *Yogāṅgānuṣṭhānāt aśuddhikṣaye jñānadīptiḥ āvivekakhyāteḥ* (*Y.S.*, II.28) i.e., by regular and devoted practice of the eight petals of yoga, the impurities of the *sādhaka's* body, mind and intelligence are consumed, the causes of afflictions removed, and the crown of spiritual light or wisdom is bestowed. What are these eight petals? They are *yama*, *niyama*, *āsana*, *prāṇāyāma*, *pratyāhāra*, *dhāraṇā*, *dhyāna* and *samādhi*.

Yama is self-restraint, or the don'ts of life, and *niyama* is the fixed practices, or the do's of life. These form the framework of rules on which the individual and society are based. They are the core of every culture and the foundation of every society. *Yama* helps to restrain the organs of action. The rules of *yama* are clearly laid down for us to live in the midst of society and at the same time remain as yoga practitioners. They are conducive to social harmony and integration. Great souls like Buddha and Mahavira were known for their uncompromising practice of *yama*. In our own lifetime, we have seen what a tremendous moral and social force Gandhi was. He practised non-violence, continence and truth with devotion. The components of *yama* are called the "mighty universal vows", as they are not limited by class, place, time or concept of duty. They have to be followed unconditionally by all in general and students of yoga in particular, irrespective of one's station or situation.

As *yama* is a universal social practice, *niyama* evolves from the individual's practice. Both are meant to culture oneself. The observances of *niyama* are not only meant to culture the senses of perception but also the five sheaths *(kośa)* of man, the anatomical, physiological, mental, intellectual and spiritual.

The first *niyama*, cleanliness *(śauca)* is of two types, external and internal. Both are necessary. Taking a bath is external purification; performing *āsana* and *prāṇāyāma* is an internal bath. Contentment *(santoṣa)*, linked to friendliness, compassion and indifference towards dualities or extremes is a pillar in the observance of *niyama*. Penance *(tapas)* is done to control the body, senses and mind, which frees the *sādhaka* from desire, anger, greed, infatuation, arrogance and jealousy. Most people undertake *tapas* because they are discontent with their lack of control and its ensuing vices. *Santoṣa* enables us not to suppress our weakness and vice, but to abandon them without regret.

Self-study *(svādhyāya)* is the re-examination of one's thoughts and habits of mind, involving the subtle and finer parts of yoga, *pratyāhāra*, *dhāraṇā* and *dhyāna*. By this we reduce our tendency to err. Surrendering to God *(Īśvara praṇidhāna)*, transforms the consciousness to allow the radiation of the purity of Self. There cannot be freedom without discipline. Without morality and discipline, spiritual life is an impossibility. Mastery of yoga would be unrealisable or unreliable without the observance of the ethical disciplines of *yama* and *niyama*.

It is important to note that *yama* and *niyama* pervade all spheres of life. In each limb of yoga, one has to practise *yama* and *niyama*. I often say that balancing of violence with non-violence and non-violence with violence is necessary. One has to study what is a violent *āsana* and what is a non-violent *āsana*. In a non-violent *āsana*, there is neither aggression nor laxity, neither overdoing nor underdoing. If overdoing is a deliberate action of destroying the cells, underdoing can bring stagnation and starvation. Thus, both overdoing and underdoing result in the premature death of cells. The study and balance of body cells lead to the preservation of energy and of seeing the self in the cells. This is *brahmacarya*, as the self moves with the cells as well as with the *āsana*. This way of practice transforms the *sādhaka* from sensual stimulation towards unbiased spiritual joy.

Each *āsana* is a *niyama* in itself. One should learn to observe cleanliness both externally and internally. Each *āsana* calls for critical intuitive observation from the body to the self, and from the self towards the body. While performing each *āsana*, one has to switch the intellectual vision inwards *(antardṛṣṭi)*, and draw attention to the cells to act at once, judiciously and harmoniously.

Patañjali says that the consciousness becomes favourably disposed and serene by contemplating an object that helps to maintain steadiness of mind. *Viṣayavatī vā pravṛtti utpannā manasaḥ sthiti nibandhani* (*Y.S.*, I.35).

This *sūtra* of Patañjali is one example of an explanation of *dhāraṇā* in *āsana* as *āsana* is made to become the object of interest and attention. If we get totally engrossed in practice of *āsana*, the mind develops steadiness, and then the penetration begins from that steadiness.

We can thus measure how deeply the *āsana* reaches into the unfathomable self inside. This is the process of self-study *(svādhyāya)*. Finally, when the *āsana* is done perfectly, as it should be done in accordance with the principles of *yama* and *niyama*, surrender of effort sets in. The body, mind and self become things in themselves. As the *āsana* reaches its zenith, the practitioner's individuality becomes universal. This is *Īśvara praṇidhāna*.

Āsana is basic to strengthening and cleansing the body and purging the impurities of the mind. I emphasise perfection in *āsana*, because the body is the means through which we perceive and act. Therefore, a healthy and strong body is an incomparable asset in yogic *sādhanā*. In the *Upaniṣads* it has been said that the search for the sight of the soul is not for weaklings.

Āsana strengthens and purifies each and every limb, fibre, and cell of the body. The range of *āsana* is infinite. Traditional books mention that there are as many *āsana* as living species.

Each *āsana* has a great depth and each one is a science and art in itself. *Āsana* helps us to proceed from the external to the internal, from the gross to the subtle, from the known to the unknown and from the skin to the soul. Patañjali's *sthira sukham āsanam* has not been understood by many. They interpret it as if it applies only for the purpose of meditation. I define *āsana* as firmness in the body, steadiness in intelligence and majestic benevolence in consciousness. Whatever *āsana* one performs, it should be done with a feeling of firmness and endurance in the body, good will in the intelligence of the head, and awareness and benevolent delight from the seat of the heart. With this understanding, one feels a sense of nourishment and illumination. When infinite poise and balance are instilled in the *āsana*, the body, mind and self become one and effort becomes effortless. Patañjali observes that when the finite vehicle – the body – breaks its frontiers to be merged in the infinite, it brings the pairs of opposites like pain and pleasure, heat and cold, honour and dishonour to an end. This is beatitude, perfection in action and freedom in consciousness. If restraint of consciousness is defined as yoga, I prefer to define *āsana* as the stability and restraint of the entire cellular system of the *sādhaka*. If the cells are not controlled and restrained there is no serenity in the cells, fibres and nerves, or peace in the mind. *Āsana* is meant for *snāyuvṛtti nirodha*. *Snāyu* means sinews, which are the source of strength, power and vigour. *Nirodha* means control and restraint.

Prāṇāyāma, the fourth constituent of yoga, deals with the control of *prāṇa* and energy, grossly translated as breath. *Prāṇāyāma* does not allow the vital energy *(prāṇa)* to dissipate, but stores it in the cells for the better use of life. Hence *prāṇāyāma* is for *prāṇavṛtti nirodha* (control and restraint).

Prāṇa is a self-energising force that permeates each individual as well as the entire universe at all levels. It acts as physical energy, mental energy, intellectual energy, sensual energy, spiritual energy and cosmic energy. All that vibrates in the universe is *prāṇa*. Heat, light, gravity, magnetism, vigour, power, vitality, electricity, life and self are all *prāṇa*. It is a cosmic entity, and hence it is present in all beings and non-beings. *Prāṇa* is the prime mover of all activities. It is the wealth of life. This self-energising force is the principle of life and of consciousness. As the atmosphere carries fine ingredients of life's elixir, yogis discovered the method of *prāṇāyāma* so that profound energy is continuously earned, stored and distributed, providing needed energy to the body, mind and self.

Prāṇa and *citta* are in constant contact with each other. Mind is mercurial and moves with infinite speed. But the breath moves more slowly, and hence it is easier to control, though its flow is unrestrained, unconditioned and irregular. Svātmārāma says *"cale vāte calaṁ cittaṁ niścale niścalaṁ bhavet"* (*H.Y.P.*, II.2) "as the breath moves so the mind moves, and as the breath is stilled so the mind is stilled."

Prāṇāyāma cannot be done forcibly. One can use willpower to the optimum level while performing an *āsana*, but the same willpower has to be subdued and sublimated for the practice of *prāṇāyāma*. It needs a very delicate, subtle adjustment in the system of the lungs, quietness of the brain cells, an alert attention and observation, an even balance of elasticity and stability in the spinal muscles and nerves. Hence, it has to be learnt under the guidance of a competent teacher. Without attaining strength, stability and purity through *āsana*, one is not fit for the practice of *prāṇāyāma*. Patañjali is very emphatic about this. He expressly advises the *sādhaka* to do *prāṇāyāma* only after attaining proficiency in a number of *āsana*. For the first time, he marks a distinct step in the ascent on the ladder of yoga, whereas he has not stipulated the stages of the other components.

Patañjali sums up the effects of *prāṇāyāma*, saying that it removes the veil covering the light of knowledge and heralds the dawn of wisdom. By its practice, illusion, ignorance, desire and delusion, which obscure the intelligence, are destroyed and the inner light of wisdom is allowed to shine. As a breeze disperses the clouds that cover the sun, so *prāṇāyāma* clears away the clouds of ignorance that hide the light of intelligence. Thus, *prāṇāyāma* becomes the gateway to *dhāraṇā* and *dhyāna*.

Pratyāhāra, the fifth constituent, begins with the inner quest and acts as a foundation in the path of renunciation. The return journey towards the seer begins from here. Memory and mind are so interwoven that it is hard to distinguish between them. Memory incites the mind to seek out sensual pleasures. *Pratyāhāra* helps the senses of perception and memory to reside quietly, each in its place, and to cease importuning the mind for their gratification, making them let go the tastes and flavours to which they are addicted. The mind, which till now acted as a bridge between the senses and the seer, draws back from the contact of the senses, and turns inwards to explore spiritual wealth, and the domain of the seer. In fact *pratyāhāra* is an effect of *prāṇāyāma*. Hence, *pratyāhāra* is *manovṛtti nirodha*. It brings the restraint of fluctuations of *manas* or mind.

From *manovṛtti nirodha* the focal attention of the *sādhaka* moves on to the Self, ever fresh, unchanging and poised.

Dhāraṇā, dhyāna and *samādhi* are the last three petals *(dala)* of *aṣṭāṅga yoga.* They bring us close to the *citta.* Patañjali coins a special word, *saṁyama,* meaning integration, for the unity of the last three aspects. These three petals of yoga are encased together as fine, finer and the finest parts of *saṁyama. Dhāraṇā* is the confinement of *citta's* attention to an object or region outside or inside the body. *Dhyāna* is the attention flowing uninterruptedly, and *samādhi* is total absorption in the object of meditation. These three constituents of yoga are experiencing states. They cannot be presented with explanations. *Āsana* and *prāṇāyāma* can be explained, taught, shown and corrected, while *yama* and *niyama* are explained by stories of great men as ideal examples to build up character. If *dhāraṇā* is *buddhivṛtti nirodha, dhyāna* is *ahaṁkāravṛtti nirodha* (restraint of the 'I'). A consequence of *dhāraṇā* and *dhyāna* is grace in consciousness *(cittaprasādana),* while in *samādhi* comes the effulgence of the soul *(ātmaprasādana).*

Dhyāna is the art of bringing the complex mind to a state of simplicity, but with innocence. One who is free from doubt and confusion and has instant intuitive clarity, has reached the pinnacle of *dhyāna.*

Today, there is a craze for meditation and instant enlightenment. Meditation being a part of yoga, it cannot be separated from its parent body. However, *dhāraṇā, dhyāna* and *samādhi* are the effects or fruits of practice. To bypass other petals of yoga, and directly enter into these practices, would not only be dangerous but also an abuse of yoga. When the Lord graced Arjuna to look at His Form, Arjuna had to beg Lord Krishna to bless him with divine eyes to see the Infinite Lord. This instance is sufficient for practitioners like us to know that we have to build up that strength and vigour to face the light of the Divine when divinity graces us with its light. For this reason, Patañjali advises practitioners like us to earn and store that vital energy, in order to drink the nectar of immortality, when the spiritual light dawns through yoga.

Patañjali prescribes *Samādhi Pāda* for evolved souls and *Sādhana Pāda* for unevolved souls. However he brings them together in the *Vibhūti Pāda* for the intricate practice of *dhāraṇā, dhyāna* and *samādhi.*

In our teachings of *āsana* and *prāṇāyāma,* we prepare students for higher practices by giving them the technique to experience *dhāraṇā* and *dhyāna.* As man is made up of physical, mental and spiritual layers, so too, yoga can be divided into three tiers of practice. From *yama* to *pratyāhāra,* the anatomical, physiological and psychological sheaths are purified. *Dhāraṇā* and *dhyāna* purge the impurities of the intellectual sheath such as base motives, disingenuousness, manipulation, self-seeking and desire for power. While *samādhi* lights the lamp of the sense of conscience *(dharmendriya),* for the seer to shine everlastingly.

Patañjali says that practice and detachment are the means to restrain the fluctuations and modifications of the *citta*. Practice is action with knowledge and devotion. It is a systematic, repeated performance involving a certain methodology in order to accomplish skill or proficiency. It is helpful in building up confidence and refinement in culturing the consciousness. Renunciation is a cultivation of freedom from worldly desires and appetites. Renunciation is knowledge with devotion to God. Renunciation is the act of discharging that which obstructs the consciousness from proceeding along the spiritual path.

If practice is the path of evolution, renunciation is that of involution. Both need to be balanced for a harmonious development. Overall, one can broadly say that from *yama* to *pratyāhāra* is the evolutive path for human beings, and from *pratyāhāra* to *samādhi*, it is the involutive path through *prakṛti*. *Pratyāhāra* contains aspects of both tendencies. As a bird cannot fly with one wing, a yogi cannot ascend to a spiritual height without co-ordinating practice and renunciation. Without discriminative powers practice will only be sensual.

Yama begins with non-violence and ends with non-possession. *Niyama* starts with the practice of cleanliness and culminates in the surrender of the ego. In *āsana*, one learns to transcend dualities, while in *prāṇāyāma* one uncovers the veil that obscures the light of knowledge and takes one's consciousness nearer to the seer. Practice of *pratyāhāra* brings supreme control over the senses and mind. Without the mind being withdrawn from sense objects, *dhāraṇā* and *dhyāna* are not easy to practise or assimilate. *Samādhi* is a desireless state, a supreme state of renunciation *(paravairāgya)*.

Thus, Patañjali begins yoga with the explanation of sorrow and ends with emancipation. He recognises the importance of the aims *(puruṣārtha)* of man, namely, science of duty *(dharma)*, purpose of life and wealth *(artha)*, desire and passion *(kāma)* and emancipation *(mokṣa)*. The philosophy of yoga is not meant only for celibates or renunciates but for all. Continence is not negation, forced austerity and prohibition. All aims of man are meant for the seer to experience the pleasures of the world, or for reaching emancipation with right perception. Married life is also one of the ways of moving from human love to divine love or union with the supreme soul. Thus, yoga acts as an instrument to develop purity in thought, word and deed.

To sum up yoga, I would say that essence of yoga is the dissolution of ego, and not emotional exuberance.

Dear children of yoga: I have practised yoga by living in yoga. As I said earlier, it is a life-absorbing subject and to mature in it is a Herculean task. I love you, and you all adore me with esteem. I advise you all to gain courage and confidence to practise yoga, because for decades this art and science has been a most misconceived and misunderstood subject. The general attitude was that you only came to yoga for negative reasons, such as depression or family problems. I also faced humiliating remarks from people in my early days of practice. I was only in my teens when I embraced this noble art and such remarks were not uncommon.

Today, I am the happiest man on earth, because in spite of all the condemnation and frustration, I have not only earned name and fame, but I have brought back respect and majesty to this art and science. I made it popular by attracting all types of people to taste its flavour. I have trained lots of pupils, encouraging them to teach fearlessly and to carry on this work all over the globe.

The time has come now for me to hand over this greatest of arts. It is time for you to further explore its depth from where I leave and, as ambassadors of yoga, take its message of physical and mental health, spiritual beauty and grandeur to your brothers and sisters.

Scientists have begun accepting the moral codes of yoga as essential for health and happiness. Contentment *(santoṣa)* for example is known to strengthen the immune system. They are also clear in their thinking that 'psyche' (mind) and 'soma' (body) are interrelated, and it may not be far for them to establish a psycho-spiritual bond as well as neuro-spiritual link in man. The World Health Organisation proclaims that the 2lst century will be filled with physical health and mental well being. I do not think there is any alternative method that fulfils the ambitions of the W.H.O. As yoga blends both brain and brawn, mind and body, to become fit instruments of the soul, you have a tremendous responsibility first to give physical health and mental harmony to present and future generations before we think of taking them towards the spiritual light.

I have often said that yoga is my *guru* and I assure you that yoga is going to be your *guru.* The tenacity to stick to a regular practice is very important. It requires a tremendous tolerance, patience and mental discipline. This cultivation of discipline strengthens the willpower. Otherwise, willpower is of a short duration. I want you all to build up the culture of practice and not the cult of personality. Get established wholeheartedly in what you have started to learn, then experience its hidden wealth.

Though learning is very difficult, know that it is even more difficult to maintain a daily practice savouring the freshness and fragrance of yoga. For years there will be conflicts between body and mind. Sometimes, the body is fresh to accept but not the mind, and at other times the mind remains fresh, but not the body. When both are conducive, practise with vigour and drink the nectar of yoga.

Unfortunately, we are inclined to have too much theory and too little practice, too many words and very little work. Note that knowledge born of experience is a million times superior to acquired and accumulated knowledge. Honest, sincere, intensive and intelligent practice makes one ascend the ladder of self-realisation. Let your life in yoga be a life of self-progression, which in the true sense becomes a religious life. Let zeal in practice kindle within you all. Accept all experience as a lamplight, without anticipation of results. Then God becomes kind and compassionate, instilling in you the grace of His Divine Light.

A word for those who are teachers or would like to be teachers: there is an Indian adage, "Service to man is service to God." Hence I feel that teaching yoga is the noblest of all services as you guide your pupils from darkness to light, from ignorance to knowledge and from the cult of the mortal body towards the culture of the immortal soul. This way, you make them really become the children of God. Behave in such a way as not to go beyond your capacities. Even if you admonish your pupils, feel in your hearts that you are serving the Almighty within them. And my last request, but not a command, is, "Be an ideal example to your students." Practise with faith, practise with courage, practise with zest, practise with understanding, and practise uninterruptedly and reverentially. Be ethical in your teachings. If you see a mistake and do not care to correct the mistake, that teaching is unethical. When corrected, if a pupil does not adapt and adopt, that pupil is an unethical student. Retain integrity and purity in your *sādhanā*. The light will be brilliant and sorrows yet to come will not come. Even if they come, they too will be vanquished. *Heyaṁ duḥkham anāgatam* (*Y.S.*, II.16). The pains which are yet to come can be and are to be avoided.

May God bless you and may God shower His grace on you all. May you all prosper in yoga. Let the masters of yoga rest in your hearts, and let me wish you God speed in your endeavours. Let me take the name of Sage Patañjali, the master of all masters of yoga, to be your guide throughout your lives.

Auṁ Srimat Patañjali Mahāmunayenamaḥ

AṢṬĀṄGA YOGA: THE EIGHT LIMBS OF CLASSICAL YOGA*

WHAT IS YOGA?

Yoga is a timeless pragmatic science that has evolved over thousands of years. It deals with the physical, moral, mental and spiritual well-being of man as a whole. The first book to systematise this practical science was the classic treatise, the *Yoga Sūtra* (or aphorisms) of Patañjali, dating from 200 BC.

The word yoga is derived from the *Sanskṛt* root *yuj* meaning to bind, join, attach and yoke, to direct and concentrate one's attention upon, to use and apply. It also means union or communion. It is the true union of our will with the will of God. "It thus means," says Mahadev Desai in his introduction to the *Bhagavad Gītā according to Mahatma Gandhi*, "the yoking of all the powers of body, mind and soul to God; it means the disciplining of the intellect, the mind, the emotions, the will, which yoga pre-supposes; it means a poise of the soul that enables one to look at life in all its aspects evenly."

Yoga is one of the six orthodox systems of Indian philosophy. It was collated, co-ordinated and systematised by Patañjali in his *Yoga Sūtra*, which consists of 196 terse aphorisms. According to yogic philosophy, everything is permeated by the Supreme Universal Soul (*Paramātmā* or God) of which the individual human soul *(jīvātmā)* is a part. It teaches the means by which the *jīvātmā* can be united to, or be in communion with, the *Paramātmā*, and secure liberation *(mokṣa)*. One who follows the path of yoga is a yogi or a *yogini*.

AṢṬĀṄGA YOGA - THE EIGHT LIMBS OF YOGA

The *Yoga Sūtra* of Patañjali is divided into four chapters or *pāda*. The first deals with *samādhi* (the super-conscious state), the second with *sādhana* (the means) to achieve yoga, the third elaborates the *vibhūti* (powers or attainments) that the yogi comes across in his quest, and the fourth deals with *kaivalya* (emancipation).

---

* Published in *Review of Yoga*, Varanasi. Based on the Introduction to *Light on Yoga*, George Allen & Unwin, London.

Patañjali enumerates the means as the eight *(aṣṭa)* limbs or stages *(aṅga)* of yoga for the quest of the soul. They are: 1. *Yama* (ethical disciplines or universal moral commandments); 2. *Niyama* (self-purification by discipline); 3. *Āsana* (posture); 4. *Prāṇāyāma* (rhythmic control of the breath); 5. *Pratyāhāra* (withdrawal and emancipation of the mind from the domination of the senses and exterior objects); 6. *Dhāraṇā* (concentration); 7. *Dhyāna* (meditation) and 8. *Samādhi* (a state of super-consciousness brought about by profound meditation), in which the aspirant becomes one with the object of his meditation –*Paramātmā* or the Universal Soul.

Yama and *niyama* control the yogi's passions and emotions and keep him in harmony with his fellow man. *Āsana* practice keeps the body healthy and strong and in harmony with nature. Finally, the yogi becomes free of body consciousness. He conquers the body and renders it a fit vehicle for the soul. *Prāṇāyāma* teaches the aspirant to regulate his breathing and thereby control the mind. These first four stages form the outward quest *(bahiraṅga sādhanā)*.

To free the senses from the thrall of the objects of desire is *pratyāhāra*. It is considered as the transitional state from *bahiraṅga sādhanā* to *antaraṅga sādhanā*.

Dhāraṇā and *dhyāna* take the yogi into the innermost recesses of his soul. This stage is called *antaraṅga sādhanā*. Finally, the yogi does not look heavenward to find God, he knows that He is within, and known as the *antarātmā* (the Inner Self). This last stage keeps the *sādhaka* in harmony with himself and his Maker. This is *samādhi* or *antarātma sādhanā*, the quest of the soul.

By profound meditation, the knower, the knowing and the known become one. The seer, sight and the seen have no separate existence from each other. It is like a great musician becoming one with his instrument and the music that comes from it.

YAMA

The first limb of *aṣṭāṅga yoga* is *yama* (ethical discipline), the great commandments that transcend creed, country, age and time. They are: *ahiṁsā* (non-violence), *satya* (truth), *asteya* (non-stealing), *brahmacarya* (continence) and *aparigraha* (non-coveting). These commandments are the rules of morality for society and the individual, which if not obeyed bring chaos, violence, untruth, stealing, dissipation and covetousness. The roots of all these evils are the emotions of greed, desire and attachment. They may be mild, medium or excessive. They only bring pain and ignorance. Patañjali strikes at the root of these evils by changing the direction of our thinking in accordance with the five principles of *yama*.

•

Ahiṁsā: The word *ahiṁsā* is made up of the particle *"a"* meaning "not" and the noun *hiṁsā* meaning killing or violence. It is more than a negative command not to kill, for it has a wider positive meaning, love. This love embraces all creation for we are all children of the same Father – the Lord. The yogi believes that to kill or to destroy a being or thing is to insult its Creator. Men either kill for food or to protect themselves from danger. It does not necessarily follow that a man is non-violent by temperament or that he is a yogi merely because he is a vegetarian, though a vegetarian diet is a necessity for the practice of yoga. Bloodthirsty tyrants may also be vegetarians. Violence is more a state of mind, not of diet only. It resides in a man's mind, not in the instrument he holds in his hand. One can use a knife to pare fruit or to stab an enemy. The fault is not in the instrument, but in the user.

Men take to violence to protect their own interests, their own bodies, their loved ones, their property or dignity. But a man cannot rely upon himself alone to protect himself or others. It is a wrong belief that he can do so. A man must rely upon God, who is the source of all strength. Then he will fear no evil.

Violence arises out of fear, weakness, ignorance or restlessness. In order to curb it, what is most needed is freedom from fear. To gain this freedom, what is required is a change of outlook on life and a re-orientation of the mind. Violence is bound to decline when men learn to base their faith upon investigation and reality rather than upon ignorance and supposition.

The yogi believes that every creature has as much right to live as he has. He believes that he is born to help others and he looks upon creation with eyes of love. He knows that his life is linked inextricably with that of others and he rejoices if he can help others to be happy. He puts the happiness of others before his own and becomes a source of joy to all who meet him. As parents encourage a baby to walk the first steps, he encourages those more unfortunate than himself and makes them fit for survival.

For a wrong done by others, men demand justice; while for that done by themselves they plead mercy and forgiveness. The yogi, on the other hand, believes that for a wrong done by himself, there should be justice, while for that done by another there should be forgiveness. He knows and teaches others how to live. Always striving to perfect himself, he shows them by his love and compassion how to improve themselves.

The yogi opposes the evil in the wrongdoer, but not the wrongdoer. He prescribes penance, not punishment, for a wrong done. Opposition to evil and love for the wrongdoer can live side by side. A drunkard's wife, whilst loving him, may still oppose his habit. Opposition without love leads to violence; loving the wrongdoer without opposing the evil in him is folly and leads to misery. The yogi knows that to love a person whilst fighting the evil in him is the right course to follow. The battle is won because he fights it with love. A loving mother will sometimes smack her child to cure it of a bad habit; in the same way a true follower of *ahiṁsā* loves his opponent.

Satya: *Satya* or truth is the highest rule of conduct or morality. Mahatma Gandhi said, "Truth is God and God is Truth". As fire burns impurities and refines gold, so the fire of truth cleanses the yogi and burns up the dross in him.

If the mind is filled with thoughts of truth, if the tongue speaks words of truth and if the whole life is based upon truth, then one becomes fit for union with the Infinite. Reality in its fundamental nature expresses itself through these two aspects, love and truth. The yogi's life must conform strictly to these two facets of Reality. That is why *ahiṁsā*, which is essentially based on love, is enjoined. *Satya* presupposes perfect truthfulness in thought, word and deed. Untruthfulness in any form puts the *sādhaka* out of harmony with the fundamental law of truth.

Truth is not limited to speech alone. There are four sins of speech: abuse and obscenity, dealing in falsehoods, the calumny of telling tales and lastly ridiculing what others hold to be sacred. The talebearer is more poisonous than a snake. The control of speech leads to the rooting out of malice. When the mind bears malice towards none, it is filled with charity towards all. He who has learnt to control his tongue has attained self-control in a great measure. When such a person speaks, he will be heard with respect and attention. His words will be remembered, for they will be good and true.

When one who is established in truth prays with a pure heart, then things he really needs come to him when they are really needed: he does not have to run after them. The man firmly established in truth gets the fruit of his actions without apparently doing anything. God, the source of all truth, supplies his needs and looks after his welfare.

Asteya: The desire to possess and enjoy what another has, drives a person to do evil deeds. From this desire springs the urge to steal and to covet. *Asteya* (*a* = not, *steya* = stealing) or non-stealing includes not only taking what belongs to another without permission, but also using something for a different purpose to that intended or beyond the time permitted by its owner. It thus includes misappropriation, breach of trust, mismanagement and misuse. The yogi reduces his physical needs to the minimum, believing that if he gathers things he does not really need, he is a thief. While other men crave for wealth, power, fame or enjoyment, the yogi has one craving and that is to adore the Lord. Freedom from craving enables one to ward off great temptations. Craving muddies the stream of tranquillity. It makes men base and vile and cripples them. He who obeys the commandment "Thou shalt not steal", becomes a trusted repository of all treasures.

Brahmacarya: Brahmacarya means the life of celibacy, religious study and self-restraint. Patañjali lays stress on continence of the body, speech and mind. This does not mean that the philosophy of yoga is meant only for celibates. *Brahmacarya* has little to do with whether one is a bachelor or married and living the life of a householder. One has to translate the higher aspects of *brahmacarya* in one's daily living. It is not necessary for one's salvation to stay unmarried and without a house. On the contrary, all the *smṛti* (codes of law) recommend marriage. Without experiencing human love and happiness, it is not possible to understand divine love. Almost all the yogis and sages of old in India were married men with families of their own. They did not shirk their social or moral responsibilities. Marriage and parenthood are no bar to the knowledge of divine love, happiness and union with the Supreme Soul. Even if a human being discards society and goes into the forest, he may be away from human beings, but the love in his heart makes him closer to animals.

When one is established in *brahmacarya*, one develops a fund of vitality and energy, a courageous mind and a powerful intellect so that one can fight any type of injustice. The *brahmacārī* will use the forces he generates wisely: he will utilise the physical ones for doing the work of the Lord, the mental for the spread of culture and the intellectual for the growth of the spiritual life. *Brahmacarya* is the battery that sparks the torch of wisdom.

Aparigraha: Parigraha means hoarding or collecting. To be free from hoarding is *aparigraha*. It is but another facet of *asteya* (non-stealing). Just as one should not take what one does not really need, so one should not hoard or collect things one does not require immediately. Neither should one take anything without working for it or as a favour from another, for this indicates poverty of mind. The yogi feels that the collection or hoarding of things implies a lack of faith in God and in himself to provide for his future. He keeps faith by keeping before him the image of the moon. During the dark half of the month, the moon rises late when most men are asleep and so they do not appreciate its beauty. Its splendour wanes but it does not stray from its path and is indifferent to man's lack of appreciation. It has faith that when it faces the Sun it will be full again and then men will eagerly await its glorious rising.

By the observance of *aparigraha*, the yogi makes his life as simple as possible and trains his mind not to feel the loss or the lack of anything. Then everything he really needs will come to him by itself at the proper time. The life of an ordinary man is filled with an unending series of disturbances and frustrations and with his reactions to them. Thus there is hardly any possibility of keeping the mind in a state of equilibrium. The *sādhaka* has developed the capacity to remain satisfied with whatever happens to him. Thus he obtains the peace which takes him beyond the realms of illusion and misery with which our world is saturated.

NIYAMA

While *yama* is universal in its application, *niyama* is the rule of conduct that applies to individual discipline. The five *niyama* listed by Patañjali are: *śauca* (purity), *santoṣa* (contentment), *tapas* (ardour or austerity), *svādhyāya* (study of the Self) and *Īśvara praṇidhāna* (dedication to the Lord).

Śauca: Purity of body is essential for well being. While good habits like bathing purify the body externally, *āsana* and *prāṇāyāma* cleanse it internally. The practice of *āsana* tones the entire body and removes the toxins and impurities caused by over-indulgence. *Prāṇāyāma* cleanses and aerates the lungs, oxygenates the blood and purifies the nerves. But more important than the physical cleansing of the body is the cleansing of the mind of its disturbing emotions such as hatred, passion, anger, lust, greed, delusion and pride. Still more important is the cleansing of the intelligence *(buddhi)* of impure thoughts. The impurities of the mind are washed off in the waters of *bhakti* (adoration). The impurities of the intelligence or reason are burned off in the fire of *svādhyāya* (study of the Self). This internal cleansing gives radiance and joy. It brings benevolence *(saumanasya)* and banishes mental pain, dejection, sorrow and despair *(daurmanasya)*. When one is benevolent, one sees the virtues in others and not merely their faults. The respect which one shows for another's virtue, makes one self-respecting as well as helping one to face and fight one's own sorrows and difficulties. When the mind is lucid, it is easy to make it one-pointed *(ekāgra)*. With concentration, one obtains mastery over the senses *(indriya-jaya)*. Then one is ready to enter the temple of one's own body and see the Self in the mirror of one's consciousness.

Besides purity of body, thought and word, pure food is also necessary. Apart from cleanliness in the preparation of food, it is also necessary to observe purity in the means by which one procures it.

Food, the supporting yet consuming substance of all life, is regarded as a phase of Brahman. It should be eaten with the feeling that with each morsel one can gain strength to serve the Lord. Then food becomes pure. Whether or not to be a vegetarian is a purely personal matter, as the traditions, habits and economics of the country in which one is born and bred influence each person. But in the course of time, in order to attain one-pointed attention and spiritual evolution, the practitioner of yoga has to adopt a vegetarian diet.

Food should be taken to promote health, strength, energy and life. It should be simple, nourishing, juicy and soothing. Avoid food that is sour, bitter, salty, pungent, burning, stale, tasteless, heavy and unclean.

Character is moulded by the type of food we take and by how we eat it. Men are the only creatures that eat when not hungry and generally live to eat rather than eat to live. If we eat for the flavours of the tongue, we over-eat and so suffer from digestive disorders, which throw our systems out of gear. The yogi believes in harmony, so he eats for the sake of sustenance only. He does not eat too little. He looks upon his body as the rest house of soul and guards himself against over-indulgence.

Besides food, place is also important for spiritual practice. It is difficult to practise in a distant country away from home, in a forest, in a crowded city, or where it is noisy. One should choose a place where food is easily procurable, which is clean and protected, with pleasing surroundings. The banks of a lake or river or the seashore are ideal. Such quiet ideal places are hard to find in modern times; but one can at least make a corner in one's room available for practice and keep it clean, airy, dry and pest-free.

Santoṣa: Contentment has to be cultivated. A mind that is not content cannot concentrate. The yogi feels the lack of nothing and so he is naturally content. Contentment gives unsurpassed bliss to the yogi. A contented man is complete for he has known the love of the Lord and he has done his duty. He is blessed for he has known truth and joy.

Contentment and tranquillity are states of mind. Differences arise among men because of race, creed, wealth and learning. Differences create discord and there arise conscious or unconscious conflicts, which distract and perplex us. Then the mind cannot become one-pointed *(ekāgra)* and is robbed of its peace. There is contentment and tranquillity when the flame of the self does not waver in the wind of desire. The *sādhaka* does not seek the empty peace of the dead, but the peace of one whose reason is firmly established in God.

Tapas: Tapas is derived from the root *tap* meaning to blaze, burn, shine, suffer pain or consume by heat. Therefore it means a burning effort, under all circumstances, to achieve a definite goal in life. It involves purification, self-discipline and austerity. The whole science of character building may be regarded as a practice of *tapas*.

Tapas is the conscious effort to achieve the ultimate union with the Divine and to burn up all desires which stand in the way of this goal. A worthy aim makes life illumined, pure and divine. Without such an aim, action and prayer have no value. Life without *tapas* is like a heart without love. Without *tapas*, the mind cannot reach up to the Lord.

It is *tapas* when one works without any selfish motive or hope of reward and with an unshakeable faith that not even a blade of grass can move without His will. By *tapas* the yogi develops strength in body, mind and character. He gains courage and wisdom, integrity, straightforwardness and simplicity.

Svādhyāya: Sva means self and *adhyāya* means study or education. Education is the drawing out of the best that is within a person. *Svādhyāya*, therefore, is the education of the self, as a means to attaining knowledge of the Self.

Svādhyāya is different from mere instruction like attending a lecture where the lecturer parades his own learning before the ignorance of his audience. When people meet for *svādhyāya*, the speaker and listener are of one mind and have mutual love and respect. There is no sermonising and one heart speaks to another. The ennobling thoughts that arise from *svādhyāya* are, so to speak, taken into one's bloodstream so that they become a part of one's life and being.

The person practising *svādhyāya* reads his own book of life and at the same time writes and revises it. There is a change in his outlook on life. He starts to realise that all creation is meant for *bhakti* (adoration) rather than for *bhoga* (enjoyment), that all creation is divine, that there is divinity within himself and that the energy that moves him is the same that moves the entire universe.

To make life healthy, happy and peaceful, it is essential regularly to study divine literature in a pure place. This study of the sacred books of the world will enable the *sādhaka* to concentrate upon and solve the difficult problems of life when they arise. It will put an end to ignorance and bring knowledge. Ignorance is from time immemorial, but it has an end. By *svādhyāya* the *sādhaka* understands the nature of his soul and gains communion with the divine. The sacred books of the world are for all to read. They are not meant for the members of one particular faith alone. As bees savour the nectar in various flowers, so the *sādhaka* absorbs things in other faiths that will enable him to appreciate his own faith better.

Īśvara praṇidhāna: Dedication to the Lord of one's actions and will is *Īśvara praṇidhāna*. He who has faith in God does not despair. He has illumination *(tejas)*. He who knows that all creation belongs to the Lord will not be puffed up with pride or drunk with power. He will not stoop for selfish purposes; his head will bow only in worship. When the waters of *bhakti* (adoration) are made to flow through the turbines of the mind, the result is mental power and spiritual illumination. While mere physical strength without *bhakti* is lethal and mere adoration without strength of character is like an opiate. Addiction to pleasures destroys both power and glory. From the gratification of the senses, as they run after pleasures, arise *moha* (attachment) and *lobha* (greed) for their repetition. If the senses are not gratified, then there is *śoka* (sorrow). They have to be curbed with knowledge and forbearance; but to control the mind is more difficult. After one has exhausted one's own resources and still not succeeded, one turns to the Lord for help, for He is the source of all power. It is at this stage that *bhakti* begins. In *bhakti*, the mind, the intellect and the will are surrendered to the Lord and the *sādhaka* prays: "I do not know what is good for me. Thy will be done". Others pray to have their own desires gratified or accomplished. In *bhakti* or true love there is no place for 'I' and "mine". When the feeling of 'I' and "mine" disappears, the individual soul has reached full growth.

When the mind has been emptied of desires for personal gratification, it should be filled with thoughts of the Lord. In a mind filled with thoughts of personal gratification, there is a danger of the senses dragging the mind after objects of desire. Attempts to practise *bhakti* without emptying the mind of desires are like building a fire with wet fuel. It makes a lot of smoke and brings tears to the eyes of the person who builds it and of those around him. A mind with desires does not ignite and glow, nor does it generate light and warmth when touched with the fire of knowledge.

The name of the Lord is like the Sun, dispelling all darkness. The moon is full when it faces the sun. The individual soul experiences fullness *(pūrnatā)* when it faces the Lord. If the shadow of the earth comes between the full moon and the sun, there is an eclipse. If the feeling of 'I' and "mine" casts its shadow upon the experience of fullness, the efforts of the *sādhaka* to gain peace are futile.

Actions mirror a man's personality better than his words. The yogi has learnt the art of dedicating all his actions to the Lord and so they reflect the divinity within him.

ĀSANA

The third limb of yoga is *āsana* or posture. *Āsana* brings steadiness, health and lightness of limb. A steady and pleasant posture produces mental equilibrium and prevents fickleness of mind. *Āsana* are not to be treated merely gymnastic exercises; they are postures. To perform them one needs a clean airy place, a blanket and determination, while for other systems of physical training one needs large playing fields and costly equipment. *Āsana* can be practised alone as the limbs of the body provide the necessary weights and counter-weights. By practising them one develops agility, balance, endurance and great vitality.

Āsana have been evolved over the centuries to ensure that every muscle, nerve and gland in the body is exercised. It secures a fine physique, which is strong and elastic without being muscle-bound and keeps the body free from disease. It reduces fatigue and soothes the nerves. But its real importance lies in the way it trains and disciplines the mind.

There may be many actors, acrobats, athletes, dancers, musicians and sportsmen who possess superb physiques and have great control over their body, but it does not mean that they have control over the senses, the mind and intelligence. They might have a harmonious development of muscle and movement, but it is far from certain that they will be of a balanced character or at harmony with themselves. For them the body and its physique may be an object of cult. Though the yogi does not underrate his body, he does not think merely of its perfection but of his senses, mind and intelligence in order to reach the soul. The yogi conquers the body by the practice of *āsana* and makes it a fit vehicle for the soul. This is the necessary role of body.

By performing *āsana*, the *sādhaka* first gains health, which is not mere existence. It is not a commodity that can be purchased with money. It is an asset to be gained by sheer hard work. It is a state of complete equilibrium of body, mind and self. Forgetfulness of physical and mental consciousness is health. The yogi frees himself from physical disabilities and mental distractions by practising *āsana* and he surrenders his actions and their fruits to the Lord in the service of the world.

The yogi realises that his life and all its activities are part of the divine action in nature, manifesting and operating in the form of man. In the beating of his pulse and the rhythm of his respiration, he recognises the flow of the seasons and the throbbing of universal life. His body is a temple, which houses the Divine Spark. He feels that to neglect or to deny the needs of the body and to think of it as something not divine, is to neglect and deny the Universal Life of which it is a part. The needs of the body are the needs of the divine self, which lives through the body. The yogi does not look heavenward to find God for he knows that He is within, being known as the *antarātman* (the Inner Self). He feels the kingdom of God within and without and finds that heaven lies in himself.

Where does the body end and the mind begin? Where does the mind end and the Self begin? They cannot be divided, as they are interrelated, yet different aspects of the same all-pervading divine consciousness.

The yogi never neglects or mortifies the body or the mind, but cherishes both. To him the body is not an impediment to his spiritual liberation, nor is it the cause of his fall, but is an instrument for attainment. He seeks a body as strong as a thunderbolt, healthy and free from suffering so as to dedicate it in the service of the Lord for which it is intended. As pointed out in the *Muṇḍakopaniṣad,* the Self cannot be attained by one without strength, nor through heedlessness, or without an aim. Just as an unbaked earthen pot dissolves in water, the body soon decays. So bake it hard in the fire of yogic discipline in order to strengthen and purify it.

The names of the *āsana* are significant and illustrate the principle of evolution. Some are named after vegetation like the tree *(vṛkṣa)* and the lotus *(padma);* some after invertebrates like the locust *(śalabha)* and the scorpion *(vṛśchika);* some after aquatic animals and amphibians like the fish *(matsya),* the tortoise *(kūrma),* the frog *(bheka* or *maṇḍūka)* or the crocodile *(nakra).*

There are *āsanas* called after birds like the cock *(kukkuṭa)*, the heron *(baka)*, the peacock *(mayūra)* and the swan *(haṁsa)*. They are also named after quadrupeds like the dog *(śvāna)*, the horse *(vātāyana)*, the camel *(uṣṭra)* and the lion *(siṁha)*. Creatures that crawl like the serpent *(bhujaṅga)* are not forgotten, nor is the human embryonic state *(garbha-piṇḍa)* overlooked. *Āsana* are named after legendary heroes like Vīrabhadra and Hanumān, son of the Wind. Sages like Bharadvāja, Kapila, Vasiṣtha and Viśvāmitra are remembered by having *āsana* named after them. Some *āsana* are also called after gods of the Hindu pantheon and some recall the *Avatāra*, or incarnations of Divine Power. Whilst performing *āsana* the yogi's body assumes many forms resembling a variety of creatures. His mind is trained not to despise any creature, for he knows that throughout the whole gamut of creation, from the lowest insect to the most perfect sage, there breathes the same Universal Soul which assumes innumerable forms. He knows that the highest form is that of the Formless. He finds unity in universality. True *āsana* is that in which the thought of Brahman flows effortlessly and incessantly through the mind of the *sādhaka*.

Dualities like gain and loss, victory and defeat, fame and shame, body and mind, as well as mind and soul vanish through mastery of *āsana*, and the *sādhaka* then passes on to *prāṇāyāma*, the fourth stage in the path of yoga.

PRĀṆĀYĀMA

Just as the word yoga is one of wide import, so also is *prāṇa*. *Prāṇa* means breath, respiration, life, vitality, wind, energy or strength. It also connotes the soul as opposed to the body. The word is generally used in the plural to indicate vital breaths. *Āyāma* means length, expansion, stretching or restraint. *Prāṇāyāma* thus connotes extension of breath and its control. This control is mainly over the three aspects of breathing, namely, (1) inhalation or inspiration, which is termed *pūraka* (filling up), (2) exhalation or expiration, which is called *recaka* (emptying) and (3) retention or holding the breath either after inhalation or after exhalation. This is termed *kuṁbhaka* (pot either full or empty). In some of the texts on yoga, *kuṁbhaka* is also used in a loose generic sense to include all the three respiratory processes of inhalation, exhalation and retention. A *kuṁbha* is a pitcher, water pot, jar or chalice. A water pot may be emptied of all air and filled completely with water, or it may be emptied of all water and filled completely with air. Similarly, during inhalation the lungs are filled with the life-giving air and after this is done *(pūraka)*, the fullness of the lungs is retained *(antara kuṁbhaka)*, whereas during exhalation *(recaka)*, the lungs are emptied of noxious air and retained without air *(bāhyabāhya kuṁbhaka)*.

The yogi's life is not measured by the number of his days, but by the number of his breaths. Therefore, he follows the proper rhythmic patterns of slow deep breathing. These rhythmic patterns strengthen the respiratory system, soothe the nervous system and reduce craving. As desires and cravings diminish, the mind is set free and becomes a fit tool for concentration. It has been said by Kariba Ekken, a seventeenth century mystic: "If you would foster a calm spirit, first regulate your breathing; for when that is under control, the heart will be at peace; but when breathing is spasmodic, then it will be troubled. Therefore, before attempting anything, first regulate your breathing on which your temper will be softened, your spirit calmed".

Prāṇāyāma is thus the science of breath. It is the hub around which the wheel of life revolves. "As lions, elephants and tigers are tamed very slowly and cautiously, so should *prāṇa* be brought under control very slowly in gradation measured according to one's capacity and physical limitations. Otherwise it will kill the practitioner", warns *Haṭhayoga Pradīpikā*. Often people attempt to start the practice of *prāṇāyāma* alone by themselves, without having the proper base and without knowing their physical and mental limitations. For it is essential to have the guidance of a *guru*.

In the practice of *prāṇāyāma* the nostrils, nasal passages and membranes, the windpipe, the lungs, the diaphragm and the spine are the only parts of the body which are actively involved. These alone feel the full impact of the force of *prāṇa*, the breath of life. By its proper practice, though one is freed from many diseases, yet by its improper practice respiratory diseases will be invited and the nervous system will be shattered. Therefore, one should not choose to learn or do *prāṇāyāma* in a hurry, as one is playing with life itself. The *sādhaka* may introduce several disorders into his system like hiccough, wind, asthma, cough, catarrh, pains in the head, eyes and ears and nervous irritation. It takes a long time to learn slow, deep, steady and proper inhalation and exhalation. One needs to master this before attempting *kuṁbhaka*.

As a fire blazes brightly when the covering of ash over it is scattered by the wind, the divine fire within the body shines in all its majesty when the ashes of desire are scattered by the practice of *prāṇāyāma*. *Prāṇa* in the body of the individual is part of the cosmic energy. In *prāṇāyāma* an attempt is made to harmonise the individual breath *(piṇḍa-prāṇa)* with the cosmic breath *(brahmāṇḍa-prāṇa or viśva caitanya śakti)*.

THE CHARIOT OF MAN

The consciousness is like a chariot yoked to a team of powerful horses. One of them is breath *(prāṇa)*, the other is desire *(vāsanā)*. The powerful horse pulls the chariot in its own direction. If breath prevails, the desires are controlled, the senses are held in check and the mind is stilled.

If desire prevails, breath is in disarray and the mind is agitated and troubled. The yogi masters the science of breath and, by the regulation and control of breath, he controls the mind and stills its constant movement. In the practice of *prāṇāyāma* the eyes, the gateways to the mind, are kept shut to prevent the mind from wandering. "When the *prāṇa* and *manas* (mind) have been absorbed, an indefinable joy ensues". (*H.Y.P.*, IV.30).

Emotional excitement affects the rate of breathing; equally, deliberate regulation of breathing checks emotional excitement. As the very object of yoga is to control and still the mind, the yogi first learns *prāṇāyāma* to master the breath. This enables him to control the senses in order to reach the stage of *pratyāhāra*. Only then will the mind be ready for concentration.

PRATYĀHĀRA

If a man's reason succumbs to the pull of his senses, he is lost. On the other hand, if there is rhythmic control of the breath, the senses, instead of running after external objects of desire, turn inwards and man is set free from their tyranny. This is the fifth stage of yoga, namely, *pratyāhāra*, where the senses are brought under control.

When this stage is reached, the *sādhaka* goes through a searching self-examination. To overcome the deadly but attractive spell of sensual objects, he needs the insulation of adoration *(bhakti)* by recalling to his mind the Creator who made the objects of his desire. He also needs the lamp of knowledge of his divine heritage. The mind is in truth the cause of bondage and liberation; it brings bondage if it is bound to the objects of desire, and liberation when it is free from those objects. There is bondage when the mind craves, grieves or is unhappy over something. The mind becomes pure when all desires and fears are annihilated. Both the good and the pleasant present themselves to men and prompt them to action. The yogi prefers the good to the pleasant. Others, driven by their desires, prefer the pleasant to the good and miss the very purpose of life.

The yogi feels joy in what he is. He knows how and where to stop and therefore lives in peace. At first he prefers that which is bitter as poison, but he perseveres in this practice knowing well that in the end it will become as sweet as nectar. Others, hankering for the union of their senses with the objects of their desires, prefer that which at first seems as sweet as nectar, but do not know that in the end it will be as bitter as poison.

The yogi knows that the path towards satisfaction of the senses by sensual desire is broad, but that it leads to destruction and that there are many who follow it. The path of yoga is like the sharp edge of a razor, narrow and difficult to tread, and there are very few who follow and realise its value. The yogi knows that the paths of ruin or of salvation lie within himself.

Consciousness manifests with three different qualities. For man, his life and his consciousness, together with the entire cosmos, are the emanations of one and the same *prakṛti* (cosmic matter or substance), emanations that differ in designation by the predominance of one or other of the *guṇa* (quality or attribute), namely *sattva, rajas* and *tamas. Sattva* is the illuminating, pure or good quality, which leads to clarity and mental serenity. *Rajas* is the quality of mobility or activity, which makes a person active and energetic, tense and wilful. *Tamas* is a quality of delusion, obscurity, inertia and ignorance, which obstructs and counteracts the tendency of *rajas* and *sattva*.

The quality of *sattva* leads towards the divine and *tamas* towards the devilish, while in between these two stands *rajas*.

The faith held, the food consumed, the actions done, the sacrifices performed, the austerities undergone and the donations given, the thoughts conceived and deliberated by each individual vary in accordance with his predominating *guṇa*.

The yogi, who is human, is also affected by the three *guṇa*. By his constant and disciplined study of himself and of the objects that his senses tend to pursue, he learns which thoughts, words and actions are prompted by *tamas* and which by *rajas*. With unceasing effort he weeds out and eradicates such thoughts as are prompted by *tamas* and he works to achieve a *sāttvic* frame of mind. When the *sattvaguṇa* is preponderant, the human soul has advanced a long way towards the ultimate goal.

DHĀRAṆĀ

When the body has been tempered by *āsana*, when the mind has been refined by the fire of *prāṇāyāma* and when the senses have been brought under control by *pratyāhāra*, the *sādhaka* reaches the sixth stage called *dhāraṇā*. Here he concentrates wholly on a single point or on a task in which he is completely engrossed. The mind is stilled in order to achieve this state of complete absorption.

The mind is an instrument that classifies, judges and co-ordinates the impressions from the outside world and those that arise within oneself. Thoughts are the product of the mind. They are difficult to restrain for they are subtle and fickle. A thought that is well guarded by a controlled mind brings happiness. To get the best out of an instrument, one must know how it works. The mind is the instrument for thinking and therefore it is necessary to consider how it functions. Mental states are classified in five groups. In the *mūḍha* state the mind is foolish, dull and stupid. It is confounded and at a loss to know what it wants and here the *tamō-guṇa* predominates. The second of these is the *kṣipta* state, where the mental forces are scattered, being in disarray and in a state of neglect. Here the mind hankers after objects, the *rajō-guṇa* being dominant. The third is the *vikṣipta* state, where the mind is agitated and distracted. Here there is a capacity to enjoy the fruits of one's efforts, but the desires are not marshalled and controlled.

The fourth state of the mind is the *ekāgra* (*eka* = one; *agra* = foremost) state, where the mind is closely attentive and the mental faculties are concentrated on a single object or focused on one point only, with the *sattva-guṇa* prevailing. The *ekāgra* person has superior intellectual powers and knows exactly what he wants, so he uses all his powers to achieve his purpose. At times the ruthless pursuit of the desired object, irrespective of the cost to others, can create great misery. It often happens that even if the desired object is achieved, it leaves behind a bitter taste.

The last mental state is that of *niruddha*, where the mind *(manas)*, intelligence *(buddhi)* and ego *(ahaṁkāra)* are all restrained and all these faculties are offered to the Lord for His use and in His service. Here there is no feeling of 'I' and "mine". As a lens becomes more luminous when strong light is thrown upon it and seems to be all light and indistinguishable from it, so also the *sādhaka*, who has given up this mind, intelligence and ego to the Lord, becomes one with Him, for he thinks of nothing but Him who is the creator of thought.

DHYĀNA

As water takes the shape of its container, the mind, when it contemplates an object, is transformed into the shape of that object. The mind that thinks of the all-pervading divinity, which it worships, is ultimately, through long-continued devotion, transformed into the likeness of that divinity.

When oil is poured from one vessel to another, one can observe the steady constant flow. When the flow of concentration is uninterrupted, the state that arises is *dhyāna* (meditation). As the filament in an electric bulb glows and illumines when there is a regular uninterrupted current of electricity, the yogi's mind will be illumined by *dhyāna*. His body, breath, senses, mind, intelligence and ego are all integrated in the object of his contemplation – the Universal Soul. He remains in a state of consciousness that has no qualification whatsoever. There is no other feeling except a state of Supreme Bliss. (Plate n. 7)

The signs of progress on the path of yoga are health, a sense of physical lightness, steadiness, clearness of countenance and a beautiful voice, sweetness of odour of the body and freedom from craving. One has a balanced, serene and tranquil mind. The aspirant is the very symbol of humility. He dedicates all his actions to the Lord taking refuge in Him, frees himself from the bondage of *karma* (action) and becomes a *jīvana mukta* (a liberated soul).

SAMĀDHI

Samādhi is the end of the *sādhaka's* quest. At the peak of his meditation he passes into the state of *samādhi*, where his body and senses are at rest as if he is asleep, his faculties of mind and intelligence are alert as if he is awake, yet he has gone beyond consciousness. The person in a state of *samādhi* is fully conscious and alert.

The *sādhaka* is tranquil and worships Brahman as that from which he came forth, as that in which he breathes, as that into which he will be dissolved. He realises that all creation is Brahman and the soul within the heart is smaller than the smallest seed, yet greater than the sky. The *sādhaka* enters into this state with fully matured and ripe intelligence. Then for him there remains no sense of 'I' or "mine", as the working of the body, the mind and the intelligence has stopped as if they have gone into deep sleep. When the *sādhaka* has attained an ultimate or final state, there is only the experience of being, truth and unutterable joy. There is a peace that passeth all understanding. The mind cannot find words to describe the state and the tongue fails to utter them. Comparing the experience of *samādhi* with other experiences, the sages say: *"Neti! Neti!"* – "It is not this! It is not this!" The state can only be expressed by profound silence. The yogi has departed from the material world and is merged in the Eternal. Then there is no duality between the knower and the known for they are merged like camphor and the flame.

There wells up, from within the heart of the yogi, the *Song of the soul*, sung by Shri Adi Shankara in his *Ātma Ṣaṭakam*:

I am neither ego nor intelligence, I am neither mind nor thought,
I cannot be heard nor cast into words, nor by odour nor sight ever caught:
In light and wind I am not found, nor yet in earth and sky -
Consciousness and joy incarnate, Bliss of the Blissful am I.

I have no name, I have no life, I breathe no vital air,
No elements have moulded me, no bodily sheath is my lair:
I have no speech, no hands and feet, nor means of evolution -
Consciousness and joy am I, and Bliss in dissolution.

I cast aside hatred and passion, I conquered delusion and greed;
No touch of pride caressed me, so envy never did breed:
Beyond all faiths, past reach of wealth, past freedom, past desire,
Consciousness and joy am I, and Bliss is my attire.

Virtue and vice, or pleasure and pain are not my heritage,
Nor sacred texts, nor offerings, nor prayer, nor pilgrimage:
I am neither food, nor eating, nor yet the eater am I -
Consciousness and joy incarnate, Bliss of the Blissful am I.

I have no misgiving of death, no chasms of race divide me,
No parent ever called me child, no bond of birth ever tied me:
I am neither disciple nor master, I have no kin, no friend -
Consciousness and joy am I, and merging in Bliss is my end.

Neither knowable, knowledge, nor knower am I, formless is my form
I dwell within the senses but they are not my home:
Ever serenely balanced, I am neither free nor bound -
Consciousness and joy am I, and bliss where I am found.

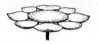

SVĀTMARĀMA SHAKES PATAÑJALI'S HAND*

Children of yoga,

I am indeed pleased to see that the seed of yoga that I sowed in San Francisco in 1974 has grown very well. I see the zeal and interest you all have. The reception I received just now shows how delighted you all must be at having me here with you.

The yoga we practise is a noble and majestic subject, but sadly misinterpreted and misrepresented. It was this challenge that helped me to strive to prove the critics and detractors of yoga were wrong. Today's gathering proves that my work is going in the right direction and gaining momentum.

Many people practise yoga. However few have a clear picture of the value of this famous subject, so better I say a few words about it and use more time for the practical presentation.

According to the scriptures, *ha* means the "sun" – solar energy – and *ṭha* means the "moon" – lunar energy. These two energies function in us at physiological, psychological and mental levels. When these two energies unite and are wedded together, they become one. Thus the merged energies together become the divine energy which ignites the spiritual light in the practitioner of yoga. As these energies basically cleanse the nervous system of the *sādhaka*, one should not mistake of thinking that *haṭha yoga* deals with the physical and physiological level only. It begins but does not end here. It takes one further than the known physical level. It brings the *sādhaka* to mental equilibrium as well as to spiritual contentment and delight.

Ha, the "sun", stands for the *ātman* or the Self. The sun or the Self never fade. The moon draws the energy from the sun to cool this planet of ours by reflecting the glory of the sun.

The rays of the sun cause the moon to shine and in turn the Earth is benefitted. The Earth maintains its environmental and atmospheric balance. In our body too we have this provision. Whatever exists in *Brahmāṇḍa* (Universe) exists in *Piṇḍāṇḍa* (individual) too.

* Address at the Palace of Fine Arts, San Francisco, June 1990.

The sun and moon both exist in us. The Self is the sun, and the consciousness is the moon. The consciousness draws the light from the Self and it is reflected on the entire human system. So consciousness or *citta* is dependent on the light of the Self. In turn our entire body is benefitted by the contact of sun and moon. Hence, *haṭha yoga* is the energy of the nervous system uniting consciousness and Self. The nervous system including the brain is a kind of bridge, or a link between the body and consciousness. *Haṭha yoga* is a means to strengthen this bridge. Thus the energy of the body and consciousness, which of course is *prakṛti*, is united with *puruṣa*. *Haṭha yoga* calls *puruṣa* (the *ātman)*, as Shiva, and *prakṛti* as *śakti*. *Haṭha yoga* thereby brings the union of *puruṣa* and *prakṛti*. It is the union of Shiva and Shakti.

We human beings are covered with five sheaths, called *pañcakośa*. They are *annamaya, prāṇamaya, manomaya, vijñānamaya and ānandamaya kośa* (Table n. 4). These sheaths encase the indweller. *Prakṛti* ensheaths the *puruṣa* in us. They are the anatomical, physiological, mental, intellectual and blissful sheaths. They blend together, becoming one to dwell with the indweller, creating spiritual bliss.

In human beings *citta*, the consciousness, is the pinnacle of all the elements of nature *(prakṛti)*. The consciousness has three components called mind, 'I'-ness or ego and intelligence. When the *citta* is pervaded with intelligence, it becomes illumined. When such enlightened intelligence is brought into contact with the fineness of the Self, it is known as the divine marriage of the *puruṣa* and *prakṛti*, or the Self with the body. This is the teaching of *haṭha yoga*. Without knowing the depth of the subject, if we stigmatise *haṭha yoga* as physical yoga, then it shows nothing but the poverty of our intelligence. It is mere propaganda by those who are too unprepared to train their bodies and transform them into a holy shrine for the Self.

Often *haṭha yoga* is equated with *āsana* and the *āsana*-aspect is reduced or degraded to physical exercise. Let us see what Patañjali says about *āsana*, one of the eight petals of yoga.

The *Yoga Sūtra* defines *āsana* and its effects in three aphorisms (*Y.S.*, II.46-48). The first is, *Sthira sukham āsanam* (*Y.S.*, II.46). Steady and comfortable posture is an *āsana*. Its effect is to take one beyond the disturbances of duality. We are caught up in our own comfort and joy, and consequently fail to open our eyes. We do not see what Patañjali meant when he defined the *āsana*. He wanted each one to derive not only steadiness and comfort, but also unity in body, consciousness and self from the practice of *āsana: Tataḥ dvandvāḥ anabhighātaḥ* (*Y.S.*, II.48). Here Patañjali says that *āsana* makes one not only experience an undisturbed, non-dual state, but at the same time indicates the wealth that the yogi gains through its practice. According to him, the wealth of the yogi is beauty and charm in body, grace in approach, compactness, elephantine strength, impenetrable willpower, loveliness in mind and liveliness in mental attitude, firm as a diamond and soft as a petal.[1] Many of you will have read these aphorisms hundreds of times without noticing the implication of the value of *āsana* as he deals with them.

The *Haṭhayoga Pradīpika*, on the other hand, explains that the body is inert and cannot work on its own, but that its functions depend on the senses and the mind. The mind, being vibrant, moves fast. *Haṭha yoga* guides each practitioner to take the inert body to the level of the vibrant mind. By intensifying the practice, awareness, the power of attention and the intelligence increase for further interpenetration, which in turn develops the potential of the cells throughout the body and the mind to reach the level of the serenity of the Self.[2]

Does not this definition of *āsana* from the *Haṭhayoga Pradīpika* convey the same meaning as Patañjali's three aphorisms? It is important that you go through the text, otherwise you can only believe what others say and be misled. *Haṭha yoga* texts say, use the body as a springboard to unveil the coverings of the Self, so that the Self shines in a pure naked mind. That naked mind is nothing but absolute consciousness. If coal is covered by ash, we have the illusion that it is only ash, but the moment you touch the ash, your fingers get burnt. Similarly the practice of yoga makes the intelligence like a live wire, so that impediments, fluctuations or changes *(vṛtti)* are noticed by the consciousness, which carries the message to its master, the Self. Then the master directs and guides the consciousness on how to counteract the disturbances by practical means. This is the technique of yoga.

Some individuals who have reached the zenith may say that these practices are not essential but we are not all so blessed as they are. We have to be prepared to work from scratch. You and I are in the same boat, facing sorrow, despair and disease. We have to cross these bridges of sorrow and illness one by one to reach the last bridge, the space between the intelligence and Self, and cross over that bridge so that the intelligence and the Self commune with each other and become a single instrument. Thus the impediments and disturbances are counteracted, and the pure, uncontaminated intelligence and the Self remain in harmony with each other. Patañjali calls this communion "exalted intelligence" *(vivekaja jñānam)*. When this exalted intelligence reaches the culminating point, the *prakṛti* unites with *puruṣa* and both become one.

Kṣetra is *prakṛti* or the field or the body. *Kṣetrajñā* is the knower of the field, the *ātman* or *puruṣa* or the Self. You may have read in *Light on Yoga*[3] the analogy of the chariot and the charioteer. The body is the chariot. The senses are the horses. The *ātman* is the charioteer. This

---

1 *Rūpa lāvaṇya bala vajra saṁhananatvāni kāyasampat* (*Y.S.*, III.47).
2 See *H.Y.P.*, I.17, *Jyotsnā* (Brahmananda's commentary), Adyar Library and Research Centre, Chennai.
3 Published by Harper Collins, London.

chariot has to be maintained like your car: you send it for servicing and lubrication so that when you drive, it runs smoothly. Similarly, yoga keeps the body healthy so that the senses are ready and move with smoothness for the journey towards Self-realisation. In order to build this strength in the mind and consciousness, the yogic steps of *āsana* and *prāṇāyāma* are given.

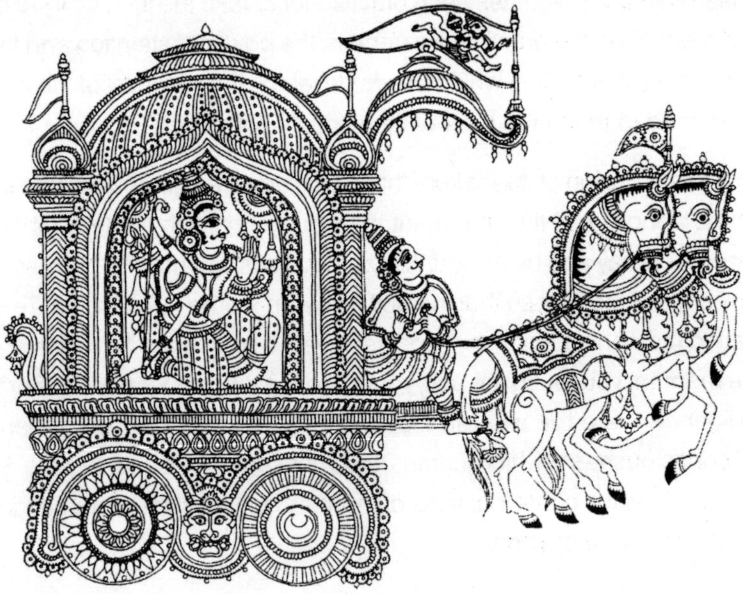

This is the background for us to start yoga from first principles, i.e.; cleansing the body, clearing the dust inside it that is in our way of thinking, acting and comportment. By practice, the external attributes of Self are cleansed and the mind is made free to send messages to the intelligence. The intelligence communicates with the Self and the Self in turn guides us to act in a right way. When the practice of yoga becomes internal, we use the body and the mind as complementary and supplementary instruments of the Self. When mind, intelligence, ego and consciousness are yoked together to move in unison, the experience of oneness or equipoise is felt within us.

However when the internal journey begins, the intricacy of the yogic method is understood more deeply and clearly. We humans are time-bound. We lose sight of eternity as time ensnares us. Art is eternal, not bound by time. But when you and I sit here and discuss, time is involved. As time gets involved, we lose sight of eternity. No philosopher has explained time as beautifully as Patañjali. Time is the movement of moments. The movement of moments rolls on like a wheel and the moments move constantly like spokes of the wheel. This movement of spokes of moments is time as past, present and future. If you do not get enticed or disturbed and do not get caught by the movement of moments, and give your attention to observing the moment only, then you experience the virgin state of timelessness[1].

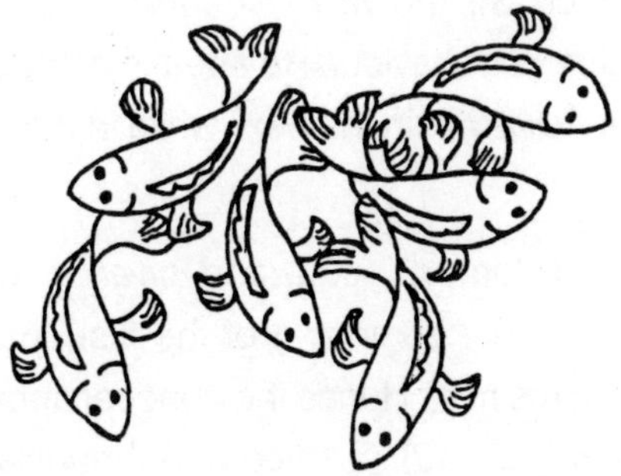

The mind is like a fish in water which is constantly moving. Motion and movement are its inherent nature. It tosses on the movements of the moments. Every present and future moment turns into a past moment. The mind is carried off on the rushing stream of moments and does not remain in the single, still and present moment. When intelligence reaches the exalted state, then the turbulent *citta* is silenced. Only then does one understand moments and live constantly in the purity of the moment. When the moment changes into movement, the present is forgotten and mind becomes sullied by past thoughts and future planning. In order to see through the mentally created construct of time, we need to be pure. We need to be unpolluted. The practice of yoga brings this purification in ourselves – in our *prakṛti* from the outer sheath to the inner sheath. The exalted yogi teaches one how to observe and live in the *āsana*, or even when one is walking, how one has to live in the moment. Such a person would definitely be a highly sensitive intelligent human being. The practice of *āsana* and *prāṇāyāma* can lead us to this lofty condition.

For everyone the practice of yoga has to begin from the very first step of the ladder. Naturally one has to face a lot of ups and downs in the practice. Some trees are healthy; they give fruits earlier than one anticipates. Some trees grow very healthy but bear no fruit. Some seeds take ten or fifteen years to sprout. Some sprout in two or three days. Therefore nobody can decide when the seed of yoga will sprout in one and when the tree of yoga will give fruit. (Plate n. 4)

You have begun well. Now lots of dedicated pupils are there with teachers to guide them. I feel and say, "Where there is dedication, the method always grows in the right direction". As a dedicated pupil of yoga, doubt should not arise in your mind. So let there be no misconception about *haṭha yoga* and *rāja yoga* being separate and different.

---

1 See *Light on the Yoga Sūtras of Patañjali*, Harper Collins, London.

Let me once again return to Patañjali. All of you know that yoga means *citta vṛtti nirodhaḥ*. This is the second *sūtra*, but how many think about what the first *sūtra* conveys? It says, *Atha Yogānuśāsanam*. All translators say, "Now the exposition of yoga". *Anuśāsana* is not "exposition". *Śāsana* is a code of conduct for human beings, something that has to be followed. Is it just an exposition? Or is it an exposition on the code of conduct? So, the very first *sūtra* of Patañjali involves *abhyāṣa* – practice. What is practice? It is a code of behaviour. He speaks of practice *(abhyāsa)* in the first *sūtra* and restraint and detachment *(vairāgya)* in the next, while in the third, he describes the zenith of *abhyāsa* and *vairāgya*.

Practice is imbued with codes of conduct in the form of *yama* and *niyama*, which Patañjali explains later. He speaks of renunciation in the very beginning of the first chapter because the people of his time were capable of observing restraint. Hence the concept appears early in the text as *abhyāsa vairāgyābhyām tannirodhaḥ* (*Y.S.*, I.12), practice and renunciation restrain the movements of consciousness. His introduction of restraint in the first chapter is meant for the enlightened ones, known as *uttamābhyāsi* (intensively intense practitioners), or those who have the seed of yoga in their hearts. Through intense practice, their intrinsic genius rapidly germinates and grows to the highest level.

The fourth *sūtra* of the first chapter says that the self is drawn by mind to sweet waves of pleasure and fluctuating mood. Patañjali does not want the *sādhaka* to be caught in the web of thought, but to cut his way to freedom. That is why *abhyāsa* (practice) and *vairāgya* (renunciation) were dealt with so early in the text for those who are intensely intense.

Knowing that it is not possible for all to keep the self away from the net of the mind, Patañjali has divided the practice into four stages according to the level of the *sādhaka* known as *mṛdu, madhya, adhimātra* and *tīvra* (mild, middle, intense and intensely intense). In the first chapter he is speaking for the intensely intense *sādhaka* and not for the other levels.

The second chapter is for the mild, the average and the intense students. There he begins, with *tapaḥ svādhyāya Īśvarapraṇidhānāni kriyāyogaḥ* (*Y.S.*, II.1), which means, practice with zeal, study to know about the Self, and devotion towards God. For an average intellect, this yoga filled with action is easier than jumping straight into renunciation. In *tapas*, *karma* is involved. *Tapas* builds up cleanliness of the body, of the senses and mind. Only when the mind is cleansed is the *sādhaka* able to understand something about the Self; so *svādhyāya*, or study of the Self, begins externally as acquired knowledge *(jñāna)*. If *tapas* is action, *svādhyāya* is knowledge. *Karma* leads towards *jñāna*. When knowledge dawns, we understand the functions of the inner self. When this understanding becomes ripe and exalted, the time has come to learn to surrender everything, including ourselves, to God *(Īśvara praṇidhāna)*. This is *bhakti*.

We use the expression "surrender to God". Patañjali explains who is a fit person to surrender. A person who has perfected his body, senses, mind, and whose intelligence is utterly clear and exalted; only that person is able to surrender to God. Where *karma, jñāna* and *bhakti* meet, that is *kriyāyoga* or the foundation of *aṣṭadaḷa yoga.*

For you and me, he has given the name *aṣṭāṅga yoga,* so that we may easily understand and then climb the ladder, step by step, of *yama-niyama-āsana-prāṇāyāma-pratyāhāra-dhāraṇā-dhyāna-samādhi.* As a common principle, all ancient Indian philosophers begin from the top and then come down to the bottom; whereas today writers start from the bottom and take one towards the essence of the subject.

Patañjali comes to the base in the second chapter and shows different ways for an average person to understand the subject. He begins the second chapter by explaining what one has to do, what one has to observe, and how one has to reflect and live. He connects the first *sūtra* of the first chapter, *anuśāsanam,* with *yama (karmendriya vṛtti staṁbhana)* and *niyama (jñānendriya vṛtti staṁbhana),* since one has to bring stability and control in the organs of action and senses of perception respectively, before bringing restraint in one's behaviour. *Yama* and *niyama* teach us the ways of building our behavioural patterns, *anuśāsanam.*

Āsana cultures our sinews, fibres and tendons and brings sensitivity of intelligence in these. Though I often defined it as *snāyuvṛtti nirodha* (restraint of the fluctuations of the cells), or more precisely as *snāyuvṛtti sthiratā* (to bring a state of firmness to the cells) and *snāyuvṛtti samādhāna* (to bring the equipoise to the cells), its more appropriate definition would be *śānta snāyuvṛtti pariṇāma* (transformation towards tranquillity of the cells). *Snāyu* stands for the sinews, the cellular and the nervous systems. The practice of *āsana* keeps them in a state of concord.

Then comes *prāṇāyāma. Prāṇāyāma* is *prāṇa vṛtti staṁbhana*[1]. The vital energy is controlled, stabilised, sustained and retained before it is restrained. It prevents the vital energy from dissipating and deviating unnecessarily. By this the system retains power and vigour.

Through *yama* and *niyama* the mind is indirectly stilled, whereas in *pratyāhāra* it is brought under direct control. Hence in *pratyāhāra, śānta manovṛtti parināma*[2] takes place. We must always be on guard that our senses do not entice our mind into the pastures of pleasure, but that it remains in a pacified state.

---

[1] And more precisely *samādhāna prāṇavṛtti pariṇāma* (transformation towards equipoise through calming the fluctuation of energy).

[2] Transformation towards tranquillity of mind.

After mastery in these aspects of yoga, Patañjali says, "mind *(manas)* is now fit for concentration, *dhāraṇā*". Here, he uses the word *manas* since it is a constituent of *citta. Pratyāhāra* transforms the mind for concentration. Focussing the mind *(dhāraṇā)* on a given subject or a given thought, frees the mind from fluctuations, modifications and modulations, and puts an end to its wanderings. When the mind is stabilised by the practice of *dhāraṇā*, then comes *dhyāna*.

In *dhyāna* or meditation, not only is the intelligence kept stable, sharp and dynamic, both inside and outside, from inner to outer and outer to inner, but also the *ahaṁkāra* (the impostor of the Self) is reduced to insignificance. Prolonged continuation of this non-egoistic state is *samādhi*. In *samādhi*, the *ahaṁkāra* dissolves, as does the *citta*, because the *sādhaka* loses the feedback from their accessories. As they are silent, so the consciousness becomes silent. In this state of silence, the consciousness loses its identity and the Self shines in an absolute state. This is the end of yoga. The search for the Self culminates.

Patañjali says that the search and the feeling of the Self fade out and disappear. *Ātma bhāva bhāvanā nivṛttiḥ* (*Y.S.*, IV.25). There is no place for I, Me and Mine. The barriers are removed, the Self shines, and there is no room for separateness. The conceptions of "I am different from this", "I am different from that", vanish. One hears that body is different, mind is different and Self is different. When the feeling of the Self or *ātma-bhāva* does not exist, where is the body, where is the mind, where is the goal? The soul and the goal become one. It may take several years of persistent, patient and persevering yogic practice. We may have to wait for years, or for the next life or lives to come, to live in the state of oneness of body, mind and soul.

WHY PRACTISE *AṢṬĀṄGA YOGA?**

I have been a practitioner of yoga for the last sixty years and with a background of teaching for fifty-eight years.

Five decades ago, yoga was not as popular as it is today. In those days, many in India were under the impression that yoga was meant for those who leave their homes breaking away from their family. In the early days of my *sādhanā* I was considered as such. People were pointing their fingers at me as a madcap!

In those days, knowledge on yoga was not widespread as it is today. It was then a Herculean task for me to ignite interest in it and explain how its practice could culture both the physical and mental well-being of man.

The only way to impress people and to arouse interest was to give lecture-demonstrations so that they could directly see and perceive the art.

There is no doubt that yoga structure plays an important role in maintaining the body as well as keeping the respiratory, circulatory, nervous, digestive and hormonal systems in perfect balance, besides providing mental uplift and intellectual clarity.

Nowadays, health clubs have sprouted everywhere and yoga has gone into these clubs as both health building and remedial therapy. This is how yoga has gained popularity.

Is yoga meant only to remove structural disorders such as backaches, physiological disorders such as indigestion and psychological disorders such as emotional stresses and strains, or has yoga something more to offer?

In the beginning, each one of us has some motivation to get rid of physical or emotional problems. When relieved, why do we continue the practice? Is it just to tone the body, or is it to

---

* Talk by *Gurujī* on Hanuman Jayanti, April 1992.

tune the mind? We have now some understanding of the importance of a healthy body and a healthy mind. Ultimately, the aim of yoga is to make the seeker become the seer. This is *ātma-darśana*, and then the yogi proceeds towards *paramātma-darśana*.

Normally we practise as doers. Then we begin to see and observe the changes in our attitudes and we begin to feel something hidden. This hidden feeling of something becomes the source for our transformation from the physical and mental levels towards the spiritual level.

The *Viśiṣṭādvaita* philosophy of Shri Ramanuja is practically based on the performance of pure *karma*. Shri Ramanuja insists on actions throughout the spiritual endeavour as being moral and ethico-religious, as well as psycho-spiritual practice. According to him, *bhakti* is undoubtedly the ultimate goal, but the *bhakti* he propounds is not a blind one. *Bhakti* is attainable through *jñāna* derived from *karma* or actions done without attachment to their fruits. Patañjali, in the Sādhana Pāda of the *Yoga Sūtra*, expresses the purport of this methodology of Shri Ramanuja. It is recognised as *kriyāyoga*. *Tapaḥ svādhyāya Īśvarapraṇidhānani kriyāyogaḥ* (*Y.S.*, II.1)[1]. *Aṣṭāṅga yoga* is structured in the scale of *kriyāyoga* based on *karma, jñāna* and *bhakti*. This *sūtra* imports the very approach of Shri Ramanuja, that *karma* done with *jñāna* takes one towards *bhakti*. *Tapas* is *karma*, *svādhyāya* is *jñāna* and *Īśvarapraṇidhāṇa* is *bhakti*.

BHAKTI

Patañjali speaks of God as one who is unaffected by actions and untouched by cause and effect. He is represented in *auṁ* as *praṇava japa*. As He is the seed of all knowledge, omniscient and omnipresent, Patañjali advises the yoga *sādhaka* to meditate on Him by constant repetition of *auṁ (japa)* and to contemplate its meaning *(artha)* and feeling *(bhāvana)*, as a form of *bhakti*. It is similar to the *bhakti* cult of Shri Ramanuja.

Patañjali has no place for dullness, inactivity or inertia. Shri Ramanuja also does not allow his devotees to become victims of idleness or indolence. For him the performance of ritual is *jñānapūrvaka karma (karma* filled with *jñāna)* leading towards *bhakti*. *Bhakti* is the means as well as the goal for Patañjali and Shri Ramanuja. Their emphasis on *Īśvara praṇidhāna* is to cleanse the consciousness *(citta)* so that it becomes a means towards emancipation *(kaivalya)*.

Self-realisation cannot come without emancipation and emancipation cannot come until one frees oneself from the law of cause and effect. Patañjali's method of yoga is such that

---

1 Discipline, study of the spiritual scriptures and surrender to God are the base of yogic *sādhanā*.

it leads one to freedom. He uses the word *puruṣārtha śūnya* (devoid of four aims of life) in the last aphorism. According to *Viśiṣṭādvaita, mokṣa* (freedom or liberation) does not differ from the concept of Patañjali, since liberation from sorrow is liberation from the wheel of life and death.

KARMA

Our present life is nothing but the product of *saṁcita* and *prārabdha karma*. The seed of the present life is formed according to the *karma* of these two. When we grow, we build up *kriyamāṇa karma*.

Saṁcita karma is the accumulated effect of past actions, which affect one in the present life, without rhyme or reason: the reason cannot be traced, but it is stored within as subliminal impressions.

Yatamāna or *prārabdha karma* is the oscillation of pleasure and pain, which affects us in our day to day life.

Kriyamāṇa karma is the action of the present life that builds up to be the seed of the next life.

The need for yogic practice is the necessity to overcome *karma*. Conquest of *karma* is in order to move the intellect and consciousness closer towards Self-realisation.

It will be interesting to observe that there is very little room in the correct practice of yoga for us to generate actions which build up reactions. Consciously and deliberately, while we are doing yogic practices we minimise actions so they will not rebound on us as reactions or fruits. As practitioners of yoga we cultivate tolerance and patience as well as equanimity to face the onslaught of the laws of *karma*, so that subliminal thoughts and impressions gradually fade out.

In a metal rod, a good conductor carries electricity fast and a bad conductor slowly. Yogic practice acts as a good conductor to burn out the past *karma* of the *sādhaka* and keep the effects at a minimum level, whereas in non-yogic persons the law of *karma* will be fiercer, sapping their energies to the maximum.

Patañjali begins with the exposition of yoga and says that the restraint of movement in consciousness makes the Self shine in its own glory. But in both *sūtra* of the fourth chapter, he brings out the hidden effects of yoga. He says, "Through perfection in yoga, cycles of action and reaction which cause pain and sorrow come to an end".[1] This indicates that sorrow and pleasure sprout from *karma* and hence one should work to restrain those actions which boomerang on one, and to perform those which lead towards freedom.

As long as there is sorrow or mixed pleasure, there will be mental wavering *(vṛtti).* The moment one is free from sorrow, the waves of the *citta* recede. This recession of the thought-waves in *citta* is *nirodha* or restraint of *citta* or consciousness. This restraint should come naturally and not by force. Then the afflictions and mental wavering are either minimised or eradicated. When the actions that bring about fluctuations and afflictions come to an end, then the consciousness becomes silent and the actions that generate afflictions culminate *(kleśakarma nivṛtti).* From then on, no effort is required to restrain the consciousness and its movements. With this natural restraint, the Self shines and the search for Self-realisation comes to an end.

THE SECRET OF *SĀDHANĀ*

Sādhanā does not mean just a ritual practice. Both habitual and mechanical practice cannot lead one towards spiritual knowledge. While doing *sādhanā* we need to learn to watch the state of the *citta* along with the quality of mind, intelligence and 'I'-consciousness and find out how the *citta* is transformed in the beginning, in the middle and at the end of practice. Day by day observing the subtle changes and spacing that take place in the cells of the body, mind and intelligence, and storing that in the seat of the memory, the *sādhaka* filters, cleanses and refines it and ultimately retains the ripe memory to meditate upon.

Otherwise we remain eternally at square one. Though each one at the beginning practises with a motive for health and peace, one should proceed further towards the seat of the intellectual and ethereal sheaths *(vijñānamaya kośa* and *ānandamaya kośa).* We have to learn to connect all these sheaths of the Self while we do *āsana* or *prāṇāyāma.* This is the diffusion of the consciousness as well as the Self.

We should know that Shri Ramanuja points out *dharma bhūta jñāna.* We are made of five elements *(pañcamahābhūta):* earth, water, fire, air and ether. The counterparts of these elements are: odour, taste, shape, touch and sound *(pañcatanmātra).* Earth and odour represent *annamaya kośa*; water and taste represent *prāṇamaya kośa.* The development of these two leads to physical health and coolness or calmness in the cells of the body. Fire and shape represent the mental sheath *(manomaya kośa).* The fire burns the impurities and develops poise in mind through yoga. Air and touch belong to *buddhimaya* or *vijñānamaya kośa,* which

---

[1] *tataḥ kleśa karma nivṛttiḥ* (IV.30)

shapes the intelligence to spread in the body as well as the core of being. Touch of intelligence and its contact throughout the self enliven it. This enlivening of the self belongs to ether, producing vibrations to stir up total action in the practice of yoga. This brings the self *(asmitā)* in touch with its sheaths. This touch of the *asmitā* dynamises and atomises all the sheaths and all appear as Self. Therefore, real yogic practice begins from the intelligence. Intelligence *(vijñānamaya kośa)* moves and spreads in both directions, either to bind or liberate one. This pervasiveness of intelligence is the exact progress required in the practice of *āsana* and *prāṇāyāma* to make the seer spread himself over the entire body. One needs to practise *āsana* and *prāṇāyāma* to interact with *yogāgni* and *jñānāgni*, and discover that hidden, blazing divine force.

There is often variance in our thoughts and actions. We get afflicted in merit and demerit and this determines our class of birth, span of life and what experiences are to be undergone, which again produce pleasant or unpleasant feelings or both. Thus the cycles of birth and death continue.[1]

Some may not believe in rebirth, but life is progressive. Each one wants to improve – to become better than what he or she is. This is a natural phenomenon. Similarly, continuity of life is a natural phenomenon.

If there were no law of cause and effect, then all men and women would have the same intelligence, same mind and same psychological poise. But you find no one who is the same or equal to another. All are not from the same mould. Everyone's mental state, psychological behaviour and intellectual capacity differs. For example, in a class, there may be about forty students with one teacher. All hear the same words of the teacher, and note down the points according to their mental calibre. Even if all make the same notes, their exam results will be different. Even if they get the same rank, they do not get the same type of work. This is enough for us to understand that though as human beings they are all the same and kept under the same conditions and circumstances, facing the same situations, yet fate leads them in different directions. Why does this happen? Two persons might have scored the same marks in their examinations yet fate leads them to work at different levels. The fate is hidden in *karma* and *karma* is rooted in afflictions. As long as the roots of *karma*, the afflictions *(kleśa)*, exist, *karma* cannot vanish. One *karma* leads to the next *karma* and therefore life also does not end. The chain of life continues, the afflictions get compounded and the cycle of *kleśa* and *karma* continues.

---

1 *Kleśamūlaḥ karmāśayaḥ dṛsta adṛṣṭą janma vedanīyaḥ* - The accumulated imprints of past lives, rooted in afflictions, will be experienced in present and future lives (*Y.S.*, II.12). *sati mūle tadvipākaḥ jāti āyuḥ bhogāḥ* - As long as the root of actions exists, it will give rise to class of birth, span of life and experiences.(*Y.S.*, II.13). *te hlāda paritāpa phalāḥ puṇya apuṇya hetutvāt* – According to our good, bad or mixed actions, the quality of our life, its span and the nature of birth are experienced as being pleasant or painful. (*Y.S.*, II.14).

Karma has to yield fruit, therefore future lives are needed for *kārmic* consequences to be worked out as accumulated actions come to fruition *(karma phala)*. This gives a clear indication that we have existed in the past, we exist in the present and we shall live in the future also until the *kleśa karma* comes to an end. Patañjali explains the change of understanding in each individual in *sūtra* 12, 13, and 14 of the *Sādhana Pāda*.

In the *Viśiṣṭādvaita* philosophy, it is said that at birth, air *(vāyu)*, known as *shaṭha*, engulfs us and makes us forget our past lives. The example is given of Sage Shaṭagopan, the founder of this philosophy, who discarded this *vāyu* at the time of his birth and hence could remember all his previous lives. Later, Shri Ramanuja expounded this philosophy.

The first evolute of nature (cosmic intelligence or *mahat)* stirs *prakṛti* to function. So does *citta*, as the first evolute within us, creating action by stirring the five elements, their counterparts, the five senses of perception, five organs of action, mind, intelligence and 'I' into activity. The yogis of yore understood that the first evolute of man being *citta*, it has to be controlled; hence *cittavṛtti nirodha* became an axiom.

We have lost that degree of intellectual control, so we are forced to begin on the other evolutes of nature in order to come back into contact with our first evolute *(citta)*. When maturity sets in, all our practice begins from the source; then *cittavṛtti* cannot take place. This is the conquest of *karma*.

Many of you must have read the *Bhagavad Gītā* wherein Lord Krishna presents his universal form for Arjuna to see. It is known as *viśvarūpa darśana*. The Lord wanted to prove to Arjuna that He exists in all things. He is within each of us as *Paramātman*. *Ātman* means the Self and *Paramātman* means the Supreme Self.

The practice of yoga is meant for the discovery of the Self through the discipline of our body, senses, mind, intelligence, ego and consciousness, so that we become worthy and ripe to have that sight. Till then we cannot perceive or see that divine force.

Now, let us begin our practice in such a way that the *vijñānarūpa ātmā* (expansion and diffusion of the Self) touches us from the core to the periphery and from the periphery to the core. By this way of thinking in practice, dualities disappear and infinity emerges. Like a river that joins the sea and becomes one with it, so do all the *kośas* become one with the Self.

This is *viśvātma-darśana* (sight of the Self), a stepping stone to God-realisation. This is the spiritual *abhyāsa* of *āsana* and *prāṇāyāma*. When the practices of *āsana* and *prāṇāyāma* are done from the understanding of the elements of air and ether, spiritual life begins.

Mind is like mercury. Mercury cannot be held by the hand, but it can be stored in a capsule. The body is like a capsule in which the mind is bound. As mercury spreads when it is spilled, so does the mind. It spreads in every nook and corner of the body. Fire blazes. As mind belongs to the element of fire, through yoga it is set ablaze to engulf the entire body. Otherwise the fervour of the mind diminishes and loses its inflammable quality. Then the mind contracts and loses its power to ignite the cells of the body and the intelligence.

Let us forget for a moment *sthira sukham āsanam (Y.S.,* II.46) or active and passive *āsana.* These are explained on the anatomical and physiological levels. You have to pour the power of *tejas* (fire) while doing *āsana* so that it triggers and enflames the sheath of intelligence *(vijñānamaya kośa)* to penetrate the body with rhythm and harmony. It is not like focussing at one point and changing the point every now and then. One has to focus on all parts of the body throughout the practice of each *āsana* so that awareness *(prajñā)* may bring out the discriminative power of the mind as fuel to enflame the intelligence. Use the mind as fuel to generate power in the intelligence in order to experience the splendour of the Universal Self *(viśva-puruṣa).*

Here the 'doing' ends and the 'observing' begins. So begin yoga at an intellectual and conscious level in such a way that the radiant light that is within blazes and eradicates darkness. When we practise with this zeal, then there is no room for actions to generate or create reactions. Hence, no room for *karma phala* or effects of *karma* to bear fruit. Hence no room for the seen or the unseen; for pleasant or unpleasant feelings or for troubling and non-troubling stress to play on us. This way, one can put a stop to *kriyamāṇa karma* also.

Aṣṭāṅga yoga is like a single chain with eight links. We who practise yoga cannot separate the links of the chain of yoga, because we get subjectively involved. It is those arm chair speakers who see yoga at a distance and separate the chain from the links. When the links are removed, the chain does not exist. In the same way, if the links of the chain of yoga are separated, there will be no yoga. As all links of yoga are interwoven, we, as practitioners, have to be in contact with all the links of the chain.

The theories and values of yoga are fine to grasp but they do not help unless they are adopted and adapted along with their disciplined practice. One can cook food but only the one who eats can taste and relish it. Yoga also can 'cook' the mind, but to taste and relish it, one has to undergo daily practice and make the fibres, cells, mind, intelligence, ego and consciousness ripe in order to taste its essence.

As I said earlier, yoga definitely helps in this life to free oneself from the effects of actions and at the same time prepares a cool and collected mind to face the *saṁcita* and *prārabdha karma* with patience. Practice keeps one away from anger, hatred and speaking ill of others, and builds in us the quality of forgiveness *(kṣamā).*

Just as an actor plays various roles based on one theme, so does the consciousness moment to moment play various roles in one. It becomes active with the thoughts of the world and submissive when it does not want to play. If overextended, it wants restraint. At other times, it wants to focus on a given thought or object. On account of these modes, the fissures in consciousness occur, oscillating, creating dejection, hatred, anger and greed. Practice of yoga makes the *citta* realise its true nature and helps it to be no longer an actor or a witness, but to be both at the same time. This way of transforming the *citta* helps one to wash off all the past *karma* and keeps the present life free from generating actions.

As the water of a river ripples when hitting a stone, thought-waves disturb the intelligence. This causes ripples in the consciousness. The practice of *āsana* must be done in such a way that the intelligence holds the consciousness without any obstruction or restriction. This leads to *ānanda*, a state free from motivation.

Prāṇāyāma too, cultivates the intelligence to act as a bridge between the core of being and the body. Observe the source that initiates inhalation and feel how it spreads and covers its frontier; similarly, see in exhalation how the peripheral body recedes and reaches the core and at the same time feel the union of the core with its sheaths as a single unit, during retention.[1]

If the practice of *aṣṭāṅga yoga* is done with this approach, purification of *karma (karma śuddhi)* takes place and through this the purification of the consciousness *(citta śuddhi)*. The exalted intelligence *(viveka jñāna)* shines and actions and the fruits of actions come to a standstill[2]. This is emancipation, liberation and freedom from the fruits of *karma*.

The *vivekaja jñāna* not only illumines the objects of the world but also the very source of all objects, the *paramātman*. This exalted intelligence leads one towards *parama bhakti*.

Patañjali, in his last *sūtra*, points out that when the yogi is devoid of all the aims *(puruṣārtha śūnya)*, then all the vehicles of nature, the *karmendriya* (organs of action), the *jñānendriya* (senses of perception), the *pañcamahābhūta* and *pañcatanmātra, manas* (mind), *buddhi* (intelligence), *ahaṁkāra* (ego) and *citta* (consciousness) along with the *triguṇa*[3] return to the very source, and the seer, as a *śeṣan (jīvātman)*, merges in the *śeṣin* (*citiśakti* or God), the Supreme Lord. The *ātman* coexists with the Supreme Soul. Here, he has a *paramātma-darśana*. This is Supreme Beatitude.

---

1 See the article entitled *Practice of prāṇāyāma*, pp. 274.

2 *Yogāṅgānuṣṭhānāt aśuddikṣaye jñānadīptiḥ āvivekakhyāteḥ* (*Y.S.*, II.28). Practice of various aspects of yoga removes the cause of afflictions so that the crown of wisdom radiates in its own glory.

3 Luminosity, vibrancy, inertia.

VARṆĀŚRAMA AND *YOGA*

According to the Indian cultural and spiritual heritage, our society is divided according to the qualities *(guṇa)* of man, into four classes. This later became the caste system. The four qualities or classes are known as *brāhmaṇa* (priest class), *kṣatriya* (warrior class), *vaiṣya* (mercantile class) and *śūdra* (labouring class). Nowadays these divisions are disappearing, but they unconsciously exist in all vocations. Take for example yoga. Even in the discipline of yoga, a beginner of yoga has to labour hard and sweats to learn. From this stage he moves on to demonstrating or teaching and earning a living through yoga. This state of mind is the character of the mercantile class. Then he wants to compete with his colleagues or teach with pride and superiority. This is nothing but martial character in the *sādhaka*. It is the quality of a *kṣatriya*. The final one is the *brāhmaṇa* class where the learner or the teacher delves deep in the field of yoga to drink the nectar of spiritual realisation. This is the religious fervour of yoga and if one acts with this feeling, one becomes a *brahmin* in yogic *sādhanā*.

Man's life too, is divided into four strata of religious order known as *āśrama* or stages of life. These are known as *brahmacarya* (educative and religious studentship), *gṛhastha* (householder's life), *vānaprastha* (preparation to learn non-attachment while living as a householder) and *sannyāsa* (detachment from the affairs of the world and attachment to the service of the Lord).

The sages of yore having established the class and stages of life according to man's behavioural patterns, divided the span of his life of one hundred years into four parts, each running for twenty-five years. They advised that we follow the rules of the four *āśrama* to fulfil the aims of life *(puruṣārtha)*.

The aims of life are four: *dharma* (science of ethical, social and religious duties), *artha* (acquisition of wealth), *kāma* (pleasures of life) and *mokṣa* (freedom or liberation).

Spiritual attainment without *dharma*, the observance of ethical duty, is an impossibility. This is learned in *brahmacaryāśrama*.

Artha or the acquisition of wealth is to become free from the parasitic life. It is not meant to accumulate wealth but to earn so that the body is kept healthy and the mind free from wants. Otherwise a poorly nourished body becomes a fertile ground for disease and worry. In this stage not only does one acquire money, but also a partner to lead a householder's life. This second stage gives a chance to experience human love and happiness and prepares the mind for divine love through friendliness and compassion. This helps one to develop universality so that one soon realises divine love. One is never allowed to shirk one's responsibilities towards the upbringing of one's children and towards fellow beings. Hence there is never any objection towards marriage and parenthood and, at the same time, they are not considered as a bar to the knowledge of divine love, happiness and union with the Supreme Soul.

Kāma is to have the pleasures of life. It depends largely on a healthy body and a balanced harmonious mind. As the body is the abode of man, it has to be treated as the shrine of the soul. Practice of *āsana, prāṇāyāma* and *dhyāna* purifies the body, stabilises the mind and brings clarity in intelligence. This is the reason why the sages said that the body is the bow, *āsana* the arrow and the *puruṣa* (the Self at the core of being), the target.

Mokṣa means freedom from the bondage of worldly pleasures and sorrows. It is liberation, emancipation, freedom and beatitude. This liberation is possible only if one is free from the obstacles of physical disease, languor, doubt, carelessness, physical laziness, self-indulgence and sensual gratification. Illusiveness, failure to maintain willpower, inability to maintain steadiness in practice, despair, tremor of the body and irregular breathing are no longer a hindrance to the yogi. It is also freedom from poverty, ignorance and pride. When one is free from all these, emancipation sets in and divine beauty shines. This is *mokṣa*. In this state one realises that power, pleasure, wealth and knowledge do not bring freedom or aloneness *(kevalāvasthā)*. One learns to go beyond the qualities of *tamas, rajas* and *sattva* and frees oneself from the aims of life to become a king amongst men and second to none. One is a *guṇātītan* (above the qualities of nature). This is the path of life, worth attempting and living.

To come back to the explanation of the *aśramas, brahmacarya* plays an important role.

It means celibacy, religious study, self-restraint and chastity.

All the yoga texts say that the loss of semen leads to death and its retention to life. By the preservation of semen, the yogi's body develops a sweet odour. As long as it is retained, there is no fear of death, says *Haṭhayoga Pradīpikā* (III.88).

Patañjali too, lays stress on continence of body, speech and mind. He conveys that the preservation of semen establishes in one valour and vigour, strength and power, courage, fortitude and energy, and the elixir of life. Hence his injunction that it should be preserved by concentrated effort of will. This does not mean that the philosophy of yoga is meant only for celibates. The *smṛti* (codes of law) recommend marriage. Almost all the yogis and sages of old in India were married men with families of their own. For example, Sage Vasiṣṭa had one hundred children, yet he was called *brahmacārī* because he did not indulge in sex for the sake of pleasure only. In olden times, courtship took place under the conjunction of auspicious stars, the day, the time and so forth which might not coincide even once a year. That is why they were called celibates *(brahmacārī)* though they were married.

The concept of *brahmacarya* is not one of negation or forced austerity and prohibition.

According to Shri Adi Shankara, a *brahmacārī* is a man who is engrossed in the study of the sacred *vedic* lore, who moves constantly in *brahman* and who knows that *brahman* exists in all. In short, one who is in contact with the very core of being is a true *brahmacārī*, as he sees the spark of divinity in all.

Brahmacarya can be observed even by married men and women provided they have controlled sexual relations.

Today, in the name of freedom, everyone behaves wantonly. This libertine life is not freedom. The five principles of *yama* are social ethics. Social freedom is not reaction against social ethics. Every one has a certain discipline to follow in society. Hence, freedom to behave as one likes is not freedom. It is liberty without discrimination. Freedom with discipline alone is true freedom.

Today I say, a married and contented life is *brahmacarya*, as the married practitioner learns to love his partner with his head and heart, rather than the one who claims to be a celibate but lets his evil eyes stray for sensual gratification. Married people are united together whereas those who are unmarried may stray and become mere pleasure seekers.

Lord Krishna says that moderation in sleeping, eating and regulation in courtship is the path of *brahmacarya* followed by a yogi[1]. This is the way of a yogi's life where he blends with his *sādhanā* without casting his wanton eyes around lecherously.

---

1 *Yuktāhāra vihārasya yukta ceṣṭasya karmasu* |
yukta svapnāvabodhasya yogo bhavati duḥkhahā || (*B.G.*, VI,17).
(For him who is moderate in eating and recreation, temperate in his actions, who is regulated in sleep and wakefulness, yoga becomes the destroyer of pain.)

DUAL FUNCTION OF *ĀSANA**

Āsana performs dual jobs. It works on the body externally as well as internally. When there are lots of obstacles in our system, then the practice becomes external. These obstacles may be in the joints, the muscles, the nerves, the organs, the mind or the memory. Similarly, desires and temptations may arise in the brain or in the mind. In the beginning, an average student naturally will be in the external level for years and may take many, many years to internalise his *sādhanā*. These impediments come in his way to tie him mentally and sap his energy and intelligence. In the beginning, the practice of *āsana* creates now and then sensations on the nerves of our system, giving a certain feeling of exhilaration which later imprints on the consciousness. This encourages us further to feel and experience what may arise even later.

As you are practising, if the mind is not co-ordinating with the flow of your movement, flow of your thinking, flow of your energy, the electrical impulses do not trigger. They do not imprint the feelings. It may take months or years (God alone knows) for that power to reproduce that feeling, unless and until one strives for consciousness to integrate actively with the practice. When integration of practice with consciousness takes place, your body, your mind and your nerves get acclimatised to stay longer in the *āsana* and you like to penetrate inwards. The feeling that is experienced by this inward penetration of the intelligence is not from the sensory organs but from the intuitive intelligence only.

The principle of memory is to absorb and store the gathered experience. Patañjali says that if the memory is unripe, intelligence remains immature, and if memory is ripe, intelligence also gets rightly matured. This ripeness of intelligence and memory transforms one's practice from *bahiraṅga sādhanā* into *antaraṅga sādhanā*, as an inward journey to find the source tapped at the start, middle and end of each *āsana* or breath. The moment the movements in *āsana* create unalloyed bliss in heart and head, know that the sign of *pratyāhāra* has begun to set in. Till then, your practice is like that of a street performer whose main aim is to earn a few

---

* Talk given on 14th December, 1982.

coins and not to know how the intelligence functions or for what purpose it is done. As his intelligence is limited for gaining his livelihood only, similarly, our intelligence is also limited to getting rid of pains.

The inward journey starts when *anuṣṭhāna* or reverential practice begins. Mechanical repetitive practice without giving a thought to its purpose is commonly called *abhyāsa*. *Abhyāsa* and *anuṣṭhāna* are two terms commonly used for *sādhanā*. *Abhyāsa* is general practice, whereas *anuṣṭhāna* is done with heart and head mingling attentively throughout practice. In *anuṣṭhāna* the awareness of the *sādhaka* is demanded from moment to moment and phase to phase, attentively living from movement to movement in each *āsana*. Like the movement of the river, which moves from its source towards the sea and not back, similarly the same movement cannot be repeated. But our intelligence *(jñānavāhini)* can move both ways. It penetrates from its source to reach the periphery and then returns from periphery to its source. When we learn and observe these phases, there is oneness. Subject, object and the instrument used unite as one, and that is *dhyāna*. *Dhyāna* is not a thing to recall or recollect sitting in a corner of our house or in a remote place, or making ourselves empty and living in loneliness. Our intelligence may be sleeping while we are sitting, or our intelligence may be alert but our body might have gone to rest. This is not *dhyāna*. *Dhyāna* is the single flow of energy in body and attentive intelligence from the source towards the periphery and vice versa (Plate n. 7). Even from the chronological point of view, from the time we are awake till the time we go to sleep, maintenance of intelligence without any fickleness in all activities of life is *dhyāna*. When I teach or you teach, if the intelligence is maintained steadily throughout in the classes, we are practising and preaching *dhyāna*. But we are brainwashed through books or by listening to people into believing that there is no activity at all in *dhyāna*, and get confused. If that is the case, then deep sleep must be a state of *dhyāna*. Practice of *āsana* keeps the thread of our intelligence steady on a single string without any breaks.

Know that a *guru* wants his pupils to do their best and he tries to help them even though he has not reached that pure unalloyed state.

Today seekers choose their *gurus* according to their taste as you choose your food.

You say, "I have found a very good *guru*". Unfortunately you have not found a good *guru*, but have only found one to suit your taste, that is all. The real *guru* is the one who will not care for your taste but will evaluate you and will take care to uplift and bring evolution in you. He will improve your way of living qualitatively.

Patañjali says that in this world we have so many avenues for our attention to run after pleasures and get disturbed. Second to second the mind moves and strays away from attention. So he begins at the source of the problem with *cittavṛtti nirodha*. As you use a pin or a needle to remove the thorn that is stuck in your foot, so also you have to bring the quality of *rājasic* nature to achieve *cittavṛtti nirodha*. He has not said we should just surrender or sit in a corner with closed eyes. Patañjali's suggestions are of a high order to restrain the wandering mind. Actually this is *pratyāhāra*. In *pratyāhāra*, the organs of action do not function and so the senses of perception naturally get merged in the mind, losing their potency. As they lose their potency, they recede and *citta* surfaces with *ahaṁkāra*, the ego or 'I'. This *ahaṁkāra* plays the role of recharging the battery of the mind to get back those satisfactions. If the ego is not brought under control, you are caught up in illusion. So, to quieten the senses, one has to go back to the principles of *pratyāhāra* through the practice of *āsana* and *prāṇāyāma* to subdue the ego or 'I'.

Without mastery of *pratyāhāra* we cannot think of *samādhi*. As beginners, we naturally do *bahiraṅga sādhanā* in the form of *yama, niyama, āsana* and *prāṇāyāma*, and then start *antaraṅga sādhanā* in the form of *dhāraṇā* and *dhyāna* after the mastery of *pratyāhāra*. *Dhāraṇā* and *dhyāna* are *antaraṅga sādhanā*. *Samādhi* is called *antarātma sādhanā*. Spiritual practice commences only when the attention does not waver at all under any circumstances. Till then, we are all caught in the web of external need. That is why *pratyāhāra* is *bahiraṅga* cum *antaraṅga sādhanā*, because the senses of perception, organs of action and memory, which are all part and particles of *manas*, are *bahiraṅga*. They have to be conquered first. Unless and until we have control over them, we cannot jump to *cittavṛtti nirodha*. *Pratyāhāra* is the beginning of *vairāgya* (renunciation). *Vairāgya* is also *abhyāsa*. The external quest comes to an end with the practice of *vairāgya*. After *pratyāhāra*, the internal journey or the return journey begins. Reversing the use of the external *(bahiraṅga)* parts towards *citta* serves to trace its source – the *ātman* or the soul. This inversion of *bahiraṅga* movements towards the *ātman* is *antaraṅga sādhanā*. Hence, *pratyāhāra* is both *bahiraṅga* and *antaraṅga sādhanā*, being a pivotal state between them.

Then commences *anuṣṭhāna* of *vairāgya*. It is not renouncing the world. But it has certain ways, certain methods and certain disciplines to practise. In order to achieve and realise the highest aim or goal in life[1], you have to conquer the *rājasic* nature of the *citta*. When this *rājasic* nature of *citta* is quietened, the search of the seeker comes to an end. From then on the seeker is transformed as the seer. This is the goal of *aṣṭāṅga yoga*.

---

1 *Tadā draṣṭuḥ svarūpe avasthānam* (When consciousness is silent, the Seer – *ātma* – radiates in his own grandeur) (*Y.S.*, I.3). See the author's *Light on the Yoga Sūtras of Patañjali*, p. 104, Harper Collins, London.

This is the spirit in which *āsana* is done. If one performs this way, the dual job of blending the head and the heart develops to unite as one, which ripens the *buddhi-tattva* (intelligence) towards *viveka-khyāti*, the discriminative intelligence or the crown of wisdom.

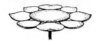

ĀSANAJAYA – A SEARCH FOR THE INFINITE

Āsana means a posture, a pose. *Āsana* is about adjusting each and every part and cell of the body to maintain such a state as to permit us to reach the Lord within.

Lord Patañjali lays *āsana* before us in the second chapter, the *Sādhana Pāda*. First he defines *āsana*: *Sthira sukhaṁ āsanam* (*Y.S.*, II.46). *Āsana* is perfect firmness of body, steadiness of intelligence and benevolence of the heart. In the next aphorism he explains the path of endeavour indicating where the *sādhaka* has to reach. He says, *Prayatna śaithilya ananta samāpattibhyām* (*Y.S.*, II.47). Perfection in an *āsana* is achieved when the effort to perform has ceased on its own and the *āsana* is performed effortlessly so that the being within is reached.

Finally, he explains the fruit of *āsana*, *Tataḥ dvandvaḥ anabhighātaḥ* (*Y.S.*, II.48). The practitioner is undisturbed by dualities.

Patañjali finishes the section on *āsana* in three *sūtra*. But this third step on the eightfold path is an extensive one, and its ramifications expand well beyond this short passage.

Āsana is summed up in two words, *sthira* and *sukha*, both of which are likely to mislead the *sādhaka* if he is not keen to find out their truth. A *sādhaka* requires keenness along with devotion. Keenness is an intellectual state of consciousness and devotion is an emotional one. Patañjali wants these two states of man to be balanced so that the *āsana* does not tend or tilt one either towards an emotional or intellectual aspect.

Patañjali uses the word *sthira* first and *sukha* later. He could have reversed the order and said *"Sukha sthiram āsanam"*, but he does not. *Sthiratā* is given first place as endeavour of the body and *sukhatā* for the mind is second. Human psychology is such that we want comforts first and make efforts later. Patañjali knows this weak point, so he demands effort first, since comfort follows effort.

Sukha means happiness. It is an enchanting word. Every one wants pleasure. The question is, is the word *sukha* used from a hedonistic point of view? No, certainly not! The psychology of pleasure-seeking man is to search for comfort. So he wants *sukha*. Patañjali refers to *sukha* as one of the afflictions. *Rāga* (attachment) follows pleasurable experience and *dveṣa* (aversion) follows unpleasant experience (*Y.S.*, II.7-8).

In this *sūtra*, if we mean pleasure by *sukha*, then the state of comfort that is pleasurable for the mind will lead towards attachment and strengthen the afflictions rather than reducing them. Comfort and attachment go together. The effect of *āsana* cannot be an adverse one. The state of discomfort is painful for the mind, which leads towards aversion and again adds to the afflictions. Discomfort and aversion go together. Then how can an *āsana* be measured by the scale of comfort and discomfort, pleasure and pain, attachment and aversion, or happiness and sorrow? The word *sukha* is certainly not used to indicate pleasant or unpleasant states.

Tukarām, being a saint, says, "Like a soldier, we have to face war every day and night because it is unknown when and which enemy will invade us". He means the six enemies of mind, namely desire, anger, greed, infatuation, delusion and jealousy. Even while doing or being in *āsana*, one has to guard oneself from these enemies, otherwise the body will be in *āsana* and the mind will be engaged in desire, anger and greed.

One cannot practise the *āsana* for the sake of pleasure or *sukhatā*. Then the question arises, what is this *sukha* if it is not that which brings pleasure? By *sukha*, Patañjali certainly means that *sukha* or joy which is free from afflictions.

Patañjali explains the cause of the very existence and the contact of *prakṛti* with *puruṣa* in *Sādhana Pāda*. The nature or *prakṛti* has three qualities or attributes, namely, *sattva*, *rajas* and *tamas*. The evolutes of nature such as mind, senses of perception, organs of action, are composed of the same three attributes. All these exist to serve the seer. *Dṛśyam* exists to serve *dṛṣṭā*. In other words, nature exists to serve *puruṣa* and this service is of two kinds, i.e. for enjoyment and emancipation. It functions either by providing enjoyment or by leading one towards freedom from sorrow and affliction.

The body, the mind, the organs of action, the senses of perception, the ego, the intelligence and the consciousness have *sāttvic*, *rājasic* and *tāmasic* qualities. While doing an *āsana*, we use our body and its faculties in order to be within the altar of the *sāttvic* nature of the heart.

If we practise *āsana* for the sake of emancipation, then it is called *yogāsana*. If we perform it for the sake of pleasure, then it is *bhogāsana*. Therefore, a *sukhāsana* has to be necessarily a *yogāsana* and not a *bhogāsana*. However, it is easier to convert the *sukhāsana* into *bhogāsana* than into *yogāsana*. In that case the downfall of the practitioner is certain.

If the *āsana* has to be *sukhāsana* in the "right" sense, then how should the *abhyāsa* be? While explaining *abhyāsa* (practice), Patañjali says that since it is a steadfast effort, it has to be done for a long time without interruption along with devotion and dedication. If the practice of *āsana* is meant for enjoyment *(bhogāsana)*, it cannot be done with dedication. It is devoid of devotion and dedication. *Sa tu dīrghakāla nairantarya satkāra āsevitaḥ dṛḍhabhūmiḥ* (*Y.S.*, I.14).

These two words, *dīrghakāla* (for a long time) and *nairantarya* (without interruption), have to be applied to *sthiratā* in *āsana*. The word *satkāra* stands for auspicious action and this has to be applied to *sukhatā* in *āsana*. *Abhyāsa* is also of three types, namely, *sāttvic*, *rājasic* and *tāmasic*. If the *āsanābhyāsa* is *sāttvic*, the *prāṇa* (energy) and *citta* (consciousness) unite in order to lead one towards *apavarga* (emancipation). Therefore, the instruments such as the *bhūta* (elements in body) and *indriya* (organs of action and senses of perception) have to be purified in order to bring them to the state of *sāttvic* nature. Otherwise, *rajas* and *tamas* dominate these two and the *āsana* becomes a *bhogāsana*. In *bhogāsana* the *prāṇa* and *citta* do not unite but the body, mind and senses unite and lead one towards *bhoga* alone.

Let this word *sukha* not mislead you. *Vairāgya* is freedom from desire. This is *sukha* in the real sense. The practice of *āsana* should strengthen the mental attitude of detachment. See that you involve the *bhūta*, *indriya*, *prāṇa* and *citta* in the practice of *āsana*. *Sukhāsana* done in this right sense of involvement leads you automatically towards *prāṇāyāma* and *pratyāhāra*. In fact, while practising the *āsana*, *pratyāhāra* acts as a fence for the mind, warding of the six enemies of the mind so that the afflictions start to be attenuated. *Pratyāhāra* protects *yogāsana* from conversion to *bhogāsana*.

The word *sthira* has a twofold meaning: firmness and steadiness. The body has to be firm and the intelligence has to be steady or stable. The word *sthira* indicates *vṛtti nirodha* whereas *sukha* indicates freedom from afflictions.

While defining what *abhyāsa* is, Patañjali says: *Tatra sthitau yatnaḥ abhyāsaḥ* (*Y.S.*, I.13). Practice is the steadfast effort to still the fluctuations of *citta*. *Abhyāsa* is a continuous effort to bring steadiness. Patañjali does not expect an impotent, dull and sterile steadiness, but demands a potent, active and fertile steadiness. Though it appears static, stable and steady it is filled with advertent intelligence and dynamic consciousness. Try to understand this contrast of a static state with a dynamic force. The practice of *āsana* should be such that one has to invest the static state *(sthiratā)* with a dynamic force. The word *sthira* indicates the firmness of the body and from *sthiratā* comes a qualitative advertent steadiness of intelligence *(sukhatā)* because of the repose that comes out of the pose. When we perform the *āsana*, it is a process of posing. After posing one has to reflect. There comes reposing. A steady and static posture is not achieved unless one reflects on it and balances the intelligence with energy concurrently and simultaneously. One can force the body to do the *āsana*, but when the body rebels and opposes, then the question arises, "what next"? If one gives up the practice, then one fails in steadfast effort as well as *sthirāsana*. Yogic practice cannot be done according to the fanciful wishes of the body or mind. While in an *āsana*, if the body rebels and the mind is in turmoil, then the practitioner has to correctly re-adjust, bringing co-ordination between body and mind. He thereafter has to observe the equipoise in the corrected adjustments and the rhythmic balance of energy in that state. When such a repose is attained, consciousness gets quietened, and energy is not dissipated. Rather, it is stored and directed towards *dhāraṇā* or concentration.

Patañjali says, *Deśa bandhaḥ cittasya dhāraṇā* (*Y.S.*, III.3). He defines concentration *(dhāraṇā)* in the third chapter, *Vibhūti Pāda*. Fixing the consciousness or focussing the attention on one point within the body or outside of it is *dhāraṇā*. The *sukhāsana* in a real sense gets converted into *yogāsana* at this stage when *sthiratā* through *dhāraṇā* leads towards spiritual discipline. At this stage the *abhyāsa* has to be intensified internally so that one progresses from *dhāraṇā* to *dhyāna*. This journey from *dhāraṇā* to *dhyāna* is parallel to the track of *prayatna śaithilya* – exalted effort, cessation of effort.

What is *prayatna śaithilya?* It is not just releasing one from efforts. It does not mean letting loose the energy of the body or severing the string of intelligence. It is neither more effort nor less effort. Less or more effort disturbs and spills the feel of balance and fullness in the *āsana*. *Śaithilya* (laxity) here, is connected to the outer structure of the body and not at all to the grip of the inner body. Laxity has its own discrimination, where the release of tightness and hardness is transformed into softness in the muscles and joints whilst holding onto the inner intellectual grip. The root meaning of lax in English is also to release and to set free, but not to flop or become flaccid.

Actually, *prayatna śaithilya* is experienced when the pinnacle of intelligence *(buddhi-tattva)* holds the body on its own, without the help of the muscles and joints, a hold or grip without effort. The laxity in effort is without losing the *sthiratā* – the steadiness. This point is very important. After putting all the effort into *sthiratā*, how can one just give up the efforts? Is it not a waste of time, waste of effort, waste of energy?

So, *prayatna śaithilya* means the exact and even weighing of effort and effortlessness. It must be a zero state of tension, that is, no more and no less is required. This state is full only when one has reached the brim or fullness in the *āsana*.

Āsana is not a process of at one time putting in effort and at another, releasing the effort. That would be absurd. It would be an illogical act. The disturbances or modifications of consciousness cannot be checked with laxity. One cannot ask to control the mental modifications in *Śavāsana*. Asking to control the modifications of the mind is a deliberate effortful process. Body and mind, both have to be made to reach a passive and pensive state in *Śavāsana*. Similarly, in the practice of all other *āsana* the same state has to be reached.

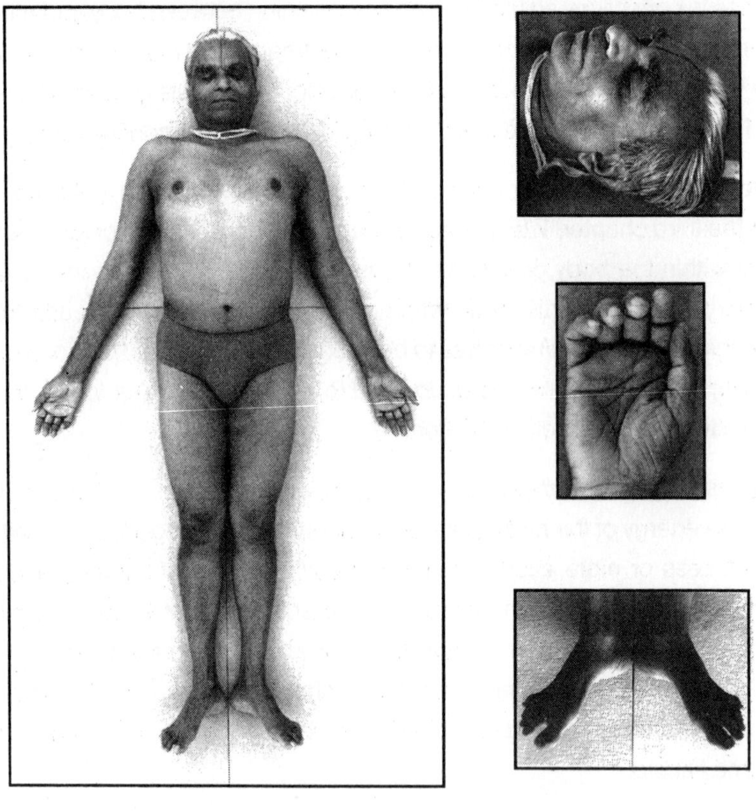

Plate n. 3 – Passive and pensive *Śavāsana*

Then the second part of the *sūtra* says, *ananta samāpattibhyām*. The *āsana* has to result into *ananta samāpatti*. *Ananta* means Infinite. *Samāpatti* means transformation. The Infinite that is residing within is called the Self. While doing or being in the *āsana* all the sheaths of the body along with *asmitā* have to reach the Self. The *citta* has to get transformed totally so that it sees the Self and nothing else. This is *ananta samāpatti* where *aliṅga* (noumenal), *liṅga* (phenomenal), *aviśeṣa* (unspecified) and *viśeṣa* (specified with marks) of *prakṛti*, merge with the Self. Therefore, one needs to ponder over these words *prayatna śaithilya* and not take them lightly.

Patañjali gives four types of favourable disposition of consciousness, namely friendliness, compassion, joy and indifference in respect to pleasure, pain, virtue and vice. This *citta prasādanam* (clemency of mind) has to be adopted in *āsana* to bring *prayatna śaithilyatā*. From whichever parts of the physical body such as muscles, bones, joints, spine or senses of perception such as eyes, ears and nose, the movements or actions occur, or when the disturbances occuring in the physiological functioning, lead one towards heavy breathing, choking, belching or yawning, or whenever one feels heavy, shaky or pain, these movements, disturbances or impediments have to be sifted through with the mental dispositions of friendliness, compassion, gladness and indifference.

The *yogāsana* that leads one towards the very core of being is a *sukha* or a contented state, and a practitioner should feel friendly towards that state. The consciousness should gravitate towards that state. When there is a painful or sorrowful state, then one should have compassion to adjust and correct but not to be indifferent. The practitioner should know the difference between *bhogāsana* and *yogāsana*. He should realise that he is standing on the edge of a cliff. He should be unmoved by the pleasures of *āsana*. If it is a *yogāsana,* he should accept it and feel the spiritual joy in it. If it is leading towards *bhogāsana,* then he should discard it. One cannot be indifferent to these feelings. If the *sādhaka* does not take the trouble to bother about this, pleasures *(bhoga)* will overpower him. One has to avoid this sort of "don't care" attitude. One has to convert the *bhogāsana* into *yogāsana*, and practise real indifference to the attachments, since the attachments to pleasure are hidden in *bhogāsana*. One should discard the *bhoga* element from *yogāsana*. That is a real and required indifference. It is the secret of *yogāsana*. One should not remain in an anaesthetised, sedated state while doing *āsana*. Then one loses sharpness and sensitivity. Sensitivity is blunted by excess, whereas *prayatna śaithilya* brings clarity and purity leading one towards *ananta samāpatti*.

Often the firmness of mind, steadiness of body and sharpness of intelligence are forgotten and the aspirant lives in a state of suspended animation. The aim of *āsana* is to steer away from the pairs of opposites and hence there is no ricochet effect between extremes.

In *Y.S.,* I.35, *Viṣayavatī vā pravṛttiḥ utpannā manasaḥ sthiti nibandhanī*, Patañjali suggests we contemplate an object conducive to maintaining steadiness of mind and consciousness. An *āsana* is a highly suitable object, external to the Self, but close to it. By absorbtion in *āsana* we feel the emanation of inner calmness. Pursued to its further limits, he says in *Y.S.,* III.49, *Tataḥ manojavitvam vikaraṇabhāvaḥ pradhānajayaḥ ca*, by this technique we may even penetrate, or as it were, conquer, *mahat*, the first evolute of nature.

Mahat has a capacity to be in a state of quietness. This silence must not be mistaken for equipoise of the Self. Therefore, the *āsana* certainly cannot lead one towards the state of dullness and stupor. The practice of *āsana* is to build up sensitivity and intelligence in order to know qualities such as the quickness to register imprints or the state of "all-knowingness" and yet at the same time remain pure.

When *Triṣikhibrāhmaṇa Upaniṣad* (verse 52) says that the one who has mastered *āsana (āsana jaya)* has in his hands the three worlds, it does not merely mean the earth, space *(antarikṣa)* and heaven. As far as our existence is concerned, these three worlds are our own *indriyas, manas* and *citta*. In other words, these are our body, mind and consciousness. The conquest of *āsana* is recognised when one conquers the organs of action, the senses of perception and the consciousness.

Therefore, *ananta samāpatti* in *āsana* is possible when one travels from the *asmitā* (individuated sprout of self) to the body and from the body to the self. It is a journey around three worlds, namely, body, *citta* (pure illuminative consciousness) and self.

Just sitting in a posture cannot be taken as the conquest of *āsana*. Patañjali explains how *dhyāna* (meditation) has to be done. He says, *Tatra pratyaya ekatānatā dhyānam* (III.2). Thus a steady, continuous flow of attention directed in depth towards the same point or region is meditation. This would only take place in an established perfected *āsana*.

Ekatānatā means a continuous and an uninterrupted flow of attentive awareness. The consciousness *(citta)* has to have one pointed attentiveness throughout. The seer has one specific characteristic (*Y.S.,* II.20), i.e. he witnesses the seen *(citta)* but does not rely on it. In this process of witnessing, the seer does not get contaminated. The *ātman,* being the seer, just sees without losing his purity. If we stand on the street and watch every one and everything with all the traffic moving, then our mind, from second to second, gets polluted, since we are watching and witnessing several things: we hear the sound, the noise and at the same time ponder on them; we have our own thoughts, our own reactions and we participate in all we see and hear. But as far as the seer is concerned, he has no reaction of his own except as a neutral witness. It is the consciousness *(citta, dṛśya* or seen) which gathers, reacts and gets polluted.

The practice of *āsana* can be of great help for one who aims to experience the characteristic of the seer. The "art of witnessing" is learnt by the practice of *āsana*. *Āsana* teaches us how to overcome the identification of the body with the mind and the mind with the self. Though everyone thinks that the performance of *āsana* is a physical action instigated by the body, actually it is the body which is the object. We witness its actions from moment to moment and therefore, the body's different sheaths get integrated with the seer.

Patañjali says that the identification or association of the seer with the seen *(puruṣa* with *prakṛti)* is the main cause of sorrow (*Y.S.,* II.17). *Draṣṭṛdṛśyayoḥ saṁyogaḥ heya hetuḥ.* He says that dissociation is the remedy. How to dissociate? No layman can separate the body from the mind or mind from the body. If one is disturbed, the other gets disturbed. If one collapses, the other loses courage. We experience the potency of this union in our day to day life.

The union or identification of the seer *(puruṣa),* through *citta,* with the seen *(prakṛti)* is a known fact. Neither of them can be eliminated, so the dissociation has to be experienced positively. The body, the organs of action, the senses of perception, the mind, the intelligence, the 'I'-consciousness and *citta,* all have to work unitedly and judiciously so that there is no place for any fragmentation. One has to know that the conjunction is meant as a challenge for us. The seer and the seen both have the potential power to realise their own true natures.

Though Patañjali claims that the identification of *puruṣa* and *prakṛti* is the cause of sorrow, yet he appreciates the conjunction of these two entities in *Y.S.* II.23. Conjunction is God-made, whereas identification is man-made. Patañjali warns us not to misidentify the *puruṣa* and *prakṛti,* though their conjunction is strong. They are separate but conjoined entities. If a man and a woman are walking on the street, one cannot take it for granted that they are husband and wife. They could be brother and sister too. Again, even if they are husband and wife, they are separate individuals. They have their own identity. Similarly, *puruṣa* and *prakṛti* are two separate entities but they function as one. In spite of their conjunction one has to recognise their separate existence and the practice of *āsana* offers this *svarūpopalabdhi* –obtaining one's own form.

Dvandva means duality, the duality between *preya* (pleasure) and *śreya* (auspiciousness or goodness). It is not only the dualities like hot and cold, pain and pleasure or honesty and dishonesty that bother us. With the practice of *āsana* we are able to face them. But this is only a part of the whole experience. According to yoga philosophy, the real conjunction between the seer and the seen is for developing and going towards the cosmos and not chaos. If the seer (the master) constantly watches the seen (the servant), then the servant leads the master towards freedom. Both entities in their conjunction should have the same goal so that dualities vanish. What is the point if *prakṛti* wants *bhoga* and *puruṣa* wants yoga? The seen *(prakṛti)* can lead one either to *bhoga* or *apavarga.* The decision is in the hands of the *sādhaka* whether he wants enjoyment or emancipation. If he wants enjoyment, then he is in ignorance *(avidyā),* and if he wants emancipation, then that is knowledge *(vidyā).*

One may remain steady and comfortable in *āsana* but if *āsana* leads towards *bhoga* (pleasure), then the duality is inherent and so the *śreya* (auspiciousness) is lost. The purity in approach is important. One may cheat the outside world but one cannot cheat the inner Self. The Self witnesses every movement of the mind, every thought of the mind. Therefore, the mind and consciousness have to be careful. The servant has to be careful since the master is watchful.

The practice of *āsana* is *tapas*. *Tapas* means self-discipline. This self-discipline is meant to destroy the impurities of the body and of the eleven *indriya* (five organs of action + five senses of perception + mind).

Ṛṣi Viśvāmitra did *tapas* and had great self-control. He was a perfectionist and very strict with himself. But his *tapas* broke the moment he saw Menaka. Why was Viśvāmitra attracted by Menaka? The tinge of *bhoga* somewhere in his *prakṛti* had left its imprint. The flow of his *prakṛti* led him towards *bhoga* and not *apavarga*. As the *āsana* can become *bhogāsana* instead of leading to *yogāsana*, the *tapas* can also become *bhoga* oriented, instead of *apavarga* oriented. That is how Viśvāmitra's downfall came about. Hence, each aspirant must be aware of Viśvāmitra's fall in *tapas*. Patañjali introduces *tapas* as that which burns the impurities of the body, the organs of action, senses of perception and mind. As the body gets purified, it becomes an attractive vehicle. The body becomes wealthy with *rūpa* (appearance), *lāvaṇya* (radiance), *bala* (strength) and *vajra samhananatva* (diamantine compactness). Obviously such a body attracts and may lead towards attachment. So the very purpose of *kāya siddhi* and *indriya siddhi* will be lost. Even the senses of perception may give way. Occult powers can be destructive. To avoid this danger, it is essential to complete the transformation of the elements, senses and mind so that Self-realisation may take place. The cultured and cultivated consciousness should not be wasted. It should be transformed from its potential state to the zenith of refinement so that it leads on towards liberation. When the *sādhaka* finds that he is undisturbed and unperturbed by dualities, the foundation is laid for this supreme state. *Tadā draṣṭuḥ svarūpe avasthānam* (*Y.S.*, I.3). The seer dwells in his own true splendour when the mental modifications are restrained. Similarly, an *āsana-sādhaka* remains in his true state since he restrains himself from the onslaught of sensual pleasures. No more does the achievement of the wealth of the body disturb him. Unlike Viśvāmitra, he will have no breach in *tapas (tapobhanga)*.

Let us therefore engage in the transcendance and resolution of dualities in the most profound sense, that of *āsana sādhanā*, in which the conquest of *āsana*, *āsana jaya*, will conduct us to the goal and the end of yoga.

ĀSANA: PHYSICAL, MENTAL OR SPIRITUAL PRACTICE?*

No one knows when the world came into existence, nor does anyone know the timeless primeval absolute one. Both nature and God existed before man knew about them. As man developed, it gradually dawned on him what the culture of man should be. Through this building of culture came civilisation. Words were evolved to express man's deepest feelings. As he developed, the concepts of *dharma* (religion), *prakṛti* (nature), *puruṣa* (Self) and yoga dawned upon him.

It is very difficult to explain in precise terms these concepts, for they defy definition. Each man gives his own interpretation according to his understanding. Perhaps the word yoga came into usage as there was *vi-yoga* (separation, delusion, disunion) and *dharma* was felt to be necessary when man lived not for *śreya* (the good and auspicious), but for *preya* (the pleasant, coupled with sorrow). Sorrow and happiness follow each other like the spokes of a wheel. Man, as he underwent pleasure and pain, good and evil, love and hatred, experienced the permanent and the transient and seeing the constant struggle between these opposites, gave thought and felt the need of a Supreme Entity (*Īśvara* or God). The word God conveys the idea of primeval force that generates, organises and destroys all creatures and creation, the force that stands for birth, growth and death.

God is free from such oscillations, unaffected by afflictions and untouched by actions and reactions, or by sufferings and joys such as man experiences. He is omniscient and knows the beginning and the end of all. As human beings we are from an unmanifested form; we appear as distinct and clear entities, then again merge into the infinite. This emergence and fading away of all beings is the cycle of life.

An analytical approach on emergence and fading away of life might have led an aspirant to aim at the highest ideal embodied in the *puruṣa viśesa* or *Īśvara* or God. Thus *Īśvara* – the Eternal Being, whom man calls God, the *guru* of all *gurus* – becomes his focal point of attention,

---

* Address at the Fifth Conference of the International Yoga Teachers Association, on Christmas day, December 1976, at Panchgani (Maharashtra, India). Excerpts also published in *Yoga Journal*, May-June 1977.

concentration and meditation, and hence, life's search is centred around the question of all questions: how to reach Him? In his search for an answer, man devised a code of conduct whereby he could live in peace and harmony.

He sought to distinguish between right and wrong, good and evil, virtue and vice, morality and immorality. From this arose a comprehensive concept of *dharma* (religion), or the science of duty. Dr Sarvepalli Radhakrishnan aptly explains *dharma* as "That which upholds, sustains and supports one who is falling, who has fallen or who is about to fall, physically, morally, mentally and spiritually." This suffices to clarify that *dharma* is for the whole of mankind irrespective of race, caste, class or creed or the faith one follows.

A man should desire to accomplish his *dharma* well and experience the divine state of oneness known as the perfect state. For that, he has to keep his body *(kṣetra)* clean, healthy, strong, pure and divine for the *puruṣa (kṣetrajña)*, the *ātman* or the Self. Therefore, he discovered the science of yoga. Even the *Upaniṣads* have laid down that it is impossible for a weakling to experience Supreme Self-realisation *(nāyamātmā balahīnenalabhyaḥ)*. So man discovered certain norms of behaviour. Sage Patañjali explains these norms as *yogānuṣāsanam*, or "the disciplines of yoga". When the disciplines terminate, the aspirant experiences integration within himself (freedom from the dualities of body and mind and mind and self), termed *saṁyama yoga*, or the "yoga of integration".

WHAT IS YOGA?

Almost all of you know what yoga is. It is a science that deals with the health and perfection of the body, harmony of the mind and clarity of intelligence. By the practice of yoga, man uncovers the difference between the body and the mind, and thereby transforms them into a state of virgin purity so that they remain as pure as crystal, uncontaminated by pleasure and desire. Yoga shows the way to the art of right living and hence it is also spoken of as being a branch of philosophy. It is the communion of the individual soul with the Universal Soul, the merging of the *jīvātman* with the *paramātman*.

Before exploring the unknown and the invisible Universal Soul, man has to learn about the known and the visible objects such as the body, and then go on to the subtle aspects such as the mind, the intelligence and the will. He has to bring together these gross and subtle parts known as the vehicles of the Self. Yoga is to train the body and the mind so that they lead man to experience the tranquillity of the Self. It encompasses the whole of man and is devised for his complete evolution, from the base, the body, to the apex, the Self.

Nature introduces man into the three qualities *(guṇa)* of *sattva* (luminosity), *rajas* (action) and *tamas* (inertia). Hence, he is caught within the circles of *guṇa* and his life cycle starts moving like the wheel of the potter. The wheel of time *(kālacakra)* moulds and remoulds man in the *guṇa* and makes him a prisoner of three kinds of afflictions: *ādhyātmika, ādhidaivika* and *ādhibhautika*. *Ādhyātmika* pain has its source within oneself, either at the physical or psychological levels or both, creating mental agony. *Ādhidaivika* and *ādhibhautika* pains are due to causes beyond one's control, like destiny or accident, allergy or viral infection.

Healthy trees and plants yield good flowers and fruits. Horticulture was evolved to make trees and plants grow healthy and fertile. Man also discovered various stages of yoga to free himself from the above three afflictions and grow healthy.

Though I have been asked to speak on *āsana*, it would be imprudent on my part to speak on *āsana* without explaining in brief all the eight aspects of the *aṣṭāṅga yoga* of Patañjali. These eight aspects are: *yama, niyama, āsana, prāṇāyāma, pratyāhāra, dhāraṇā, dhyāna* and *samādhi*.

The five great universal principles of *yama*, namely non-violence, truth, non-covetousness, celibacy and non-possession of wealth beyond necessity, discipline man's organs of action, which are his hands, legs, organs of excretion, generation and speech.

The principles of *niyama*, namely cleanliness, contentment, austerity, study of scriptures that enlighten the intelligence, and surrender to the Lord, purify the senses of perception, namely the eyes, the ears, the nose, the tongue and the skin.

Āsana sublimates these controlled organs of action and senses of perception, harmonising them with the organic functioning of the body. Besides this, they keep the channels of the entire nervous system free from impediments, so that when *prāṇāyāma* is practised, the energy or *prāṇa*, which is drawnin, in the form of inhalation, is made to flow uninterruptedly in the fibres of the body.

Prāṇāyāma quietens the tensions and stress of the body and the mind, and unfolds the brilliance of the intelligence.

Pratyāhāra is the withdrawal of the mind from the objects that attract it.

Dhāraṇā (concentration or attention) and *dhyāna* (meditation) dissolve the illuminated intelligence leading to total absorption *(samādhi)* in the Self.

Science has advanced to the extent of being able to send a man to the moon and bring him back. Medical science has progressed beyond imagination. Transplantation of the heart and kidney is performed and an artificial tongue enables man to speak. In spite of all this, physical and emotional diseases are sapping the life force of man throughout the world. Man is drifting away from his fellow men. Suspicion, doubt, competition and struggle for survival have been intensified. Stresses and strains have increased and selfishness has taken root instead of selflessness. No doubt the administration of drugs helps to relieve pain, stress and strain, but it leaves behind worry, anxiety, depression and sorrow. What is it that keeps man away from pain and sorrow? Health of the body, mind and self alone can make man live happily from birth to death, enabling him to die nobly and majestically. Health is not a commodity that is gained by swallowing pills. It has to be earned by hard work and discipline. One has to exercise judiciously in order to keep the muscles, the organs, the nerves, the glands, the flow of blood and the systems of the body in proper condition. The entire human system should be well regulated like the rising and the setting of the sun. Then the mind becomes free from the shackles of the body and detached from the dictates of the senses and gets attracted to the source of all knowledge, all actions and all emotions, which is the *ātman*.

The body is the dwelling place of the Self, but a dead body has nothing to do with realisation or ethics, moderation in food, sex and sleep. It is the living body that has to be alerted by the performance of *āsana, prāṇāyāma* and *dhyāna*, and educated and re-educated in one's modes and habits, diet and sex. The body is the only capital that the Self possesses and it has to be taken care of whether it is used for pleasure of the senses or realisation of the Self. Today new inventions and discoveries are made to enhance health as well as the span of life. In olden times man was not blessed with aids and instruments for observation like microscopes and stethoscopes, yet he had developed the faculty of observation and intuition to tackle the prevailing ills by tapping natural resources. In days gone by, man experimented subjectively on himself to test his own inventions. He copied the movements of animals and other forms of life and devised *āsana*, finding out their effects on his own body. His inventive mind discovered new *āsanas* so as to deal with different ailments. He found the Universal Soul flowing throughout all creation and started naming *āsanas* after different aspects of creation, the vegetable and animal kingdoms, heroes, sages and gods. Today we live an artificial life. We have artificial food, stimulants for sex and tranquillisers for sleep. *Yogāsana* has stood the test of time; it stimulates the system as well as tranquillising it as occasion demands.

Though men have different geographical backgrounds, historical perspectives and social strata, their basic problem of desire, pleasure and pain is the same. The difference in feelings is one of degree and this difference brings about biochemical changes in the system. *Āsana* restores the biochemical balance in the system, making the body fresh and clean. *Āsana* has to be performed to make the energy flow with dynamism so that it creates new avenues and hopes. As man looks for further expansion in knowledge and experience, he has to be ever dynamic and *āsana* should never be done mechanically. If done mechanically, then the body rusts and the mind stagnates.

There is a misrepresentation and obvious misunderstanding in the interpretation of yoga. Some say it is physical, others say it is mental, while many proclaim it as spiritual. A tree has roots, trunk and branches as separate identities, but each component cannot by itself become a tree. Only together do all these parts become the tree. Yoga too is like a tree. It is rather ridiculous to break up the tree of yoga into parts and label them separately from the whole. The universal principles of *yama* are the roots. The disciplines of *niyama* form the trunk. *Āsanas* are like the branches. *Prāṇāyāma,* which aerates the body with the breath of life, forms the leaves. *Pratyāhāra,* the bark of the tree, prevents the energy of the senses from flowing outwards and turns it within, enabling the yogi to find true happiness within himself. *Dhāraṇā* is the sap flowing through the whole body holding it firm, till it blooms with the flower of *dhyāna,* which in turn ripens into the fruit of *samādhi.* As the termination of the tree is in the fragrance of the fruit, the end of the tree of yoga is the taste of the fragrance of the Self. Why demarcate the innocence of man's intelligence by one's inflated knowledge and create doubt and suspicion in his endeavours? Why not keep the mind of the aspirant free from bias?

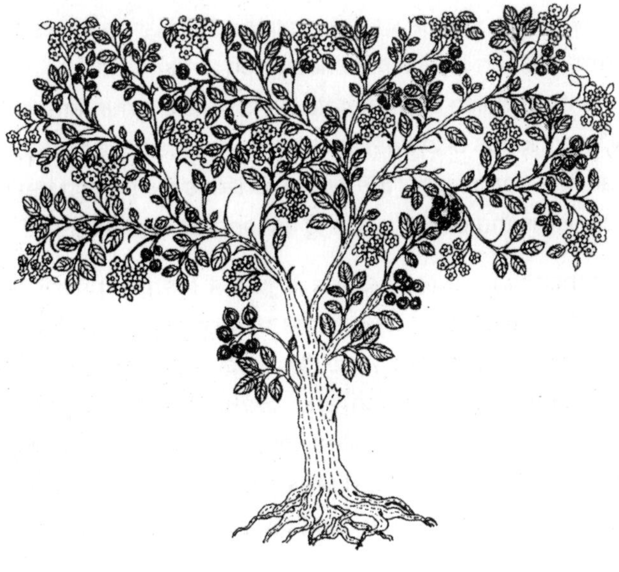

Plate n. 4 – The tree of yoga

Before proceeding further, let me quote from Sri Aurobindo's views on *āsana,* which are considered by modern yogis as pure *haṭha* (physical yoga):

"The pure *haṭha yoga* is the means of fulfilment through the body. Its processes are physical, strenuous, colossal, complex and difficult. They centre on *āsana, prāṇāyāma* and physical purification. The number of *āsanas* in the modern world is mixed and limited; in the ancient days *āsanas* were innumerable, difficult and painful, and the old yogin practised them all. The *āsana* means a simple, particular position of the body and is perfect or "conquered", in the technical language, when a man can stay in a single posture, however strained or apparently impossible, for an indefinite period without being forced by strain to remember the body.

The first objective of *āsana* is to conquer the body, for the body must be conquered before it can become divine – to be able to lay any command upon it and never be commanded by it. First conquer the physical nature by developing *siddhi* such as *laghimā, aṇimā, garimā, mahimā,* and so on. Then develop the yogic force, *tāpa* (heat) or *vīryam* (the fire of yoga). Next the yogin has to become *ūrdhvaretan,* that is to draw the whole virile force in the body up to the brain to get purified and electrified so that divinity settles between the head and heart. *Prāṇāyāma* is the mastery of the vital force, the mobile energy that keeps the universe going. In the human body, the most notable function of *prāṇa,* or vital force is breathing, which is necessary to life and motion in all men. The yogin masters it and renders himself independent of it. But he does not confine his attention to the simple vital operations. He distinguishes five major vital forces and several minor ones, to each of which he has given a name, and he learns to control all the numerous *prāṇic* currents in which they operate. As there are innumerable *āsanas,* so there are a great number of different kinds of *prāṇāyāma,* and a man is not a perfect *haṭha yogin* until he has mastered them all. The conquest of the *prāṇa* confirms the perfect health, vigour and vitality gained by *āsana,* it confirms the power of living as long as one pleases."

Another misconception is that *āsana* is just a form of physical movement with no bearing on the true meaning of yoga. The same misconception prevails with regards to the terms *haṭha yoga* (the yoga of will), *rāja yoga* (the royal way of yoga), *jñāna yoga* (the yoga of knowledge), *karma yoga* (the yoga of action) and *bhakti yoga* (the yoga of devotion). *Āsana* is a part of the yoga tree and it cannot be separated from the main tree. According to Sage Patañjali: *Tato dvandvānabhighātaḥ* (*Y.S.,* II.48). The dualities in man are vanquished by the mastery of *āsana.* If the *āsana* are physical, then how can they vanquish the dualities of mind?

Let me quote Brahmānanda, the commentator. In his commentary on *Haṭhayoga Pradīpikā* known as *Jyotsnā,* He proclaims: *Tada āsanam sthairyam dehasya manas cāncalyarūpa rajodharma nāśakatvena sthiratām kuryāt. "Āsananena rajo hanti" iti vākyāt.*

Ārogyam citta vikśepaka rogābhāvaḥ. Rogasya citta vikśepakatvam uktam patañjalasūtre "Vyādi styāna samśaya pramāda ālasya avirati bhrāntidarśana alabdhabhūmikatva anavasthitatvāni cittavikṣepaḥ te antarāyāḥ" iti. Añgānām lāghavam laghutvam. Gaurāvarūpa tamodharma nāśakatvam api etena nuktam (I.17). In short it means: The fickleness of the mind due to *rajōguna* is destroyed by the practice of *āsana*. That is why it is said in the scriptures *"Āsana* kill *rajōguna"*. Thus health in the true sense is eradication of the diseases which cause the distraction of *citta*. In the *Yoga Sūtra* of Patañjali the list of these impediments which cause distraction is given. These are namely, disease, inertia, doubt, heedlessness, laziness, indiscipline of the senses, erroneous views, lack of perseverance and backsliding. The practice of *āsana* ensures lightness of the body. The heaviness of the body arises from a preponderance of *tamas*. *Āsana* removes *tamas*.

In the *Triṣikhibrāhmaṇa Upaniṣad* it is said that: *Āsanam vijitam yena jitam tena jagatrayam.* (Verse 52.) One who has mastered *āsana* has conquered the three worlds, earth, space and heaven.

When exponents of yoga make such clear statements, it is unfortunate that some people wantonly and unnecessarily divide yoga in order to promote their own views and indulge in unwarranted criticism. Let me take the examples of a few *āsanas* and deal with the effect of them on body and mind. If *Sālamba Śīrṣāsana* is done accurately and precisely, the weight of the body is not felt and the brain feels sharpness. *Dwi Pāda Viparīta Daṇḍāsana* makes one not only sharp but also alert and active. During the practice of *Sālamba Sarvāṅgāsana*, the brain remains sober, with no negative or positive changes in it, whereas in *Halāsana* or *Uttānāsana* the brain becomes empty, silent and non-creative. In *Setu Bandha Sarvāṅgāsana*, the brain becomes alert but non-oscillating, silent and 100% positive and creative. In *Paśchimottānāsana* the whole physical body feels peace and poise in every cell. If *Baddha Koṇāsana* is performed, the bodily desire for sexual union diminishes, while in *prāṇāyāma* the mental desire for sex diminishes. In this way, each aspirant can trace the effects of *āsana* by performing it religiously with an open mind to see what comes in the wake of its presentation. I think that this much of an example is enough to understand the value of *āsana*. Please do not make understatements and do not undervalue *āsana* without subjectively undergoing training and maintaining dedicated practice for years. Then, I am sure views on *āsana* will change.

As a student, there is no separate petal for me in yoga, but it was *āsana* which really tested my tenacity of will, discipline and subjugation as well as sublimation of my vanity and ego.

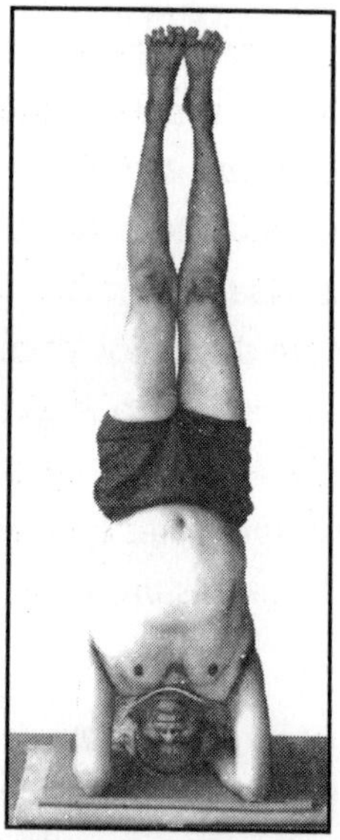

Sālamba Śīrṣāsana

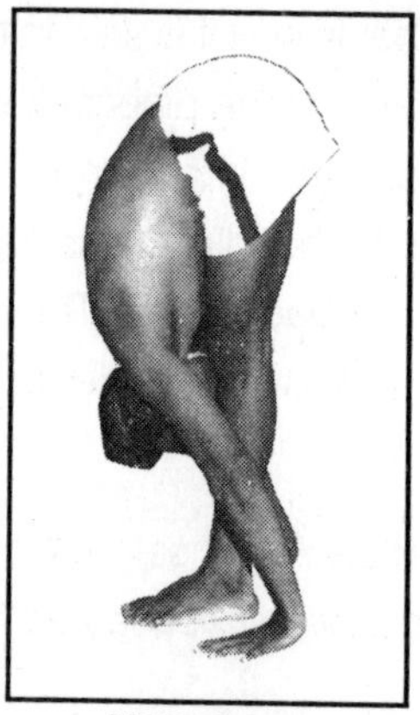

Uttānāsana

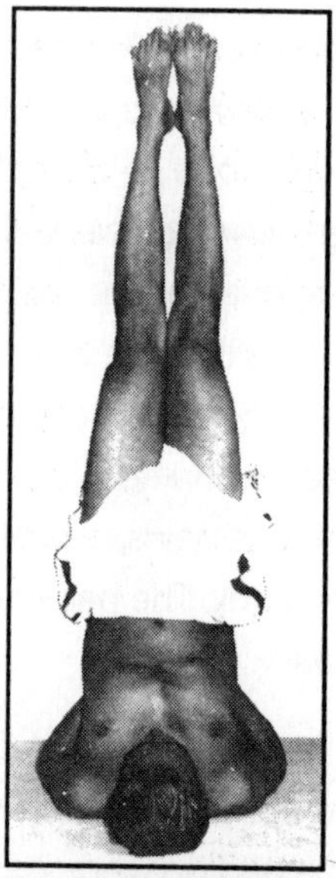

Sālamba Sarvāṅgāsana

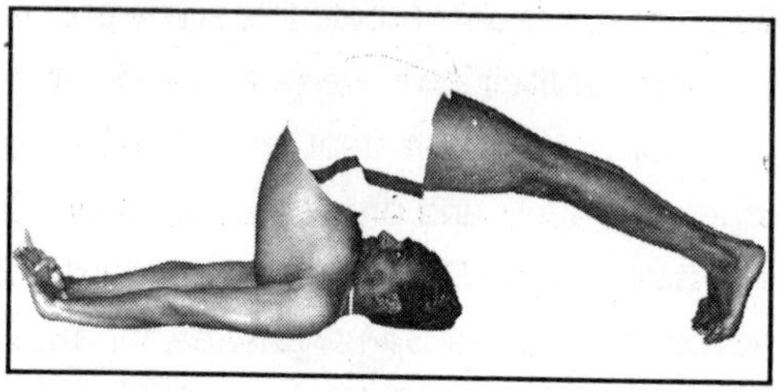

Halāsana

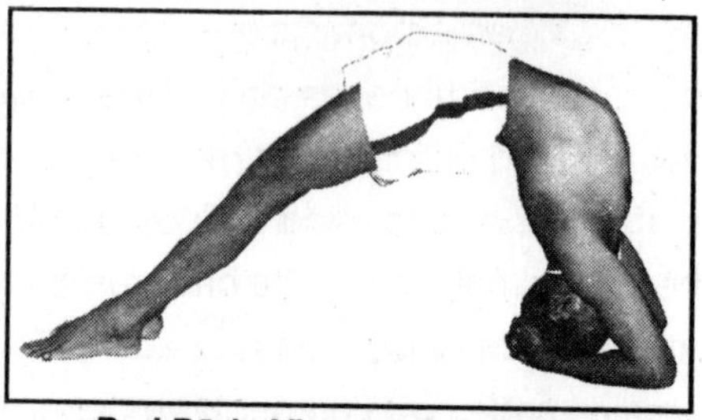

Dwi Pāda Viparīta Daṇḍāsana

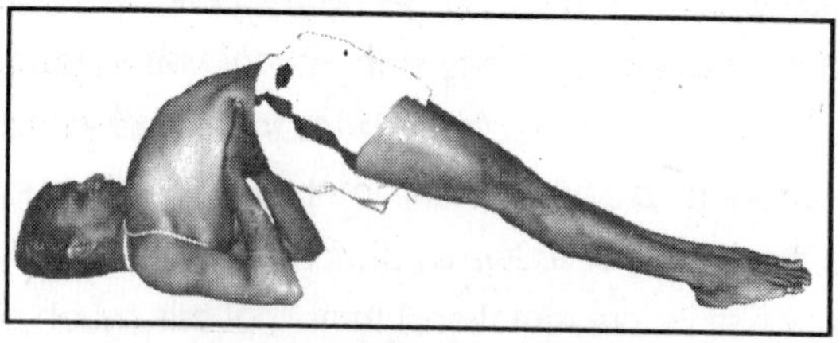

Setu Bandha Sarvāṅgāsana

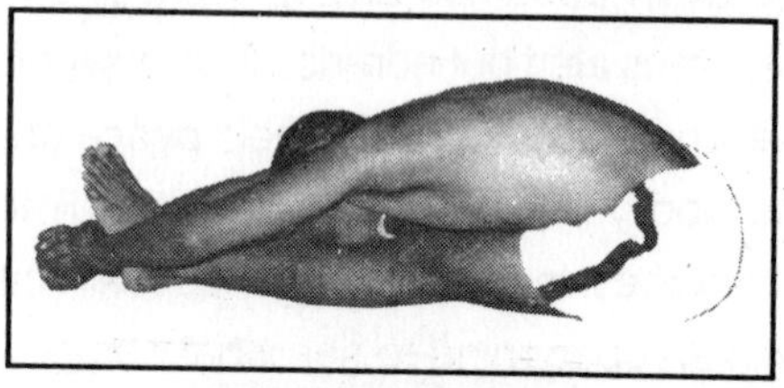

Paśchimottānāsana

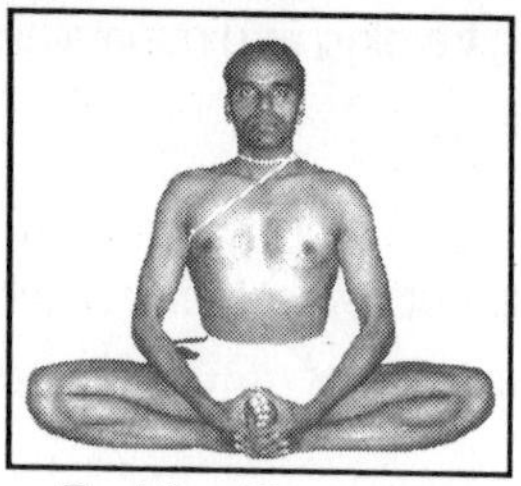

Baddha Koṇāsana

Plate n. 5 – *Sālamba Śīrṣāsana*
Uttānāsana
Sālamba Sarvāṅgāsana
Halāsana
Dwi Pāda Viparīta Daṇḍāsana
Setu Bandha Sarvāṅgāsana
Paśchimottānāsana
Baddha Koṇāsana

Where does the body end and the mind begin? Where does the mind end and the self begin? No one can answer these questions. So why demarcate, dismember and disintegrate the art and the science of yoga?

There are two ways of doing *āsana*: either without any thought *(ajñāna)* behind it or with full attention in thought and awareness *(prajñāna)*. While performing *āsana*, the spine, the arms and fingers, the legs and toes, the skin, the fibres, membranes, muscles and nerves, the organs of intelligence and the self, should be sharp, mobile, alert, alive, observant and receptive. In practising it, activity and passivity must go hand in hand to balance evenly so that one gets the best effect with receptivity. Total involvement and integration are essential while performing *āsana*.

Accurate performance of *āsana* brings peace in man's mind, poise in the body and a healthy balanced personality. Perform the *āsana* with uninterrupted awareness and undivided attention *(viveka khyāti)*. Do not perform them mechanically, with a wandering mind. Perform with total involvement. Penetrate the intellect from one end of the body to the other end, vertically, horizontally, circumferentially as well as diagonally. This will bring uniformity and harmony to the body and sculpt the body to bring out its latent beauty. Just as a goldsmith beats and melts gold to remove the impurities, so the yogin performs *āsana* to remove the toxins that are accumulated in the body. This gift of *āsana* acts to dissolve all types of complexities and enables man to come to simple living and high thinking.

Gazing at a burning candle, uttering a prescribed *mantra*, cultivating good thoughts, concentrating on a noble personality or reading sacred books and texts are normally regarded as spiritual practices *(ātma sādhanā)*. If a practitioner considers each *āsana* while performing it as his *mantra* or chosen deity, then each and every *āsana* becomes a spiritual posture. Why name some *āsana* as purely physical postures and others as meditative postures? Why not say that as long as effort is there, *āsana* is a physical posture, and with culture and refinement of them, they become meditative postures? If a right attitude and aptitude for performing them is cultivated in the mind and soul, the practitioner will gain mastery, and when efforts and refinements cease, light will dawn on him from the core of his being, extending the core's frontier.

Āsana practices effect not only physical, physiological and biological changes, but also psychological ones. The *sādhaka* does not take up the practice of the *āsana* for the sake of sensual pleasure or showmanship. But he directs his practice towards the self. It is fallacious to believe that maintaining a posture in comfort for a given length of time means mastery in yoga, for a sitting posture alone will not eradicate the scores of impediments and infirmities man is heir to. Nor is health to be mistaken for mere existence. Health is the delicate balance in harmony of body, mind and self where physical disabilities and mental distractions vanish and the gate of divinity opens.

The most important effect from performing *āsana* is that it brings the mind closer to the core of being, whereas its natural tendency and liking is to remain attached to the body, senses of perception and organs of action.

According to Patañjali, mastery of *āsana* leads towards freedom from dualities. The dualities between the body and the mind, and the mind and the self vanish; this results in tranquillity. This is the result of *yogāsana*. This happens only when the *sādhaka* attempts to make his *sādhanā* become effortless. Though he gains in health, strength, firmness and lightness, his knowledge becomes sharper, the ego dissolves and humility takes the place of 'I' or ego.

I conclude that perfect performance of *āsana* does not bring one to body consciousness as some people think but it frees one from the limitations of the body and sets one free, sublimating the mind with the self. As a devotee surrenders his all at the feet of the Lord, the practitioner surrenders and merges himself, and becomes one with the *āsana*. Then there is no difference between the knowable, the knower and the knowledge. There is only experience of that which is true *(satyam)*, auspicious *(śivam)* and beautiful *(sundaram)*.

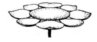

TRACE OF *PRĀṆA**

Most of us get excited when we hear the words *prāṇāyāma* and energy. But what is *prāṇa?*[1]

God is one, but He is called by different names. Energy is one but is called by different names. Let us study and know how *prāṇa* is produced in our systems. We are made up of five elements. The base is the earth, expansion is ether, and in between are the other three elements – water, fire and air. The saying that one cannot live without breath is as old as civilisation. I have pondered over this idea that normal breathing is like a thin layer of water flowing in a river. Though it has a current due to the flow, does it produce electricity? Does water, which has no current, produce electricity? Take for example just ordinary running water. It has a current but cannot produce abundant force with which to create energy.

How is electricity produced? We build a reservoir and then direct the water so that it falls down with speed on to a turbine and the turbine revolves. Similarly, the spindles of the muscles in our body act as turbines. Normal breath cannot produce electricity although it does produce a current. There is life in running water whereas water in a pond is stagnant. Compared to stagnant water, running water is better. If there is no movement of breath in the body, it is like a pond. A normal movement of the breath helps produce a minimum sufficiency of electricity or life force. This is termed as *prāṇa* or energy.

Right practice of *prāṇāyāma* makes the air go deep into the lungs like a waterfall. The air, which is drawn in, brings into fusion the element of fire and the element of water. Fire and water are contra-elements. Water cools fire, fire evaporates water. The fusion between the element of water and the element of fire produces life force as *prāṇa*. When we do *prāṇāyāma,* this stream of air activates the spindles like a turbine, and in that activation the fusion between the elements of water and fire in the body takes place. The energy that is produced as *prāṇa* triggers the nervous system and spreads in the bloodstream.

---

* From *Victoria Yoga Centre Society - Newsletter* - February 1987.

[1] For details read *The Tree of Yoga,* pp. 124-128, Harper Collins, London

In *prāṇāyāma*, the element of water and fire come together with the help of the element of air. The body, element of earth, is the place of production of energy. For production, as there must be a place, for distribution also there must be a space. If the earth element is the place for production, then the ether element is the space for distribution. In between the earth and ether are the three important elements functioning as raw materials, namely, water, fire and air. We draw on the five elements that exist in the external atmosphere in the form of breath. *Prāṇāyāma* refines our inner elements through an energy of bio-nuclear nature that we drawin from the outer atmosphere in the form of breath. We filter that bio-nuclear energy through our human system so that it may revitalise the inner elements.

Why should we do *prāṇāyāma?* The breath is taken deep so that the ions, which exist in the air, are taken by the air cells like the iron-filings which are attracted by a magnet. The ions which are attracted in this way, are brought closer to recharge the blood. Unless the ions move near these magnetic air cells, the lungs cannot grasp them. Just as a magnet slowly taken closer to iron-filings grasps them, similarly does deep breathing make the ions go nearer where the air cells can absorb and grip them to produce life's nectar.

That is why *prāṇāyāma* is essential, provided the lungs are clear. The *cakras* are nothing but various transformers. They store the energy *(prāṇa)* in various places so that it gets distributed whenever the system urgently needs it. This is the summum bonum of *prāṇāyāma,* showing what *prāṇa* is, and how it is produced in our system by the fusion of water and fire comparable to the relation of negative and positive currents of electricity. These two coming together produce a new lightning fire: *prāṇa* or *kuṇḍalinī.*

When this *prāṇa* becomes divine it is called *kuṇḍalinī* and when it flows abundantly all over the body and mind of the *sādhaka*, we say that his *kuṇḍalinī* is awakened. That is why I consider that, though the latent or dormant *kuṇḍalinī* is believed to be at the base of the spine, the awakened *kuṇḍalinī* is present everywhere.

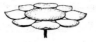

PRĀṆĀYĀMA[*]

Each and every individual strives to experience peace. Peace belongs to the domain of the heart, the field of the mind, or the seat of the emotional environment. Peace comes only when one conquers the conflicts between joy and sorrow, pleasure and pain and lust and malice through the efforts of yogic discipline and divine grace.

God, being without beginning or end, is designated as Eternal and Infinite. In the same way, conflict and peace exist from time immemorial, and they too are eternal. We all know that life is full of conflicts. Life is squeezed between pleasant *(preya)* and good or auspicious *(śreya)*. The mind of man binds the self with deluded thoughts. The delusions are: desire, anger, miserliness, infatuation, pride and hatred.

At the very beginning, Patañjali states that when the mind is stilled and silenced, then the yogi rests in his abode (*Y.S.*, I.3), the *jīvātman*. This stilling of the mind is possible only when man understands the causes for conflict, sorrow and delusion. Patañjali explains with crystalline clarity that want of spiritual wisdom and pride in one's self, attachment to desires, aversion to sorrows and fear that life might ebb away are the source for sufferings. The moment they are analysed, understood and, through the cultivation of yogic discipline, conquered, all emotional upheavals are sublimated and peace dawns.

The conflicts cannot be conquered without discretion *(vivecana)*. To distinguish pleasant transient sensations from permanent spiritual delights, discrimination and reasoning *(viveka* and *vicāra)* are required. They have to be developed through practice *(abhyāsa)* and renunciation *(vairāgya)*. Practice involves *tapas*. *Tapas* is nothing but disciplining the mind through the eight aspects of yoga. This practice is not complete or thorough without faith *(śraddhā)*, courage *(vīrya)*, the study of sacred texts and of one's own behaviour *(svādhyāya)*, determination *(dṛḍhatā)* and profound meditation *(dhyāna)*. In order to be victorious over the six causes of delusion, one

---

[*] For more details, see the author's *Light on Prāṇāyāma*, Harper Collins, London Rupa, India.

has to use the six spokes of the wheel of peace. They are *viveka, vicāra, śraddhā, vīrya, abhyāsa* and *vairāgya*. Then wisdom dawns on man through this refined culture *(saṁskāra)* whereby his head gains clarity and mind earns calmness.

In particular it is the practice of *prāṇāyāma* that has the power to calm the ruffled mind. The sages have termed *prāṇāyāma* as the "hub" of the wheel of yoga. It is the heart of yoga, a touchstone of peace and spiritual prosperity.

Prāṇa, though one, has many ramifications. *Prāṇa* means energy at all levels, physical, mental, intellectual, sexual, nuclear, spiritual or cosmic. *Prāṇa*, as energy, vibrates as heat, light, gravity, magnetism and electricity.

It is said in the *Upaniṣads*, that *prāṇa* permeates in us as well as in the life-giving sun, moon, stars, plants, clouds, winds, rains, earth, water, fire, and so on. It is in each and everything that exists in the universe.

In *Chāndogya Upaniṣad* (VII.15, 1-4) it is said that life is greater than hope; life breath is fastened as the spokes are fastened to the hub of the wheel; breath gives life to a living creature. Life breath is one's father, one's mother, one's brother, one's sister, one's teacher, and one's Brahman. Life breath is all this. He who sees this, he who thinks this, understands this, becomes an excellent orator[1].

Kauśiṭaki Upaniṣad (III, 3-4) mentions that one can live deprived of speech for we see the dumb, one can live without the eyes for we see the blind, one can live without hearing for we see the deaf, we see another without his mind and we also see people living without legs and arms. See that it is the breathing self alone that holds the body and seizes the intelligence of the seer. Thus whatever is breathing self, that is the intelligence of the seer. What is the intelligence or the seer, that is the breathing self; these together dwell in the body and together they depart.

The *Haṭhayoga Pradīpikā* also emphasises that as long as there is breath in the body, there is life. When breath departs, life too departs (*H.Y.P.*, II.3). Therefore, Svātmārāma, the author of *Haṭhayoga Pradīpikā*, says, regulate breath. He says, where there is breath, there the mind is and where the mind is, there the breath stays. Patañjali suggests alternative methods to still the consciousness. One of the means of quietening the consciousness is the control of the outflowing breath. From these, it can easily be inferred that consciousness *(citta)* and energy *(prāṇa)* are like the two banks of a river or the two wings of the seer. If the breath is irregular, the mind wavers and when the breath is steady, the mind is quiet. So long as the breath and mind are calm, tranquil serenity flows in man.

---

[1] His speech is full of truth.

PRĀṆA AND *PRĀṆA VṚTTI*

Cale vāte calam cittam, niścale niścalaṁ bhavet (*H.Y.P.*, II.2).

"As breath flows, so the mind moves, when the breath is stilled, mind too becomes still and silent".

Our normal movement of breath is not rhythmic. The inhalation may be long and the exhalation may be short, or the inhalation short and the exhalation long. If one pays attention to this inhalation and exhalation, one experiences a neutralising effect of the mind. This reaction on the mind by the regulation of breath must have led Svātmārāma to conclude that the control of *prāṇa (prāṇavṛtti stambhana)* is the key to emancipation.

Patañjali also states that mastery of *prāṇāyāma* removes the veil that covers the flame of intelligence and heralds the dawn of wisdom (*Y.S.*, II.52). He says further that the mind acquires the competence to move on towards concentration for the realisation of the seer (*Y.S.*, II.53). Thus, *prāṇāyāma* becomes the touchstone for Self-realisation.

Life exists as long as the energy drawn from the breath permeates man's whole system. Death is when breath departs (*H.Y.P.*, II.3). Regular practice of *prāṇāyāma* shields one from disease, old age and death. All *yogācāryas* of yore maintained that correct practice of *prāṇāyāma* lubricates the system and rectifies disturbances of the humours: *vāta* (wind), *pitta* (bile) and *śleṣma* (phlegm). *Prāṇāyāma* builds up tremendous power in the practitioner to face the infinite light when grace dawns on him.

As the sun radiates light evenly and uniformly on earth, so too *prāṇa* radiates evenly in all creation. *Prāṇa* is called bio-energy or vital energy or life-force. *Prāṇa* is loosely called breath or *vāyu*. Through *prāṇa*, respiration is possible; vitality or strength is gained. Life gets extinguished when *prāṇa* departs. The breath we draw in carries very powerful oxidising agents in an ionic form, invigorating the cells to recharge and discharge their current for proper and smooth functioning of the various systems of man.

For the sake of convenience, the same *prāṇa* is designated according to the locations and functions in the body. They are called *prāṇa, apāna, samāna, udāna* and *vyāna*. *Prāṇa* is located in the region of the chest. It controls the movement of breath and absorbs vital atmospheric energy. *Apāna,* located at the lower trunk, helps to discharge urine, semen and faeces. *Samāna* rests in the middle of the trunk as fuel *(jaṭharāgni)* and helps in digestion and assimilation. *Udāna,* stationed in the region of the throat, makes one breathe and swallow food. It controls the vocal chords. *Vyāna* pervades the entire body and distributes the energy received from air and food through the blood currents and nerve channels. There are five more subsidiary energies *(upavāyu).* They are *nāga, kūrma, kṛkara, devadatta* and *dhanaṁjaya. Nāga* relieves pressures of the abdomen by belching, *kūrma* controls the movements of eyelids, prevents foreign matters entering the eyes and helps the muscles of the eyes to contract or dilate according to the intensity of light. *Kṛkara* does not allow unwanted matter to enter through nose or throat. If foreign matter does enter, it immediately makes one sneeze or cough it out. *Devadatta* causes yawning and induces sleep whereas *dhanaṁjaya* produces phlegm to act as cushions within our life system and it is said that this *upavāyu* remains in the body even after death and inflates and degenerates the corpse.

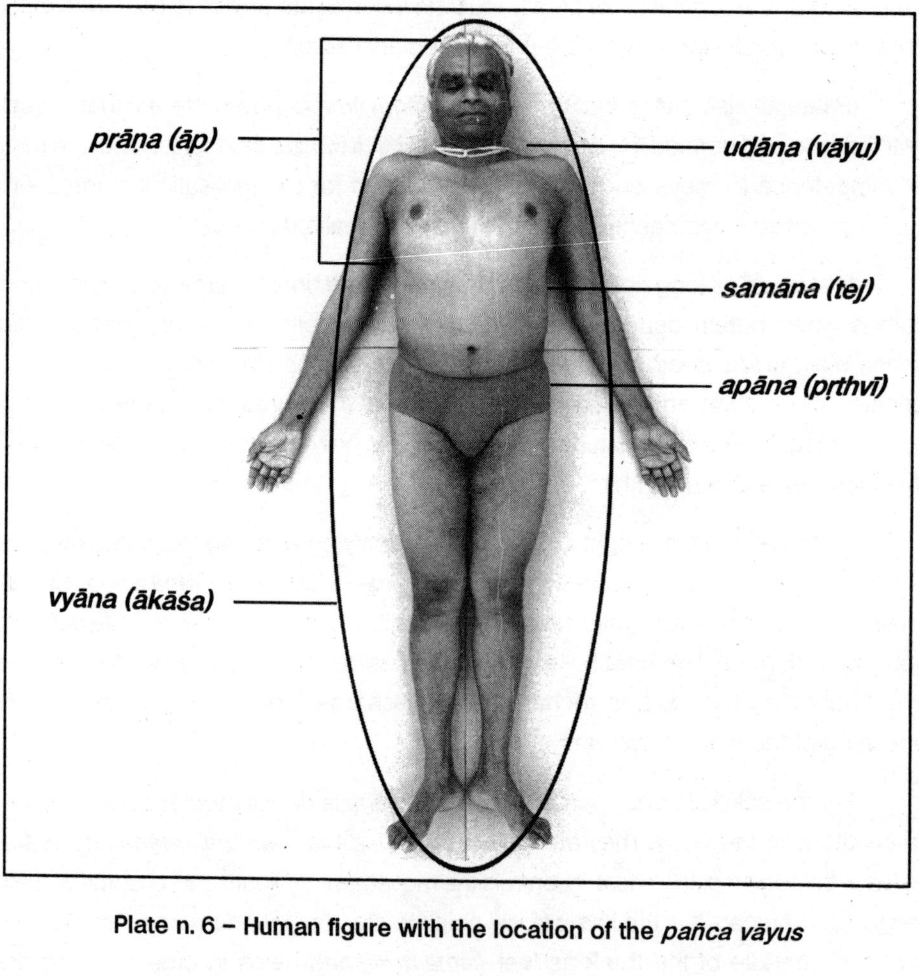

Plate n. 6 – Human figure with the location of the *pañca vāyus*

By now, you know what *prāṇa* is. But what is *prāṇāyāma? Prāṇāyāma* is a vertical ascension *(ārohatā)*, a horizontal expansion *(dairghyatā)* and a circumferential extension *(viśālatā)* of the breath for the lungs, the ribcage and the chest wall, to build up extension and expansion.

It is a compound word, composed of *prāṇa* and *āyāma*. If *prāṇa* stands for energy, *āyāma* stands for stretch, extension, expansion, length, breadth, regulation, prolongation and restraint. It consists of four aspects. They are: inhalation *(pūraka)*, internal retention *(antara kuṁbhaka)*, exhalation *(recaka)* and external retention *(bāhya kuṁbhaka)*. *Pūraka* is the long, sustained, subtle, deep, slow and rhythmic in-breath. In inhalation, the energising ingredients of the atmospheric air sensitively percolate into the cells of the lungs and rejuvenate life. This not only brings a better healthy meaningful state, but also enhances one's span of life and makes life fruitful. After deep inhalation, the second is *antara kuṁbhaka* i.e., the holding of breath. In this holding of breath, the drawn-in energy is distributed to the entire system through the blood current. The third is *recaka* or the art of slow discharge or exhalation of the vitiated air in the form of toxins through sustained slow subtle deep release of breath. After exhalation is the fourth state *bāhya kuṁbhaka*, in which a pause is maintained according to one's capacity, without the inhalation. Here all stresses are purged and drained and the mind is made to remain silent and quiet.

TYPES OF *PRĀṆĀYĀMA*

As *āsana* comes in numerous forms, so does *prāṇāyāma*. The best *prāṇāyāma* is *nāḍī śodhana prāṇāyāma*. The very name conveys to the practitioner that he has to search and trace the *prāṇanāḍī*, the channel through which the refined breath passes through the nostrils. This is done through thoughtful and skilful manipulation with the placement of the tips of the ring and little fingers and thumb. Then one derives the right benefit from *prāṇāyāma*. While dealing with *prāṇāyāma*, Svātmārāma cautions practitioners to follow the principles of *yama* and *niyama*.

He gives eight types of *prāṇāyāma* called *kuṁbhaka*. They are *Sūrya bhedhana, Ujjāyi, Ṣītkāri, Śītali, Bhastrikā, Bhrāmari, Mūrcchā* and *Plāvinī*. *Kuṁbhaka* means retention of breath. *Kuṁbha* means a pot. Here the torso represents a pot or a water jar, hence the word *kuṁbhaka*. Whatever *prāṇāyāma* one practises, one should become totally absorbed in it like a wise man who will not allow his mind to wander at all. Besides these eight *kuṁbhaka*, one more is added as *kevala kuṁbhaka*.

Though Patañjali refers to the three movements of *prāṇāyāma*, yet he speaks of *kevala kuṁbhaka* as retention of breath that takes place without deliberation. *Bāhya ābhyantara viṣaya ākṣepī caturthaḥ* (*Y.S.*, II.51). That which transcends the previous three processes of *prāṇāyāma* (*bāhya vṛtti* or outbreath – *recaka* –, *antara vṛtti* or inbreath – *pūraka* –, and *stambavṛtti* or retention – *kuṁbhaka*) and appears at once effortless, non-thoughtful, non-deliberate and natural.

The *Haṭhayoga Pradīpikā* mentions that a devoted student of yoga should practise *prāṇāyāma* four times a day, in the early morning, noon, evening and midnight. A minimum of eighty cycles of any one *prāṇāyāma* for each sitting is advocated. If one takes time into consideration, eighty cycles practised four times amounts to about four to five hours a day. It is not possible nowadays to devote so much time as one has to maintain one's life. At least once a day is necessary, giving as much time as possible or as long as the brain and lungs maintain the subtleness, the rhythm and the depth of each breath with ease. In the beginning, breathing is laborious and monotonous. One perspires and trembles. When practice becomes regular, the lungs get toned and delicacy in practice sets in.

CAUTION

While practising *prāṇāyāma*, the *sādhaka* is advised to take the example of a trainer of a tiger, lion or elephant. He studies their habits and moods, then puts them through their paces slowly and steadily. He treats them with kindness and consideration lest they turn on him and maim him. In the same way, the *sādhaka* who practises without understanding the capacity of the lungs and the art of keeping the brain passive or the proper movement of the chest wall will hurt himself (*H.Y.P.*, II.15-16).

A pneumatic tool can cut through the hardest rock. If not used properly, it may destroy both the tool and the user. Study your breath carefully and proceed step by step. If you practise *prāṇāyāma* hastily or forcibly, you may well harm yourself.

Prāṇāyāma is not just deep breathing. There is a difference between deep breathing and *prāṇāyāma*. In deep breathing the facial muscles and the brain cells are hardened. The chest walls (the intercostal muscles and the ribs) are dynamically lifted with forceful sucking of air in inhalation and with heavy expulsion of air in exhalation. If the water gushes in, very forcefully, it splashes out, damaging the container. Forceful breathing does the same. In *prāṇāyāmic* breathing the brain cells and facial muscles are kept passive and receptive. As a passive spectator, each and every fibre of the chest wall is watched and kept receptive and mobile and the breath is taken with least force. As the breath is drawn in, room is created within the chest gradually to absorb the drawn-in breath so that it is moistened and soaked to reach the remotest parts of the lungs and to feed them. The art of balancing, the effort of drawing the breath in or out should be synchronised with the receptivity of the cells of the lungs so that they respond to receive the breath.

Exhalation is when the outflow of breath is gradually released and at the same time sufficient time is given for the air cells to get full use of the energy of the drawn-in breath that remains still in the chest. This passive observation instils hope and calm in the emotional centre. Thus the effect of *prāṇāyāma* is precisely accurate in feeding the body with plenty of oxygenated energy. Then it is no more called deep breathing but actual *prāṇāyāma*.

EFFECTS OF *PRĀṆĀYĀMA*

The classical texts of yoga, while giving the effects of an appropriate practice of *prāṇāyāma*, warn the practitioners about the ill effects of the wrong practice. Svātmārāma says:

Wrong practice of *prāṇāyāma* brings hordes of maladies such as hiccough, laboured breathing, cough, itching in the ears and a burning sensation in the eyes (*H.Y.P.*, II.17), which are all the symptoms of high blood pressure.

Right practice frees one from psycho-physiological disturbances and brings a glow in the eyes, health in the body, brightness and clarity in intelligence, calmness and serenity in one's self (*H.Y.P.*, II.16).

Prāṇāyāma regulates not only the flow of energy but also restrains the movement of the mind from its fluctuations and oscillations.

Prāṇa and mind are like mercury. As mercury is bound by special processes, these two have to be bound through yoga to experience equipoise. Though these two are mingled like milk and water, yet mind is dependent on desire *(vāsanā)* and energy *(prāṇa)*. If anyone of these three, namely, mind, desire or energy, becomes inactive, then the other two also find their culmination in stillness and silence. Hence, Svātmārāma says that total absorption is achieved either by following the methods of stilling the mind or stilling the energy: If one is silenced, the other is at rest.

Thus, *prāṇāyāma* helps to suspend the movements of body, senses and mind and leads one towards *dhāraṇā, dhyāna* and *samādhi*, which are the subtle disciplines of yoga.

Prāṇāyāma clears and soothes the febrile brain which hampers right thinking and reasoning, and the mind is lifted towards meditation.

In *prāṇāyāma*, the *sādhaka* uses his body as a sacrificial altar *(yajña kuṇḍa)*. Inhalation is pouring ghee on the altar. Exhalation is the flame blazing out from the *yajña kuṇḍa*. *Kuṁbhaka* is in the form of *mantra*, an offering as oblation so that the self merges and dissolves in the Universal Soul – the God or *Paramātmā*.

IS *ĀSANA* ESSENTIAL FOR *PRĀṆĀYĀMA?*

The Self, being the core, and the body being its cover or envelope, *āsana* glues both the core and the body together so that the known (the body) merges into the unknown (the Self), and both become known as one. While performing *āsana*, certain things have to be observed in each pose. An even stretch on each side of the body is truthfulness in presentation. Co-ordination of body and mind and total absorption of the self in each *āsana* is a must. Observing the principles of *yama* and *niyama* in each movement of the *āsana,* the field or the body *(kṣetra)* connects with the knower of the field *(kṣetrajña* or the seer). While performing the *āsana,* see that both the body and the knower of the field are divinely wedded.

It is interesting to note that all the textbooks on yoga emphatically say that mastery of *āsana* is a prerequisite for *prāṇāyāma* practice. Today, this specified point is overlooked, and now it is commonly thought that any comfortable *āsana* is sufficient.

Hence practice of *āsana* is essential before one takes to the path of *prāṇāyāma*. *Āsana* helps one to keep the nervous system clear so that the drawn-in energy is moved uninterruptedly without any hindrance. If the nerves are corroded and blocked with stress, how can *prāṇa* move or how can one reach the goal? *Haṭhayoga Pradīpikā* says that the practice of *āsana* and *prāṇāyāma* lifts the veil that segregates the body and mind. It keeps one healthy and light in body, bright in head and calm in heart. It is a bridge between the mind and the Self. It is the instrument which dispels darkness and ignorance and in its place brings knowledge and immortality. It is an art by which to enjoy unconditional peace for one's inner delight.

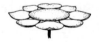

PRĀṆA AND *CITTA**

PRĀṆA

Prāṇa is an auto-energising force. This self-energising force creates a magnetic field in the form of universe in which takes place the cyclic play of creation, maintenance, destruction and further creation. It permeates each individual as well as the Universe at all levels. All that vibrates in the Universe is *prāṇa.* It is potent in all beings and non-beings and is a prime mover of all activity.

This Self-energising force is the principle of life and consciousness. It is the root-cause, the primary force of the creation of all beings in the Universe. Life and consciousness are born and live by *prāṇa* in every being. When the individual being dies, the individual breath dissolves into the cosmic breath. *Prāṇa* permeates life, providing sun, moon, clouds, wind, rain, earth and all forms of matter. It is in being *(sat)* and non-being *(asat)* as well. *Prāṇa* is the source of all knowledge and shelters everything living and non-living including human beings. It is a cosmic entity.

CITTA

In the human system, *citta* is said to be in constant contact with *prāṇa* and *prāṇa* with *prajñā.* *Citta* is composed of three categories: (a) mind *(manas),* having the faculties of attention, selection and rejection according to its own whims and wishes; (b) intelligence *(buddhi),* having the faculty of reflective awareness and discriminative power. It is able to discern and to choose; and (c) *ahaṁkāra,* which imposes itself as self *(asmitā). Prāṇa* and *citta* are inseparable twins. The yogis discovered that *citta,* however, is like a vehicle propelled by two powerful forces: *prāṇa* (the universal or cosmic breath) and *vāsanā* (desires). When *citta* follows the impelling forces of desire, the breathing is uneven and the mind is agitated. Thereby *prāṇa* loses its contact with *prajñā.* But when *citta* follows the flow of the cosmic breath, desires are subdued, the senses are held in check and the mind is stilled. Thus, *prāṇa* remains in contact with *prajñā.*

---

* From *Bhavan's Journal,* February 1, 1987; also in *Iyengar Yoga Institute Review,* San Francisco, vol. 8, no. 2 September 1988.

For most people, the *citta* is constantly disturbed by conscious and unconscious desires. The wise yogis realised that all types of vibrations and fluctuations come to a standstill when *prāṇa* or mind is quiet, steady and still.

Recognising this connection between breath and mind, they advocated the practice of *prāṇāyāma* as the means to climb the spiritual ladder. It is the fourth link of the eight-petalled system of *pātañjala yoga*. It is a powerful practice that brings *prāṇic* health, as well as quietness of mind and spiritual insight. In order to understand better the essence of *prāṇāyāma* practice, a close look at the nature of *prāṇa* and its relationship to the human system is required. *Āyāma* covers extension, ascension and expansion. Hence, *prāṇāyāma* is the extension, ascension and expansion of breath and its restraint. The constant practice of *prāṇāyāma* brings the *citta* to steadiness, keeps away conscious and unconscious desires and brings attention and awareness to the cosmic breath.

Prāṇāyāma consists of four parts. They are *pūraka*, *antara kuṁbhaka*, *recaka* and *bāhya kuṁbhaka*.

Pūraka, the life giver, is the long, sustained, subtle, deep, slow and rhythmic in-breath. Similarly, *recaka* releases the vitiated air in the form of toxin through subtle, slow and rhythmic out-breath.

Antara kuṁbhaka distributes the drawn-in energy to the entire system; while *bāhya kuṁbhaka* empties the burden of the brain, purges all strains and stresses, creating silence and quietude.

Do not mistake *prāṇāyāma* for just deep breathing. In *prāṇāyāma*, the cells of the brain and facial muscles are kept receptive and the breath is taken in pensively and released passively. In *pūraka*, the energy that is received smoothly without jerks is allowed to soak inside the lungs. In *recaka*, sufficient time is given to release the breath for the air cells to re-absorb the residual *prāṇa* to a maximum extent. This passive observation allows a full utilisation of energy, builds up emotional stability and calms the mind. Hence, *prāṇāyāma* is the refined art and science of making the respiratory organs expand deliberately and move intentionally to gain perfect rhythm and balance in effort and response. Still more, it makes the practitioner peep within himself to feel the core of life.

Before acquainting ourselves with the techniques of *prāṇāyāma*, let us see what *prāṇa* is.

According to Indian thought, *puruṣa* apart, *prakṛti* (nature) is made up of twenty-four *tattva*. *Prakṛti* evolves as *mahat* (cosmic intelligence). This *mahat*, the first evolute of *prakṛti*, transforms itself as *citta* in man. *Citta* divides itself into three parts as *manas* (mind), *buddhi* (intelligence) and *ahaṁkāra* (ego). *Prakṛti* or nature has five elements; earth, water, fire, air and ether in the ratio of 5:4:3:2:1. Each of these five has a subtle counterpart in the form of odour, taste, form or shape, touch and sound. Besides these, there are five senses of perception and five organs of action. All these combined together make up a living being, moulded by the *guṇa* of nature, *sattva, rajas* and *tamas*. Of the five elements, only one pair is antagonistic i.e., fire and water. Water cools and extinguishes fire, while heat and fire evaporate water. No other pair of elements show this dynamic polarity. In the human body the fusion of fire and water with the contact of air emits a new energy in the form of *prāṇa* (the life force of the human system). Its production is maximised during *prāṇāyāma*.

Here, the word *prāṇa* brings to my mind the epic story of *Amṛtamanthan*[1], when the elixir or nectar of life *(jīvāmṛta)* was produced by the churning of the ocean.

When the strength of the demons *(asuras)* was uppermost, Lord Shiva, Lord Brahmā and Lord Indra requested Lord Vishnu, the protector of the Universe, to help them in upholding the virtues which were disturbed by the power and strength of the demons.

Lord Vishnu thought for a while and suggested the churning of the ocean to bring out the nectar of life or immortality. He advised them to discuss with the demons the effects of *amṛita* and to impress upon them to accept the offer of churning the ocean jointly. The Lords went to the leaders of the demons and discussed with them the plan to churn the nectar from the ocean.

They decided to use Mount Meru as a churning rod and Vāsuki, one of the famous *nāga* (serpents), as the rope for whirling the mountain.

The raw materials such as plants, creepers, various grasses and herbs were cast together and dumped into the ocean so that they were churned to produce the nectar of life.

This story can be interpreted as an analogy for the production of *prāṇa* in living creatures.

The spinal column – Mount Meru – acts as a dasher or whisker of breath. *Suṣumṇā* represents Vāsuki as cosmic atmosphere while *iḍā* and *piṅgaḷā* represent Vāsuki's head and tail.

It is possible that *iḍā* represents the parasympathetic nervous system, *piṅgaḷā* the sympathetic nervous system and *suṣumṇā*, the central nervous system. As Vāsuki was used as a rope for churning, so is the breath. The inhalation and exhalation are used as two ends of the

---

1 This beautiful and symbolic story is related in *Mahabhārata (Ādi Parva), Vālmiki Rāmāyaṇa (Āraṇya Kāṇda, 35th sarga)* and in some *purāṇas* like *Vishnu-* (I.9), *Bhāgavata-* (VIII), and *Agni-* (152). For a modern explanation of the story, see the author's *The Tree of Yoga*, pp. 55-58, 115-117, Harper Collins, London.

rope to churn the rod (central nervous system) where energy is stored in seven chambers of the spine. These two ends – the inbreath and outbreath – help to churn and to generate *prāṇa* (the elixir), the *viśva prāṇa śakti or viśva caitayna śakti* (cosmic vital force).

As the churning began, the mountain sank into the ocean. Lord Vishnu, incarnated as Kūrma (tortoise), crept underneath the mountain and lifted it from the base for it to float, so that the churning would continue. Similarly, *ātman* keeps the spine floating upwards.

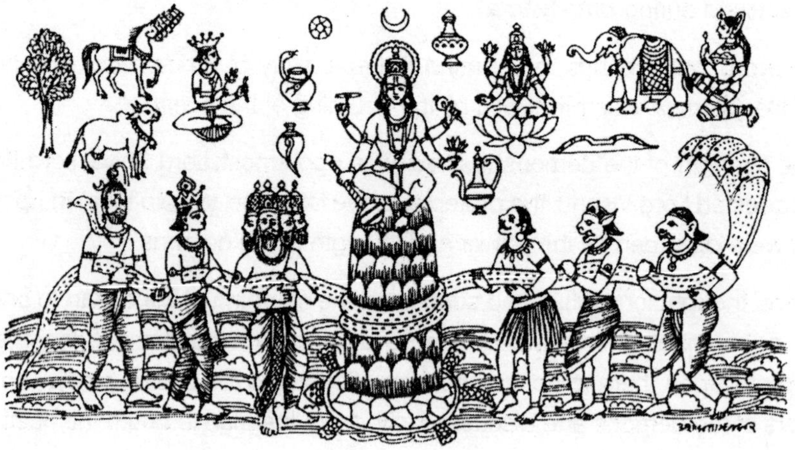

The first thing to spring out from the ocean was the poison called *Halāhala*. This was swallowed by Lord Shiva. This *Halāhala* is nothing but toxic output in the form of exhalation.

Later several gems were generated from the churning. They represent the seven constituents *(dhātu)*, namely chyle *(rasa)*, blood *(rakta)*, flesh *(māṁsa)*, fat *(medas)*, bones *(asthi)*, marrow *(majjā)* and semen *(śukra)*, and ten vital energies or *vāyu (prāṇa, apāna, samāna, udāna, vyāna, nāga, kūrma, kṛkara, devadatta* and *dhanaṁjaya)*.

The Self *(puruṣa)* is represented by Lord Vishnu and the body as nature *(prakṛti)*. The body becomes the fountainhead of production and the Lord of the body is its generative force.

The five elements and seven constituents in the body come in contact with the *ātman* and act as the raw material to produce life's elixir. The earth element acts as the base for production and the element of ether acts as distributor of energy. The element of air is the cause of respiration. The in and out-breath creates fusion between the remaining two elements, water and fire, which unite to produce electrical energy in the system as life force. By the contact of the seven constituents and the ten vital energies *(prāṇa)* and with the help of the spinal column, the life elixir is produced in the body. *Ātman* assists by acting as a supporter for blending the elements and their counterparts. In this manner the practice of *prāṇāyāma* enhances and generates more power through this self-energising force.

THE ANALOGY OF ELECTRICITY

In the practice of *prāṇāyāma*, the yogis discovered that the life sustaining energy is much more subtle and profound than the energy that is generated from normal breathing. To realise this they explored the origins and source of the production of the *prāṇa*, the bio-energy, in the living system. Their discovery can be compared to that of nuclear energy, a much more powerful source than the physical and chemical energies of the ordinary world.

In order to understand the production of *prāṇa* we have to note the difference between *prāṇāyāma* and normal breathing. Compare the flow of the breath to the flow of water (or any fluid, for that matter). Stored or pond water is stale, stagnant and lifeless, compared to running water, which has a current, a kinetic energy, a dynamism, but this energy is mostly dissipated and wasted. However, if the running water is harnessed, controlled and regulated, the energy can be used to create electricity. A reservoir is built, a waterchute is created to develop momentum and the falling water is used to turn turbines in a magnetic field. The electricity thus created, passes through accumulators and is then transmitted along the power lines to light cities and power machinery. The power is stepped up or down by transformers which regulate voltage and current. The generation and distribution of *prāṇa* in the human system may be compared to that of electrical energy.

When there is no movement of breath in the body, death supervenes. And if breathing is hard we suffocate. No doubt there is a current in normal breathing but its effect is minimal. We live with this minimal energy and assume that this is all that is possible. *Prāṇāyāma* helps to draw to the optimum level the energy that is present in air, just as the power plant uses the full energy of the falling water. The right practice of *prāṇāyāma* makes the air enter deep into the lungs, like a waterfall. The long, slow, soft breathing strengthens the thoracic area by softening, lengthening and extending the nerve fibres and tissues of the lung cells. This rhythmic extension and expansion creates internal coherence and increases space in order to develop a large magnetic field to collect energy from the drawn-in air and to store it in the lungs. There is percolation of the air current through the cells of the lungs to the extremities so that the magnetic fields of the spindles are fully exposed to the ionic energy in the breath. This is like the water current falling on and activating the turbines. Sufficient time is given during the retention and exhalation fully to absorb the energy or the essence of breath. This energy is then accumulated in the *cakra* which act as transformers to step up or down the voltage and then distribute it throughout the body along the transmission lines which are the circulatory and nervous systems. Thus, yogis of India discovered *prāṇāyāma* as a way to make full use of the energy, both inspired and inspirational, in the human system.

The word *cakra* means a wheel. A wheel rotates. As energy is rotated in the various *cakra*, they work as transmitting centres.

In *prāṇāyāma*, the carpet of the mucous membranes of the nostrils filters and cleanses the breath that enters into the lungs. At the moment of exhalation, sufficient time is given for the lungs to absorb the drawn-in energy and diffuse it in the blood. It is termed as *ratna pūrita dhātu*, "the jewel of the blood", or blood filled with optimum chemical properties.

This full use of absorption of *prāṇa* makes a man live long. The texts say that the practice of *prāṇāyāma* causes the practitioner to live one hundred years. That is why practice of *prāṇāyāma* is considered a great science *(mahāvidyā)*.

However, apart from longevity, *prāṇāyāma* makes the *citta* illuminative *(sāttvic)*. Since the *prāṇa* and *citta* are inseparable, along with *prāṇaśuddhi* (*śuddhi* = purity) the *cittaśuddhi* (purity in consciousness) too occurs. *Citta*, which often goes with *vāsanā* (desires), now embraces *prajñā*. The *citta* charged with *prāṇa* and *prajñā* becomes clean, stable and clear, achieving both *prāṇaśuddhi* and *cittaśuddhi*.

*PRATYĀHĀRA**

The precise practice of *prāṇāyāma* prepares the mind to become a fit instrument for concentration. The senses stop importuning the mind for their gratification. They lose interest in the taste and flavour of their respective objects and are drawn back from the external world in order to help the mind in its inner quest. *Pratyāhāra* is at this hinge.

It is the foundation of the path of renunciation. As the petals of a flower open in the sunlight and close at eventide, so it is in the case of a *sādhaka*. He has to follow two paths, the path of practice, from *yama* to *prāṇāyāma*, an unfolding process, and the path of renunciation, from *pratyāhāra* to *samādhi*, a centripetal one. In this way he may acquire supreme knowledge, so that he abides in his Self, seeing and perceiving things directly, without the intervention of *citta*, the conscious faculties.

The senses perceive objects with the help of the consciousness. They perceive with thoughts of acquisition, rejection and resignation. They become hypnotised by the objects of the world and are drawn towards pleasure. *Pratyāhāra* redirects the senses towards the realisation of the Self instead of seeking sensual pleasures.

The term *pratyāhāra* is composed of *prati + ang + hṛ*. *Prati* means opposite, against, in return, *ang* conveys the idea of near to or towards the self. *Hṛ*, the root word of *pratyāhāra*, means to take, to bear, to carry. So, *pratyāhāra* literally means, "to draw towards the opposite". Technically, it means withdrawing the mind from the contact of the organs of action and senses of perception, and then directing it towards the Self.

The relationship between the mind and the senses is aptly compared to that of bees following the queen bee. If the queen bee moves, the others follow. When she rests, the others rest too. They do not function independently of their queen. Similarly, whenever and wherever the mind moves, the senses move, and when the mind stops, the senses too stop functioning.

---

* Extracts from *Light on the Yoga Sūtras of Patañjali*. Courtesy Harper Collins, London.

This is *pratyāhāra*. It is the process of training the mind along with the senses to stop its outer journey so that it begins an inner trajectory. It is the beginning of man's return journey towards his Maker. *Pratyāhāra* is the science of restraining the senses and depriving them of that which energises them, that is to say, the external world and all its phenomena. Controlling the senses and mind by willpower, the *sādhaka* has to draw his consciousness towards its source - the Self *(ātman)*, and through Self to Supreme Being *(Paramātman)*. For example, while performing an *āsana* or *prāṇāyāma*, the cellular intelligence of the body extends outwards, whereas the *jñānendriya* (senses of perception), mind and intelligence are drawn inwards. This passive observation is *pratyāhāra*.

Pratyāhāra also means the freeing of the senses by not supplying nourishment to them in the form of desires and their satisfaction. Hence, *pratyāhāra* takes the ethical principles of *yama* and *niyama* directly and instantly to heart.

In order to understand *pratyāhāra*, one has to examine the principles of creation. The seer *(puruṣa)* and nature *(prakṛti)* working together stir the world into activity.

Table n. 1 – The twenty-six *tattva*

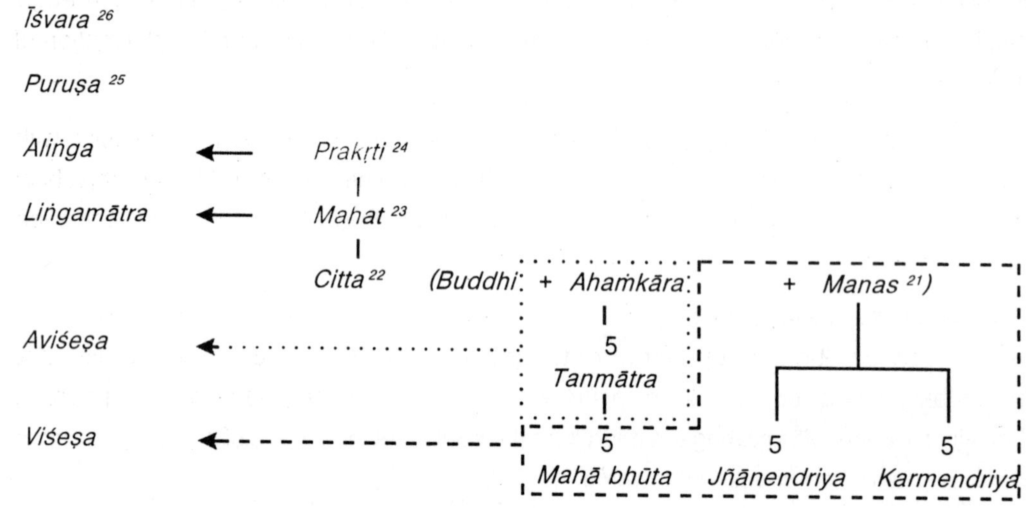

Yoga philosophy counts *ahaṁkāra* as 22nd and *buddhi-citta-mahat* as 23rd

Prakṛti consists of five gross elements with their five subtle counterparts. These ten merge with the three qualities of nature known as *guṇa*. The *guṇa* are luminosity *(sattva)*, vibrancy *(rajas)* and inertia or dormancy *(tamas)*. Then there is cosmic intelligence *(mahat)*. This cosmic intelligence has its individual counterpart in *citta*, which is divided into ego *(ahaṁkāra)*, individual intelligence *(buddhi)* and mind *(manas)*. These three form consciousness *(citta)* as the individual counterpart of cosmic intelligence *(mahat)*. *Mahat* is the primary germ of nature or the productive impulse from which all phenomena of the material world develop, including the five senses of perception and five organs of action. These are the twenty-four basic elements of which the universe is composed, according to *sāṁkhya* philosophy. *Puruṣa* is the twenty-fifth and God the twenty-sixth *tattva*[1]. (See Table n. 1).

The mind, the intelligence and the memory are encased in the brain. The five senses of perception come in contact with odour, taste, form, sound and touch and send their impressions to the mind. Through the mind, the impressions are stored in the well of memory. It is memory which longs for further experiences and ignites the mind, which in turn by-passes the intelligence and directly stimulates the senses to look for further gratification. The now hungry sensual memory triggers the mind, galvanising the organs of action to hunt for further experiences. Throughout this process, the intelligence tries to measure the advantages and disadvantages so that it may balance the memory, mind and senses of perception. They do not heed the intelligence, but with the past taste of pleasure, they thirst for more and more. Thus demands and desires augment. Weakened by this vicious addictive cycle, craving continues through past impressions and conditioned responses, but satisfaction is elusive. This brings a harvest of unhappiness. Here *pratyāhāra* enters as a true friend to rescue the unhappy *sādhaka* so that he may find happiness in the delight of the Self.

The mind, which until now had by-passed the intelligence, approaches it for guidance. Then the intelligence, with its discriminative faculty, weighs right and wrong and guides the mind not to depend completely on memory. This weighing of intelligence is *pratyāhāra*. Here, the intelligence guides the mind to swim in a right direction. *Pratyāhāra* is, a transitional state from the external to the internal quest (from *bahiraṅga sādhanā* to *antaraṅga sādhanā)*, as the senses and mind commence a return journey with the help of intelligence, towards their origin. Here detachment from the objects of the world and attachment towards the Self begins. The mind gets subdued and made to rest in the heart of the conscience *(dharmendriya)*, and the impulsive nature ends for the intuitive insight to shine. This is the real function of *pratyāhāra*.

It has been mentioned before that through perfection in *prāṇāyāma*, the clouds covering the intelligence are removed, allowing the intelligence to shine brilliantly. Due to this brilliance, the mind becomes a fit instrument for *dhāraṇā* and *dhyāna* to experience the realisation of the Self.

---

[1] Extracts from *Light on the Yoga Sūtras of Patañjali*. Courtesy Harper Collins, London. pp. 124-125.

Pratyāhāra can easily be divided into three stages as physical, intellectual and spiritual. Withdrawing the energies of the organs of action *(karmendriya)* and senses of perception *(jñānendriya)* towards the brain is physical *pratyāhāra*. Quietening the fluctuations in the four lobes of the brain and drawing the intelligence towards the stem of the brain is intellectual *pratyāhāra*. Lastly, directing the energies of intelligence and consciousness towards the seat of conscience *(dharmendriya)* in the heart is spiritual *pratyāhāra*. Thus, the journey begins from *karmendriya* and *jñānendriya*, terminates at *dharmendriya* and culminates in the vision of the seer *(ātmaṣākṣātkāra)*.

By *yama*, one develops the art of living honestly in society. By *niyama*, one cleanses one's personal impurities and purges ambition. Through *āsana*, one eliminates all physical, physiological and psychological impediments which come in the way of serenity, while *prāṇāyāma* maintains a harmonious flow of undissipated vital energy making the mind a fit instrument to go in search of the Self. *Pratyāhāra* sublimates one's senses, mind and intellect and acts as the pillar of *dhāraṇā, dhyāna* and *samādhi* for the *sādhaka* to reach the elixir of divinity in life.

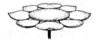

DHĀRAṆĀ

Dhāraṇā is the practice of keeping alive the mind, intelligence and consciousness in a single state of attention and recalling that intense state of attention when they get distracted.

Let us see what Patañjali says about *dhāraṇā*: *Deśa bandhaḥ cittasya dhāraṇā* (*Y.S.*, III.1). *Dhāraṇā* is a focus of attention on a particular point, region or place within the body or outside of it.

Hence *dhāraṇā* is only possible when intelligence *(buddhi)* is directed in an unshakeable, persistent state of attention to an object or a subject. When desires diminish *(vāsanakṣaya)*, the true state of being is experienced *(tattvajñāna)*. To have the knowledge of the first principle, the soul, is *tattvajñāna*. *Tattva* means principle. *Jñāna* means knowledge.

To acquire this *tattvajñāna*, cultivation of one's ethical, physical, physiological, mental and intellectual aspects is obligatory.

All over the world people think that *dhyāna* is the simplest part of the stipulated eight-fold path of Patañjali's yoga. It has even been labelled as *dhyāna* yoga.

It is unfortunate that those who are well-acquainted with the *Yoga Sūtra* of Patañjali claim that *dhyāna* is a separate yoga, when in fact it is a stage in Patañjali's yoga. *Dhyāna* is nothing but one of the petals of *Aṣṭadaḷa Yogamālā*.

Most of us mistake *dhāraṇā* for *dhyāṇa*. Patañjali says that the holding of the *citta* (consciousness) on a single-focus of attention and recapturing that intensity of attention when distracted is *dhāraṇā* and not *dhyāna*. In *dhāraṇā*, the attention has a focal point whereas in *dhyāna*, it has no point. Here the centrifugal attention and centripetal attention unite and run uninterruptedly as a single unit.

Therefore, in order to reach *dhyāna*, the *sādhaka* has to undergo practices from *yama* to *dhāraṇā* so that he earns the *jñāna* needed for *dhyāna*. When that *jñāna* (knowledge) of the highest order is acquired, *dhyāna* begins.

If *dhāraṇā* helps to eliminate desire *(vāsanakṣaya), dhyāna* quietens and humbles *ahaṁkāra.* It destroys the *ahaṁ* – 'I'-ness *(ahaṁnāśa)* and by *samādhi* one acquires the true state of being *(tattvajñāna).*

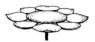

ŚUDDHI – A NEED FOR *DHYĀNA*

WHAT IS *DHYĀNA?*

Today, *dhyāna* or meditation centres and international meditation clubs are springing up like mushrooms. When I began yoga in 1934, teachers and masters would go wild if we asked about meditation.

They used to say, "First cleanse the body, speech and mind before asking for *dhyāna*". Now, we hear a lot about meditation and instant meditation, but nothing about cleanliness in word, thought and deed *(trikaraṇa śuddhi)*.

Modern thinking is filled with intellectual competition. Each one tries to reach the highest position by hook or by crook without measuring the ripeness of his own intelligence and proper understanding. This competition for position, whether it is in profession, business, science, art or in researching God is alarmingly filled with ambition.

This ambition to reap the best through short cuts has created a vacuum between one's body, nerves and mind, bringing nervous breakdown, mental depression, dejection, fear, anxiety, breathlessness, tremors in the body, and lack of confidence even to survive and live.

People afflicted in this way are searching to gain back confidence and peace and this might have been the cause for the meditation clubs to spring up everywhere.

Sage Patañjali deals with *dhyāna* as the penultimate stage in yoga whereas today we speak of *dhyāna* as an autonomous and self-sufficient practice, that can be done without following any of the basic principles of yoga namely, ethical, physical, physiological, mental and intellectual disciplines.

The very fact that Patañjali considered *dhyāna* as the penultimate stage in the path of yoga means that it must be the subtlest and the most difficult stage in which to acquire proficiency. Therefore the claim that *dhyāna* is simple is a fallacy. If so, then Patañjali must have erred in placing it where he did. He defines *dhyāna* as *ekatānatā dhyānam*. *Ekatānatā* means a single flow of uninterrupted thought where the object of attention and the power of the subject become one, losing their respective identities.

Patañjali advocates eight petals of yoga to purify the body and mind for attaining *viveka khyāti* (discriminative intelligence). The first five petals of yoga; *yama, niyama, āsana, prāṇāyāma* and *pratyāhāra* are elaborated in the second chapter, *Sādhana Pāda*. The other three petals, *dhāraṇā, dhyāna* and *samādhi*, are dealt with in the third chapter, *Vibhūti Pāda* (the chapter on attainments). Here it is to be emphasised that *dhyāna* is a natural culmination of the *sādhanā* that leads the *sādhaka* towards *samādhi*. *Samādhi* is a yoga *siddhi* or the spiritual wealth of yoga, the last petal of *aṣṭadaḷa yoga*.

Yama – ahiṁsā, satya, asteya, brahmacarya and *aparigraha* – brings about purification in the organs of action *(karmendriya śuddhi)*. *Niyama – śauca, santoṣa, tapas, svādhyāya* and *Īśvara praṇidhāna* – leads to purification of the senses of perception *(jñānendriya śuddhi)*. *Āsana* brings about purification of muscles, nerves, joints, tendons and ligaments of the body *(śarīra śuddhi)*. With *prāṇāyāma* the life-force or vital energy is purified *(prāṇa śuddhi)* and made to circulate evenly in the body. With *pratyāhāra*, the mind is withdrawn from the senses, which are attracted towards objects. This leads the *sādhaka* towards the purification of the mind *(antarendriya śuddhi)*.

Dhāraṇā is focussing or concentrating on a single point and it purifies the *buddhi* (the intelligence). *Dhāraṇā* should not be mistaken for *dhyāna*. If *dhāraṇā* has a linear flow of attention, *dhyāna* has both centripetal and centrifugal attention. *Dhāraṇā* is done to develop intelligence or *jñāna*. *Dhyāna* is done to reach the height of *jñāna*. Know that *dhyāna* without *jñāna* is no *dhyāna*.. As far as I know and understand, *dhyāna* cannot be taught. It is not an expressive subject but an individual experiential feeling where the consciousness of the *sādhaka* is diffused evenly within and without. Without seamless attention, signs of division arise.

Resolution of mind comes through *pratyāhāra; dhāraṇā* matures the intelligence so that it falls like a ripe fruit out of a tree; and *dhyāna* dissolves *ahaṁkāra* and brings humility or *vinaya* to set in permanently. This dissolution of *ahaṁkāra* is called *ahaṁ nāśa*. The three facets of consciousness, *manas, buddhi* and *ahaṁkāra*, drop away like withering leaves, and *citta* then automatically loses its identity. The loss of identity in *citta* is the resurrection of the *ātman*. This is the true meaning of *dhyāna*.

Peace of mind can be easily obtained through the layers of the other yogic petals, specifically *āsana* and *prāṇāyāma*. Hence for me, *dhyāna* is not meant merely for peace but for emancipation.

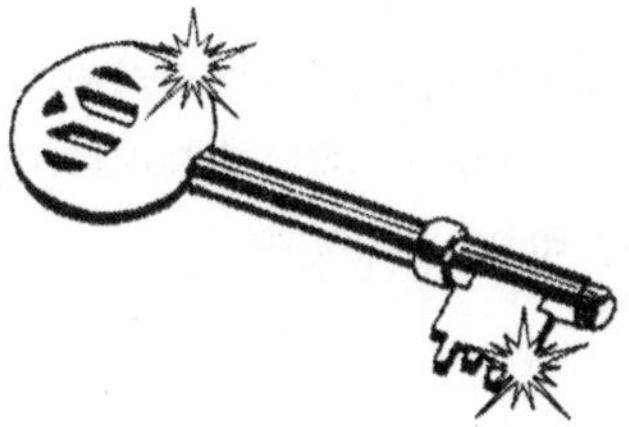

Dhyāna is a golden key to open the golden lock of the 'I'less or egoless state *(anahaṁkāra)* so that the *ātman* may emerge and spread throughout consciousness, intelligence, mind, senses of perception, organs of action and body evenly and with virtue.

IDEAL OF MAN

Man must touch the spiritual height or the sheath of bliss *(ānandamaya kośa)* at some time, for "man does not live by bread alone" *(annamaya kośa)*. Meditation is in vogue. There is a scramble for seats on the "meditation bus" but the trip to "transcendence" should not take more than five minutes. The art of meditation has been encapsulated and sugar-coated. Meditation may even be induced by drugs. An LSD or marijuana trip is supposed to give a realisation of the sublime self like that of Lord Buddha. One can easily ponder over this. Even Lord Buddha took years to reach this state. If a journey to outer space demands years of rigorous training and discipline, then it should be clear that a trip to transcendence is not that easy. The demands of meditation properly performed are more exacting than the discipline needed by the astronaut.

FIRST RESPECT

Meditation must first begin with the body, the vehicle of the Self, controlling its desires. If desire is not controlled, then true meditation is not easy. The wise people in ancient times knew this, but modern philosophers ignore the body. The body cannot be ignored because it encloses the Self. The body has to be attended to in order to attend to the Self. A mosquito bite, a stomach ache, a runny nose, is enough to wake us up to the importance of a healthy body. As far as I know, a dull body begets a dull mind and a distracted body, a distracted mind. It is easy to assert that one can meditate in the heart of Piccadilly Circus (a famous landmark in London), but has one ever tried to still the Piccadilly Circus of one's own body, nerves and emotions? The classic yoga texts proclaim that meditative wisdom begins not with the esoteric, but with the real needs of an average person. Choose a place free of insects, noise, bad smells and spread a rug and sit on it. The best time is before sunrise or after sunset, or at early dawn and late evening, when there is less dust and the Spirit of God broods over the earth like a healing benediction.

Meditation begins with the body. The correct positioning of the body with the awareness of wisdom sprouting in it from various *āsana* is itself meditation. It is like the opening of millions of intellectual eyes. The mind impregnates the body as an observer and the body becomes like the mind remaining supremely alert. Here, mind and matter are fused in the dynamism of sheer energy, active without being spent, reactive without bringing exhaustion.

IMPORTANCE OF *ĀSANA* IN *DHYĀNA*

Āsana is to be considered important, because it strengthens the nerves, lungs and other parts of the body for their role in forming a firm foundation for meditation. They are all the vehicles of meditative action.

The classical meditative pose that we find depicted even in the ruins of Mohenjo Daro is the cross-legged *Padmāsana* with the spine held straight and firm. When the ancients counselled: Sit in any comfortable position with spine straight, they certainly did not mean that slouching would do. Sitting in a loose, collapsed sort of way induces drowsiness or sleep, which should not be mistaken for meditation. Meditation does not make the mind dull, but razor sharp, vibrant, yet still and silent. This state cannot be achieved without a firm stable sitting posture, where the energy of the spine ascends and the intelligence of the brain descends and dissolves in the seat of conscience (the heart), where the true Self reveals itself. The whole body, far from being ignored, takes on this spiritual alertness, until the whole person becomes pure flame. An alert, erect spine creates a spiritual intensity of concentration that burns out distracting thoughts and the brooding over past and future, and leaves one in the virginal, pristine present.

In *dhyāna* or pure meditation, the eyes are shut, the head held erect and the gaze directed downwards and backwards as though the parallel gaze of the eyes is searching the infinity that lies behind and beyond the back of the head. Then the facial skin is relaxed and made to descend. The eyes, the ears and the root of the tongue are pacified and quiet so that the brain releases from their contact. The hands are pressed together, palm against palm in front of the chest.

SURRENDERING ONESELF

This classic pose of *dhyāna* is not only symbolic but also practical. Symbolically, the palms salute the Lord and the mind is drawn to surrender to the Holy One who is within. This surrender breaks the chain of distracting thoughts and increases the intensity of one's concentration. Practically speaking, the hands are locked by the magnetism of the human body. The increase or decrease of pressure on the palm is a sensitive gauge of one's alertness and one's freedom from distracting thoughts. The exact balance of electric current of the body can also be tested by the palms pressed against each other. If both the palms press equally against each other, then both mind and body are said to be in balance and harmony. If one palm exerts pressure more than the other does, that side of the body is more alert. By increasing the pressure of the weaker palm, a delicate adjustment is made to bring the body/mind unit back to balance. Without perfect harmony between the body, mind and intelligence, meditation becomes impossible.

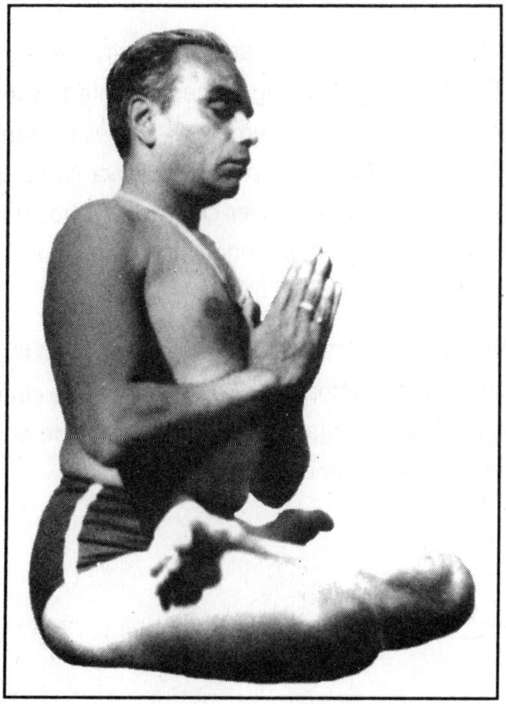

Plate n. 7 – *Dhyāna*

Many people think that yogic meditation is without content, a mere emptying of the mind. For those who have had the experience of its richness and satisfying fullness, such an assertion can only sound ridiculous. The intelligence of the mind may cease its roving but the intelligence of the heart goes out to the Lord. And in *dhyāna* it is the heart that matters. Is there really any need of the petty content of our own thoughts, when the heart is drawn to the Infinite One who is always near and ever receding, immanent and transcendent at the same time?

WITHDRAWING THE SENSES

Prāṇāyāmic breathing techniques are meditative in their origin and in their effect. Basically they consist of breath inhalation, breath retention and breath exhalation. Their rhythmic movement stills the mind, draws in the senses and helps one uncover the depth of the Self. Unlike in *dhyāna*, the head in *prāṇāyāma* is brought down to the chest with a firm chin lock *(Jālandhara Bandha* – Plate n. 20). Physically the chin lock relieves the strain on the heart. Mentally the chin lock releases the breath from the egotistical domination of the brain and makes it more gentle and impersonal. The chin lock takes one to the quiet centre of the heart where the Lord resides. But the other basic aspects of meditation such as the gaze of the eyes and the erect spine are maintained.

The techniques of *āsana* and *prāṇāyāma* are the vehicles of meditation and prayer. Inhalation *(pūraka)* is acceptance of the Lord, its retention *(kuṁbhaka)* is savouring the Lord in the full deep stillness of the self. Exhalation *(recaka)* is not simply the exhalation of breath, but it is the emptying of 'I' or the ego. Exhalation makes one impersonal and hence it is not only a fit instrument for the *sādhaka*, but the highest form of surrender to the Lord.

ŚUDDHI ŚAKTI **(CLEANSING POWERS)**

Exhalation is a cleansing process. As the breath is gently exhaled towards the heart, the heart is freed of desires and emotional disturbances. This cooling, cleansing process initiated by the lungs can be compared to *abhiṣeka* performed each morning in the temples. *Abhiṣeka* means the purificatory ablution of the idols. As the waters of the Ganga drip on the *Shiva liṅga*, so exhalation flows over the life-giving *liṅga (ātman)* within, keeping it ever clean and pure. This surrender to the Lord has to be accepted and so there is a period of silence after exhalation for the Lord to accept this surrender before inhalation begins.

Meditation is a subjective experience. No amount of description equals the delight that the first bite of the delicious mango fruit gives. Sure and safe techniques can be given, the state of the mind can be described, but the savour of the fruit is only granted to those who "taste and see that the Lord is sweet." So, one can savour *dhyāna*, but one cannot explain it.

DHYĀNA – SPARK OF DIVINITY

What is the essence of a man? Take away his education, wealth, status, emotion, intellect or achievements, and what remains is the essence, the spark of divinity, the Self within him.

Observation, reflection and absorption upon the essence of man is *dhyāna* (meditation). The search to trace that essence demands a high degree of discipline.

Sage Patañjali describes *dhyāna* as the subtlest discipline of yoga. Without the establishment of firm foundations laid down in the earlier six aspects of yoga, it is well nigh impossible to practise meditation.

The first stage, *yama* – the universal moral commandments of non-violence, truth, continence and seeing divinity in all, non-stealing and non-covetousness – provides a firm base for the edifice of yogic discipline. The practice of the second stage, *niyama,* is composed of the five personal disciplines: self-purification by cleanliness in thought, word, deed and means of livelihood and contentment, austerity, study of the spiritual texts and surrender of all of one's actions to the Lord. They calm the mind and lead to undisturbed peace within and around him. The practice of *āsana* makes the body a strong and fit vehicle for the spiritual quest. The *sādhaka* attains steadiness and stillness by practising *āsana* before moving on to *prāṇāyāma,* the rhythmic breathing techniques. Here, the *sādhaka* consciously prolongs inhalation, retention and exhalation of breath. In inhalation he receives the Lord in the form of breath. In retention, he savours Him. In exhalation, he surrenders his emotions and thoughts to the source of all energy – the Creator. Thus, *prāṇāyāma* is the cleansing of desires and emotional disturbances. It develops clarity of mind and sound judgement along with much will power. Then the practitioner becomes ready for *pratyāhāra* or quietening the senses and drawing them inwards, leading him to the divinity within himself. Finally he becomes fit for the practice of *dhāraṇā.* He remains unruffled under all circumstances and focusses the attention with awareness on a single point.

When the single pointed attention continues for a long time, it develops into *dhyāna* or meditation. Like a flower ripening into fruit, *dhyāna* matures into *samādhi.* When *dhyāna* remains uninterrupted, it merges into *samādhi*, where the *sādhaka* reaches the goal of his quest. He loses his identity in the object of his meditation, like the river losing its identity when it joins the ocean.

As dullness of the body leads to dullness of the mind, and its distractions bring about a distracted mind, meditation begins with the disciplining of the body. It is even possible to practise meditation when one is in an *āsana* with total awareness, as one regards each and every limb of the self as a part of the Self. So one works to maintain proper tension and balance. Then one becomes a living embodiment of the *āsana*, because all faculties, the body, mind and intelligence, are brought into focus over the entire range of oneself.

The practice of meditation requires complete alertness and consciousness. The mind of the practitioner is cleansed of negative and disturbing emotions like hatred and passion. The *sādhaka* conquers delusion and greed with no room for pride and envy. He comes face to face with the things he fears and remains unshaken. He frees himself from the bonds of pain and sorrow and liberates himself from the tyranny of his senses and the satisfying of their desires. Being freed from emotional disturbances and distractions, his mind and intelligence become still and sharp, silent and serene. This illumined state becomes the guiding beacon of light for others.

Meditation is the harmonious blending of the emotions and intellect. It is the secret of all creative processes of men of genius and it is the fountain or source of works of literature and art.

Meditation should be practised in an appropriate place. The best time is before sunrise or after sunset when the balm of peace is spread over the earth. The posture for meditation is equally important. It should create an intensity for concentration and at the same time be steady and comfortable. An alert spine keeps the body attentive and drives out not only dullness of the mind, but also eliminates the brooding thoughts of the past or the future.

What does one meditate upon? Here, guidance is provided by the study of eternal principles enshrined in the spiritual and sacred books of the world. By uninterrupted and devoted study of these principles for a long time, the aspirant puts them into practice in his daily life until they enter into his blood stream and merge into his thoughts, words and deeds.

To provide the aspirant with guidelines for meditation, the sages devised the symbol *AUṀ* for focal attention. This mighty *Sanskṛt* syllable, like the Latin word "omne", signifies the concepts of omniscience, omnipresence and omnipotence. The symbol consists of three letters, *A*, *U* and *Ṁ*. When the symbol is written in *Sanskṛt*, it displays a crescent and a dot on its top (ॐ). This best of prayers has been given various interpretations. The letters symbolise speech, mind and breath, and the entire symbol represents the individual self or the living self *(jīvātman)*, which is a part of the Divine Self *(Paramātman)*. They signify the three states of deep sleep, dream and full consciousness of the mind, reason and self; the entire symbol stands for the fourth state *(turīyā avasthā)*. In the realm of gender, the triad of letters symbolises the masculine, the feminine and the neuter, while the entire symbol stands for the Creator, who is beyond the confines of gender. In the form of the Lord, the symbol is worshipped as Brahmā, the Generator, Vishnu, the Protector and Rudra the Destroyer. It synthesises all the forces of matter and of life. The letters represent the phases of time – past, present and future. The entire symbol stands for the Creator, who is beyond the pale of time.

By constant focussing of his intelligence and energy upon the sacred syllable, the practitioner illumines the hidden divinity within himself. He feels the existence of the Lord everywhere. Wherever he turns, he hears the voice of the Lord from all quarters. His mind becomes still, untouched by whatever life has to offer him. His own voice is serene for the peace that he has attained is unutterable in words. From the status of a *sādhaka*, he has now evolved into a *siddha* (a seer of great purity) whose experience and wisdom has made him a mirror of his life. He is now a *jñānin* and a *dhyānin*.

SAṀYAMA

Patañjali has coined a special word, *saṁyama,* for the union of *dhāraṇā, dhyāna* and *samādhi.* *Saṁyama* means total integration. It comes as the effect or as the fruition of the *sādhanā* known as the internal quest *(antaraṅga sādhanā)* which enriches the consciousness in such a way that it moves towards the innermost being – the Self. It is a journey from *antaraṅga* to *antarātma sādhanā.*

Dhāraṇā means attention or concentration. It is a way of controlling the fluctuations of consciousness and of focussing attention on a particular chosen path, region, spot or place within or outside the body. In *dhāraṇā,* one learns to decrease the fluctuations gradually. One ultimately eliminates all waves or tides of consciousness so that, in *dhyāna,* the knower and the known, or the subject and object, become one.

When the consciousness maintains this attention from the beginning to the end in an unbroken line, without altering or wavering in the intensity of awareness, then one is in *dhyāna.*

When oil is poured from one vessel into another, it maintains a constant, steady and even flow. Likewise, the flow of attention and awareness should remain stable and constant. This steady awareness is *dhyāna.*

Dhyāna is the way of discovering the everlasting Self. It is the art of self-study, observation, reflection and the vision to see the infinite hidden within. It begins with the observation of the physical process, watchfulness of the mental state and then blending of the intelligence of the head with that of the heart and delving deep into profound contemplation. By this profound contemplation, the consciousness merges with the object of meditation and dissolves into the object. The subject, namely the meditator, loses his identity in the object. This conjunction of the subject and object makes the complex consciousness become simple, but with spiritual illumination. Arrogance, pride and ego get transformed and transfigured towards humility and innocence, leading one towards *samādhi.*

In *samādhi,* both the soul and the goal lose their identities. The seer, the seen and the seeing dissolve, and the *sādhaka* is beyond himself. He loses the awareness of time and place.

SAMĀDHI*

Samādhi is seeing the soul face to face. The purity of intelligence equals the purity of the soul. The pure illuminative consciousness shines in a similar fashion to the ever luminous soul.

Samādhi is the feeling of existing in a state of complete peace within and without and oneness with the universe and the Creator of the universe. Here the ego is annihilated. One loses the awareness of 'I'-consciousness, mind, breath or movement. What remains is Infinite Peace and Joy *(sānanda)*. This experience of Infinite Peace and Joy is the last stage in yoga, where the self becomes a fit instrument for God realisation.

Like any other artist, the yogi is creative within himself, but the experience of new creation takes him to the state where neither does time bind him, nor cause or effect touch him. His shedding of the 'I'-consciousness is at the same time an expression of a state of oneness and the awareness of an integrated personality. In him wisdom shines forth, combined with humility and simplicity. Such a person shines like the sun, which is not impeded by barriers or limitations. Not only is he illumined, but he illumines all who come to him in search of truth.

If by the grace of God, a man born blind is granted for a moment to have a glimpse of the beauty and grandeur of the world, who would be able to measure his ecstasy? In the same way, a glimpse of the Divine is worth all the pain and hard work implied in the practice of yoga.

The principles of yoga, namely, *yama* and *niyama* build up the character needed for restraint of unsocial as well as unethical practices; *āsana* builds up the potency needed fearlessly to face spiritual illumination, while *prāṇāyāma* builds up vital energy to receive that spiritual light. *Pratyāhāra* develops steadiness in the *citta* so that in *dhāraṇā*, the *citta* is made to focus on a given point or a given thought.

---

* From *Yoga News*, no. 2, March 1992.

Dhyāna is a continuous process of *dhāraṇā* for the intelligence to reach the pinnacle of *prajñāna*, while *prajñāna* automatically withdraws the veil or the screen of *ahaṁkāra*, diminishing it permanently, in order that we may experience unalloyed emancipated bliss *(turīyā avasthā)*, a state that is beyond *tamas*, *rajas* and *sattva*.

Samādhi is the process of tracing the source of consciousness. It is total absorption in profound meditation. Through the discipline of yoga, both actions and intelligence go beyond the above qualities.

The intelligence becomes pure, luminous crystal clear, and free from the attributes of nature.

The word *samādhi* is made up of two components. *Sama* means virtuous. *Ādhi* means over and above. The intelligence which has become virtuous is over and above the attributes of nature. In this state of *samādhi* the pure, virtuous, luminous and virgin-like intelligence faces the pure Soul. This state of purity is *samādhi*. Yoga is thus both the means and the goal. Yoga is *samādhi* and *samādhi* is yoga.

The yogi, in *samādhi*, experiences the fullness explained in the *Upaniṣads:*

"Pūrṇam adaḥ Pūrṇam idam Pūrṇāt Pūrṇam udacyate
Pūrṇasya Pūrṇamādāya Pūrṇamevāvaśiṣyate.[1] "

"That is full; This is full; Fullness comes out of Fullness. Even after fullness is taken from the Fullness, Fullness alone remains".

This is *samādhi* - the culmination of yoga, which brings the culmination for the search of the soul.

1 *Īśa Upaniṣad,* Introductory invocation.

SECTION II

HAṬHA YOGA

IS *HAṬHA YOGA* A MERE BODY CULT?*

There is a lot of misunderstanding of recent origin, in the minds of a great many people that *haṭha yoga* is purely a physical form of yoga and that *rāja yoga*, mainly a spiritual form of yoga. This has created a hierarchy that is very unfortunate as it does not serve the cause of yoga.

HAṬHA YOGA AND *RĀJA YOGA*

Ha stands for the positive current and *ṭha* for the negative current. They also stand for *prāṇa* and *prajñā*. The union of these two currents creates a dynamic and buoyant life.

Ha and *ṭha* also stand for the right and left sides of the body. The balance and union of these two sides is *haṭha yoga*. It also means the union of body with mind and mind with body. As *haṭha* together means volition or willpower, *haṭha yoga* means "the science of the will".

Rāja yoga has been defined as the science of the mind and the art of controlling it. I do not see any difference between the science of the will and the science of mind control as volition is the control of the mind. Sage Patañjali explains the eight petals of yoga in his *Yoga Sūtra*, while *Haṭha Vidyā Kārikā*[1] deal not only with these eight petals but also with *kriyā*, *mudrā* and *bandha*.

I have been practising yoga ceaselessly and assiduously for well nigh forty years, and such controversies not only pain but surprise me also, as it reveals the ignorance that people have on the subject.

I consider yoga to be one of the most refined forms of Indian philosophic art, based on an extremely subtle science, the science of the body and the mind. I look upon yoga as a wealth of wisdom, which not only shows the right way to live, but enables one to have an insight into one's innermost being. Is it not then the highest practical philosophy?

---

* Published in *Bhavan's Journal*, August 5th 1973.

[1] The texts dealing with *Haṭha vidyā*.

The misunderstandings and dispute must have arisen because many think that *haṭha vidyā* texts explain only *āsana* and *prāṇāyāma* in detail. But those who have even half read and half heard about this subject must know that the higher aims of man's life are never forgotten or overlooked but are dealt with in the texts. While Sage Patañjali emphasises that yoga is stilling, silencing and integrating the mind with the soul *(Yogaḥ cittavṛtti nirodhaḥ Y.S.,* I.2), he neither ridicules nor forgets the importance of *āsana* and *prāṇāyāma*, as it is not possible for an average aspirant to reach that state of stillness of the mind without making the body and the mind healthy and fit to experience that state.

Careful reasoning will make one realise that man is, in a certain sense, made up of three compartments: the head (the seat of knowledge or *jñāna*), heart (the seat of emotion or *bhakti*) and the hands and legs (the seat of actions or *karma*). As man is blessed with these organs, he is in a gifted position to follow all three paths.

If one desires the ultimate, pure and unalloyed *jñāna, bhakti* and *karma*, the path to follow is yoga. Yoga was invented by our sages in order to overcome bodily impediments, emotional and environmental disturbances of the mind and the wavering qualities of the intelligence, so that the practitioner comes closer and closer to the Self.

After teaching for more than thirty-eight years[1], I can definitely say that this much-despised *haṭha yoga* is the only way to approach *rāja yoga*. The culture of the body leads to the culture of the Self. As the body has its own intelligence, the consciousness too has its own intelligence. These two intelligences are harmonised through *āsana* and *prāṇāyāma* and prepare the *sādhaka* to experience the total awareness of Being.

When this state of Being can be realised, are we not consciously or unconsciously breeding the cult of the ego *(ahaṁkāra)* by branding one type of yoga as superior to the other? Are these not the confabulations of an intoxicated and egotistical intelligence? Is not labelling and proclaiming oneself a *rāja yogi* or a *jñāna yogi* an attempt to hoodwink society for one's own glorification?

I may be excused if I speak with strong feeling. For me this "physical" or *haṭha* yoga, which is laughed away and ridiculed as "gymnastics", "monkey tricks" or "kids' stuff", is my *dharma*, my religion. It has merged with my consciousness. Listen to what Lord Krishna says in the *Bhagavad Gītā:*

---

[1] The Author has now been teaching for sixty-five years

"Better is one's own *dharma* though imperfectly carried out than the *dharma* of another carried out perfectly. Better is death in the fulfilment of one's own *dharma*, for to follow another's *dharma* is perilous." (*B.G.*, III.35).

PRAJÑĀ

I will never waver nor turn away from yoga *sādhanā*, for it has opened the gates of *prajñā* for me. There are several states of *prajñāna:*

Table n. 2 – *Prajñā śreṇi* – ranges of *prajñā*

1. *Śarīra prajñā*	awareness and wisdom of the body
2. *Prāṇamaya prajñā*	awareness of the functioning of the physiological body, or the organic or vital body
3. *Mānasika prajñā*	understanding the intelligence of the mind
4. *Naitika prajñā*	ethical awareness
5. *Ānubhavika prajñā*	experienced awareness through direct cognition
6. *Rasātmaka prajñā*	fragrance or essence that is relished from that experienced awareness
7. *Ātmika prajñā*	awareness arising from the insight of one's being

For me, yogic discipline is meant to purge the ego, not to foster it. This ego is to be merged into the seat of consciousness within the Self. Yoga, therefore, is an art that enables one to be humble within oneself. It is the royal path to *ātma-sādhanā* – the path to spiritual tranquillity.

We are all aware that owing to felt and hidden pain, the mind, the brain and the consciousness are trapped in the body and are not free from its shackles. *Haṭha yoga* relieves the felt and the hidden pains, thereby freeing the mind from the clutches of the body. The mind thus freed is able to follow the channel to its source and to be in communion with that same source. Only in such a state does the *jīvātman* (individual soul) become a fit vehicle for God realisation.

CAKRA

There is again a feeling in the minds of many that all *haṭha vidyā* texts speak of *cakra*, whereas Sage Patañjali does not. In fact Patañjali does deal with the *cakra* in his eight-petalled path of yoga. If the *cakra* are considered as the foundation for *haṭha yoga*, then I do not hesitate to consider the *Yoga Sūtra* of Patañjali as a text on *haṭha yoga* or *kuṇḍalinī yoga*.

Patañjali explains *dhāraṇā* in a single *sūtra:* Concentration is the fixing of consciousness on one point or region *(Deśa bandhaḥ cittasya dhāraṇā, Y.S., III.1)*. While commenting on this *sūtra*, Sage Vyāsa states: "The suggested places of fixing the consciousness are: the sphere of the navel, the lotus of the heart, the light in the brain, the tip of the nose, the tip of the tongue, or any external object".

Now let me see what these places represent according to *Haṭha Yoga Kārikas:*

Table n. 3 – *Anurūpa samānatva*

Pātañjala yoga		***Haṭha Yoga Kārika***
Kūrma nāḍī	corresponds to	*Svādhiṣthāna cakra*
Nābhi cakra	"	*Maṇipūraka cakra*
Hṛdaya (puṇḍarīka)	"	*Anāhata cakra*
Kaṇṭha kūpa	"	*Viṣuddhi cakra*
Dhruva	"	*Ājñā cakra*
Mūrdha Jyoti	"	*Sahasrāra cakra*

Names may be different but the places mentioned are identical. Let me quote Patañjali:

By concentration upon the *nābhi cakra* (navel), perfect understanding of the body system dawns (*Y.S.*, III.30).

Concentration on the *kaṇṭha kūpa (viśuddhi cakra)* leads to the conquest of hunger and thirst (*Y.S.*, III.31).

Vyāsa, in his commentary on *sūtra* III.33, states: "There is a shining light in the hole which is within the skull. On integration of consciousness comes the vision of the *siddhas* who move through the ethereal space between the earth and the sky."

Again in the commentary on *sūtra* III.35, sage Vyāsa says that "the intelligence lives in that hollow which is the shrine in the form of a lotus within the city of Brahma. From *saṁyama* (integration) thereupon comes the knowledge of the mind".

SĀDHANĀ AGNI

A discriminating person realises that as long as the body and the senses experience joy, the state of tranquillity that may have been attained is essentially the tranquillity of the senses. To acquire skill and efficiency in yoga, one should not be content with this form of tranquillity. One has to go further.

The real *sādhanā* commences only when the individual self, realising the deceptive nature of this "tranquillity", commands the body and the mind to go beyond the realm of this quiet state in pursuit of the ultimate goal. The spiritual *sādhanā* begins at this point. Here the aspirant has to set about *tapas* (burning desire or zeal) with an energy that requires immense attention and hard work. Here the aspirant needs not one per cent inspiration, but 100 per cent inspiration and 100 per cent perspiration. He has to be ever watchful, moment to moment, not allowing himself to relax even for a single moment. Like a swift, ever-moving fish, his mind is ever alert, wide open and pliant, following the indications of the skill that accrue from the daily practice of yoga *sādhanā*.

In each movement of an *āsana* and in each breath of *prāṇāyāma,* the vehicles of the body such as the spine, the fibres, the membranes, the nerves, and the skin, should be steady, sharp, mobile, swift, alert and alive with total emotional poise and intellectual silence. In *āsana* the eyes are kept alert, the body as an instrument of action and the brain as the observant receiver. In *prāṇāyāma* the ears are active, receptive and observant and the eyes are kept entirely passive. In *dhyāna* (meditation) the intelligence directly acts in creating silence by arresting the inner oscillating movements of the mind.

When the body loses its alertness, the mind relapses into a state of brooding. If the body is kept fit and sharp, the intelligence remains fresh, quick and sensitive. Its sensitivity then becomes so refined that it might be compared to the fine tip of a leaf that sways to the slightest movement of the breeze. It is then that the yogi can enrich his *jñāna* and steadily retain the potentiality of the intellect. Whenever the body droops or loses its correct posture, a very gentle and graceful adjustment is required, not a sharp, violent jerk. Such a harsh movement would excite and disturb the ethics of the body and the mind.

While doing *āsana, prāṇāyāma* or *dhyāna*, one must constantly endeavour to weave the three flames: *darśanāgni* (intelligent flame of the eyes), *jñānāgni* (flame of wisdom) and *ātmāgni* (flame of the soul) into one's being. When *sādhanāgni* lights these three flames, only then do body and mind lose their identities and merge into Being. Though an inadequate description, this state can at best be compared to a piece of burning camphor and its flame, where one cannot distinguish one from the other. Or it can be compared to a glass of water, in which some sugar or salt has dissolved. Whether one tastes the water from the top, middle or bottom of the glass, the water tastes the same. This is the all-pervading state of being.

Vijñānabhikṣu (1525-1580), the commentator on Patañjali, calls this state *samāhita citta* (a state of equilibrium of the body, the mind and the self). In the *Bhagavad Gītā,* Lord Krishna terms it as *sthitha prajñā* (stable intelligence and firm establishment in wisdom).

When people speak with contempt on this branch of yoga, which is so noble, as mere physical yoga, the words of the *Bhagavad Gītā* again come to my mind:

"These acts do not bind me, Dhanamjaya, for I am sitting as if indifferent, unattached in those actions." (*B.G.,* IV.14).

The judge dispassionately gives his judgement and remains unattached and unaffected by the feelings of the parties concerned. Similarly, the Lord is indifferent and unattached to creation and destruction. Through my relentless practices, what *haṭha yoga* has given to me is that I prefer to remain indifferent to the sneers of intellectual gymnasts. My advice to those who tread this path is to ignore such remarks and follow the advice that Lord Krishna gave to Arjuna.

In conclusion I would say that the spiritual climax of the tree is the flavour of its juicy fruit, so the ultimate goal of an aspirant is to transform the body to the level of the soul which is its natural culmination. Yoga is thus a highly developed knowledge – a fount of the nectar of spiritual life.

Should we reduce this noble gift of our ancient sages to a wrangle over words and brands? This rare heritage of man surely deserves a better fate than those petty bickerings, strife and divisions!

Yoga stands for unity, making the body the temple of the self, a worthy place for the soul to dwell in. Only then is one made holy and pure. Thus yoga can be yoga only. It is neither *haṭha* nor *rāja.* It is one and the same.

HAṬHA YOGA AND *RĀJA YOGA**

I am grateful to Bharatiya Vidya Bhavan and to my pupils who have made it possible for me to stand in front of you all; it is a unique opportunity for me to address people I have not met before.

I would like to say a few words before the demonstration of my pupils, so that you get an idea of this ancient art. Let me pray to Lord Patañjali, author of the *Yoga Sūtra*, and Svātmārāma, author of *Haṭhayoga Pradīpikā*, who have shown the path of yoga to mankind.

I was of course a performing artist in yoga and some of you may have seen my demonstrations. Now that tapes and videos of demonstrations are available, you can easily tell how much interest I have created in this dry subject through my performances. Now my time is running out, hence my pupils have to learn to present yoga in an interesting and illuminating way. Yoga is fundamentally an art, which ultimately evolves into a real spiritual performing art.

I want to clarify a great confusion, which is particularly prevalent in this part of the world, that *haṭha yoga* is physical yoga. This wrong notion has now reached the East, through books by Western authors, so that the East has also begun to differentiate between *pātañjala yoga* and *haṭha yoga* as two distinct types of yoga. I want to impress upon you that this is due to a misunderstanding, so I must clarify this misconception so that you understand and realise the truth about yoga.

Patañjali begins his yoga aphorisms with *Yogaḥ cittavṛtti nirodhaḥ* (*Y.S.*, I.2). He speaks not of mind but of consciousness, which is the product of the Self. As the mind emerges from consciousness, so does the consciousness from the Self. The mind is pure and single at its source. It is known as the core of being, *ātman*. When it sprouts into a seedling, it becomes the self-conscious centre. A sense of individuality sets in there. This individuality is in a pure form up to this point. It is *sāttvic*. When this seedling begins to grow and get exposed to the world of ignorance *(avidyā)*, it develops into consciousness which branches out into 'I'-ness, intelligence

* Based on a lecture at Bharatiya Vidya Bhavan, London, 29th August 1987.

and mind. Finally, these branches have leaves, flowers and fruits which are nothing but five organs of action, five senses of perception along with gross and subtle elements. The body, senses and mind form a bridge to connect us to the external world.

Vṛtti means movement. A wandering mind is a *vṛtti*: to still it, is also a *vṛtti*. So from one movement of thought you come to another movement. Restraint of these movements is yoga. Patañjali describes this restraint in the third chapter; that *nirodha* is a base to experience *ekāgra* (*eka* = one; *agra* = base) and from it you experience the core of being.

Cittavṛtti means "movements of consciousness". First Patañjali wants us to bring the wandering consciousness to a state of stillness, then to move from stillness towards the state of silence. He calls this state "the river of tranquillity" or *praśanta vāhinī* (*Y.S.*, III.10). Then from the river of tranquillity, he wants us to proceed towards *ekāgratā*, or the state of *dhāraṇā*. When this stage of *dhāraṇā* is reached, he concludes that we are able to abide in the Self.

At other times the Self gets involved with the movements of consciousness and gets caught in attachment to the needs of the consciousness.

When there are no *vṛtti* and no movements in the consciousness, the Self rests free from the influences of consciousness. In order to keep the Self free from the influences of consciousness, Patañjali speaks of *abhyāsa vairāgyābhyāṁ tannirodhaḥ* (*Y.S.*, I.11). There are only two methods to acquire *nirodha citta*. One is practice *(abhyāsa)* and the other, restraint *(vairāgya)*. From this *sūtra* you get a clue to what *haṭha yoga* stands for. *Ha* stands for sun, the Self in us. The sun or the Self, both never fade. *Ṭha*, the moon, stands for *vṛtti* or the movement of consciousness. As the moon draws the energy in the form of light from the sun and cools the earth with that reflected light, so does the consciousness draw the light from the Self and reflect on the senses, mind and body as well as the external world. When the consciousness comes in contact with external thoughts and the world, it oscillates; then the individual being oscillates. The means of controlling this oscillation is explained in *haṭha yoga*.

Ha stands for God in the form of Shiva, Vishnu and Brahmā and *puruṣa*, *ṭha* stands for their consorts Parvatī, Lakṣmī and Sarasvatī, as well as for *prakṛti*. The Godesses are there to serve the God. They are the *śakti* of God. God is served through their *śakti*. Here consort means wife in the form of *śakti*. *Prakṛti*, in the above sense, is consort of *puruṣa* (*Y.S.*, II.18 and 19). The practice of *haṭha yoga* unifies these two.

Ha and *ṭha* yet have another meaning, as *prāṇa* and *apāna*. The union of *prāṇa* (the intake of energy) with *apāna* (the output of energy) is *haṭha yoga*. If *cittavṛtti nirodha* is the main theme of *pātañjala yoga*, *prāṇavṛtti nirodha* is the main principle of *haṭha yoga*.

The movement of breath has a certain flow, whereas the mind has no defined direction of movement. The mind travels anywhere and everywhere, whereas the breath has only one route to follow. If *prāṇa* (in-breath) is an evolutionary practice, *apāna* (out-breath) is the involutionary or the renunciatory method of practice. Hence *haṭha yoga* says that by following the channel of the breath, you still the mind so that it is drawn to savour the Self.

Haṭhayoga Pradīpikā names sixteen *āsana* but explains technically twelve or thirteen, while Vyāsa names twelve or thirteen different *āsana* in his commentary on Patañjali, without explanations. For us it is interesting to note that the practice of *āsana* was current in those days.

Abhyāsa is a continuous practical effort to control and stabilise the mind. *Vairāgya* is also a continuous practice, to keep the mind away from attachments. It is not just renunciation, as it demands a very subtle discriminative intelligence. For non-attachment and renunciation one needs to bring the senses, mind and *citta* gradually under control in order to have restraint.

These principles of *abhyāsa* and *vairāgya* are dealt with both in *pātañjala yoga* and in *haṭha yoga*, so that one can reach *samādhi*. *Samādhi* means equipoise. *Sama* means harmony and balance, while *ādhi* means over and above. It stands for the core of being, which is over and above the body and consciousness. To diffuse the core of being harmoniously within its frontier (the body) is *samādhi*. It is like water, which gets diffused evenly on any surface on which it is spread, so the diffusion of the Self takes place. In this state the experience of the Self shines forth. So I say that both *haṭha yoga* and *pātañjala yoga* guide the practitioner towards spiritual growth – *ātma-darśana* (sight of the *ātman*).

Ātma-darśana is possible only when the consciousness is restrained for *ekāgratā* to take place. Many say that Patañjali made a big mistake by putting *nirodha pariṇāma* first, *samādhi pariṇāma* second and *ekāgratā pariṇāma* last[1]. It should have been reversed as *ekāgratā pariṇāma*, *samādhi pariṇāma* and *nirodha pariṇāma*. For me *nirodha* or restraint involves the *rājasic* quality as one has to struggle with the movements of consciousness. Patañjali takes us from this *rājasic* power of restraint *(nirodha)* towards tranquillity, which is of a *sāttvic* nature and from this *sāttvic* nature towards *ekāgratā* (to be one with the self).

Patañjali uses *praśānta vāhinī* in between the moments of fluctuation and restraint. Between fluctuation and restraint, there is a pause. If one extends that space, it is *samādhi*. If one can experience and feel that flow of quietness in the consciousness, then one will be able to explore the core of being. That is why Patañjali takes us from restraint to a tranquil state and

---

[1] See Author's *Light on the Yoga Sūtras of Patañjali*, p. 180, Harper Collins, London.

from a tranquil state towards *ekāgratā*. Like the word *haṭha*, *ekāgratā* too is a compound word: *eka* plus *agra* is *ekāgra*; *eka* means one, which has no polarities, and *agra* means the base. So if we analyse the word *ekāgra*, Patañjali is not wrong[1].

Patañjali also says that in order to get the diffusion of the Self, you have to learn first the art of diffusing consciousness in your system. To do this, you have to disseminate the intelligence in each and every corner. This pervasiveness is *dhyāna*. As long as you say, "I want to concentrate on this", it means that your intelligence has to be focussed on one point, but it is not diffused. For example, right now there is no sunlight coming from the window. I can see all of you only because the light is on and focussed on you. That is *dhāraṇā*. But if I open the window, break down the wall, then there will be no difference between the light inside and outside. The rays of the sun will reach evenly or uniformly everywhere. Breaking this restriction on a focal point of intelligence is *dhyāna*. Up to this state, it is possible to guide and teach. From then on, it is a subjective experiencing *sādhanā*, where one cannot involve teaching or explanation.

Today we get lots of jet-set *gurus*, travelling all over the world, making headlines in the papers. But a *guru* is a rare product in this century and will be rarer still in the twenty-first. As a result of this, we have to rely on books by authors like Patañjali as the only true guides. If anyone claims to be a *guru*, you have to test his quality. If you are to see the light, you have to commune with the teacher and work together. Both have to see the light. As the teacher demands discipline from the pupil, it is also a need of the pupil to observe the discipline from the teacher before accepting him as his *guru*. This understanding existed in the *guru-śiṣya* relation in the olden days. There was a freedom of choice along with the bonds of discipline.

Kaivalya, according to many people, is isolation of the self. Even Krishnamurti speaks of isolation, which means quarantine. You know that if you have certain diseases you are quarantined, you cannot mix with people. Is the Soul to be quarantined or *prakṛti* to be quarantined? How we misrepresent Patañjali's *Yoga Sūtra*! If we practise yoga properly, our understanding of Patañjali will never go wrong. Therefore, experience is essential.

Patañjali also has talked about *kuṇḍalinī*, the divine cosmic energy. But he uses the word *prakṛti* – nature (*Y.S.*, IV.2), and says that the energy in a perfect yogi flows abundantly. Though this energy originates in the spine, it is everywhere in the body. When this realisation dawns, the impurities in the body are removed and the search for the Self is at an end. He explains in *Kaivalya Pāda* that where there is *ātma-nivṛtti* there is no search for the Soul, showing that culmination is certain (*Y.S.*, IV.25). There is no such culmination in our external world, but

---

[1] It should be known that Patañjali is recognised for his works on grammar as well as yoga and *āyurveda*. The choice of words in the *Yoga Sūtra* are those of a faultless grammarian.

there is such in the inner i.e., the end is *ātma-nivṛtti*. You can find this beautifully explained in the *Samādhi Prakāraṇa* of *Haṭhayoga Pradīpikā*. It compares body, mind and self to the wick, oil and flame of the lamp. When a lamp is lit, it is simply a flame. So a person who has realised the Self has reconciled the wick of the body and the fuel of the mind and is one with the flame of the Self.

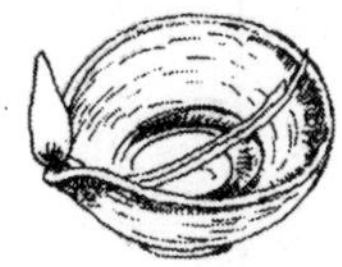

Is this a physical definition or a spiritual one? There are other definitions in the *Haṭhayoga Pradīpikā,* which I will give before the demonstration.

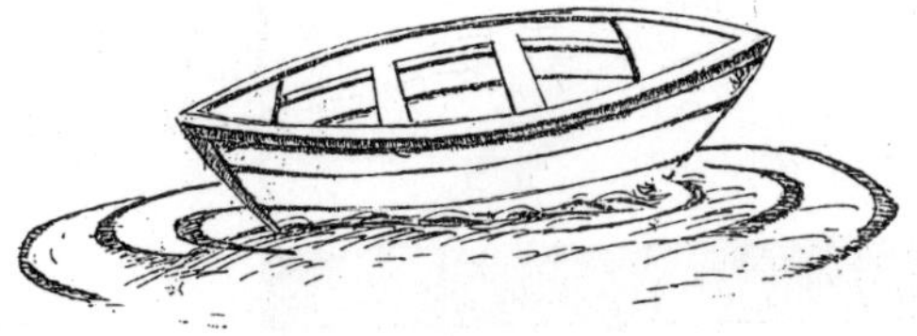

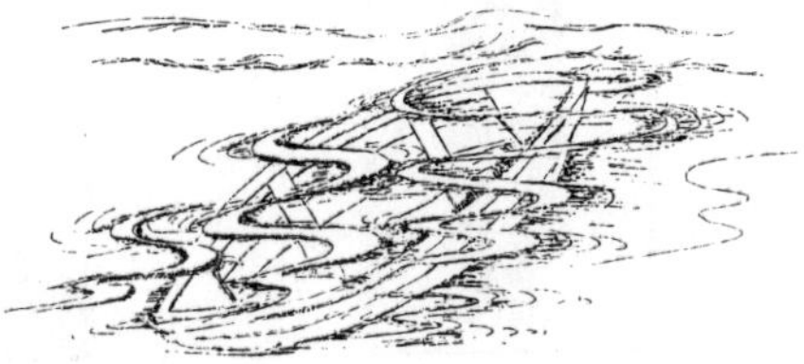

If a vessel is afloat, it is filled with air; if it is submerged in water, it is filled with water. Similarly, for a practitioner of yoga, the body and the mind can be sunk into the Self. How beautiful the analogies are in the *Haṭhayoga Pradīpikā*. See one more: salt, water and a glass are different entities. Mix the salt and the water in a glass, stir it and taste it. It is uniformly salty from top to bottom. In the same way, when you have reached that state of awareness in the Self, you cannot differentiate between body, mind and Self.

Patañjali puts it, *Prayatna śaithilya ananta samāpattibhyām* (*Y.S.,* II.47). When effortful effort ceases and effort becomes effortless or *sahaja* (natural), you are at one with the Infinite, you are one with the Seer.

The effect of *āsana* is, *Tataḥ dvandvānabhighātah.* The polarities of the body, mind and soul vanish – but only when effortful effort becomes effortless.

How is this achieved? It is often said, *sthira sukham āsanam*: sit in any comfortable pose. But after ten minutes you change the pose. A comfortable pose becomes an uncomfortable pose within a few minutes. You should go into the depth of the discomfort, convert that uncomfortable pose into a comfortable one: this is tolerance in yogic discipline, only then have you mastered the instruction, *sthira sukham āsanam*. But Patañjali does not say, "sit in any pose", he only defines the *āsana*. For example, take *Tāḍāsana* – I am standing. What is the definition of this pose, tell me. You have to find *sthiratā* (stability) and *sukhatā* (perfect balance) – perfect harmony between body and mind. If I do *Utthita Trikoṇāsana* I have to follow the same principle – how to achieve *sthiratā* and *sukhatā*. You see how we misread Patañjali's *Yoga Sūtra?* He did not mean to say, "sit in a comfortable pose", he simply defined *āsana*.

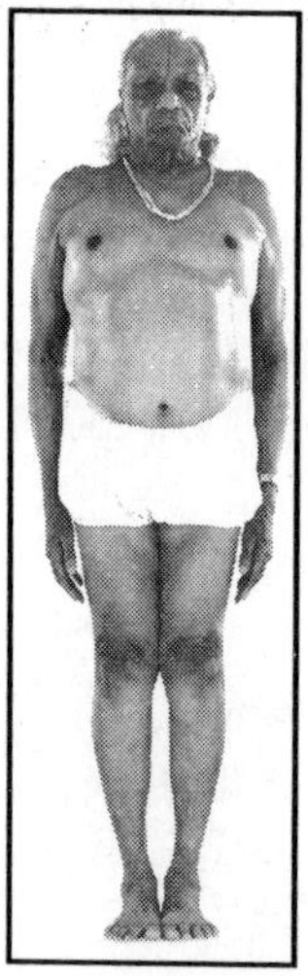

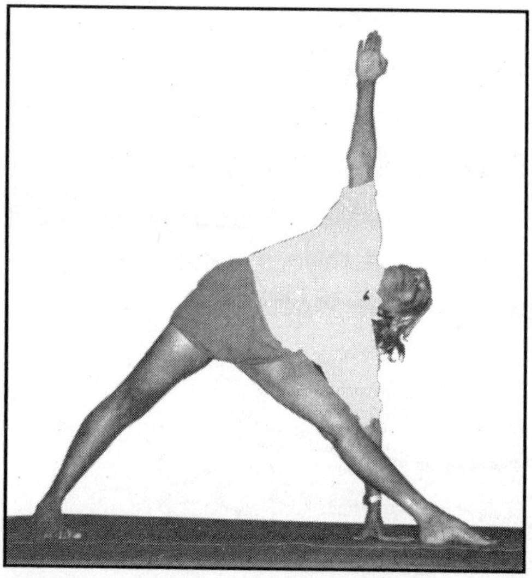

Plate n. 8 – *Tāḍāsana* and *Utthita Trikoṇāsana*

The same is true for the *Vṛśchikāsana* (scorpion pose), or for *Hanumānāsana*, the splits pose: you have to find *sthiratā* and *sukhatā*. Until you have achieved this, you have not mastered these *āsanas*. You can only claim to have mastered *āsana* in which you can stay without any discomfort: this is Patañjali's definition. He does not say that *āsana* has to be stable and comfortable. Rather you have to be stable and comfortable in *āsana*.

Modern translators define Patañjali's *Yoga Sūtra* as *rāja yoga* (mind control). This word *rāja* is borrowed from *Haṭhayoga Pradīpikā*. I quote from this text:

indriyāṇāmḥ manonāthḥ manonāthāsya mārutaḥ /
mārutasya layonātaḥ sa layo nāda māśritaḥ // (*H.Y.P.*, IV.29)

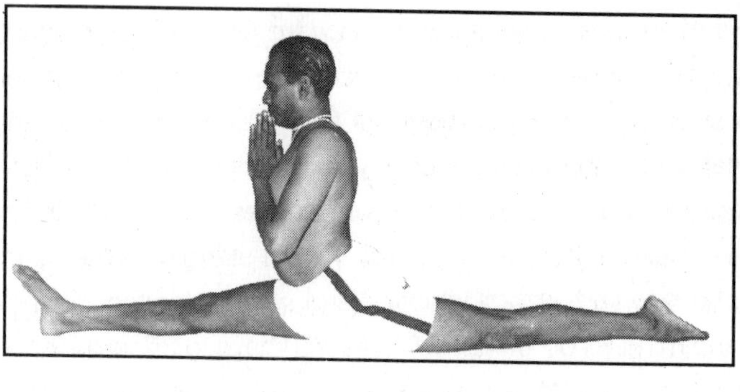

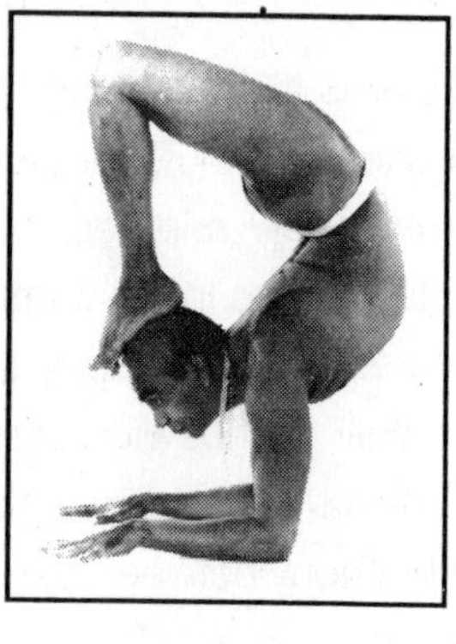

Plate n. 9 – *Hanumānāsana* and *Vṛśchikāsana*

"The king of the senses is the mind, the king of the mind is the breath, absorption is the king of the breath and that absorption has the inner sound *(nāda)*".

In fact, if you understand how to make your normal breath run harmoniously, the mind also becomes balanced. So it is the breath that is the key to silencing the mind, and when you silence the mind it can dictate to the senses of perception and organs of action how to behave.

Do not get the idea that the *Haṭhayoga Pradīpikā* omits ethical disciplines. In fact the sixteenth *śloka* of the first chapter explains it very well, listing ten *yama* and ten *niyama*, while Patañjali gives only five of each. *Haṭha yoga* has taken it for granted that *yama* and *niyama* are already well understood, so it starts with *āsana* as its first *aṅga* or limb and then proceeds with *prāṇāyāma, dhāraṇā, dhyāna* and *samādhi*.

When the author wrote *Haṭhayoga Pradīpikā*, the condition and problems of diseases that existed then must have been uppermost in his mind, more than when Patañjali was composing the *Yoga Sūtra*. Just as we are used today to new diseases and new medicines, so *Haṭhayoga Pradīpikā* introduced *mudrā, bandha* and *śaṭkriyā*. (swallowing a cloth, putting a thread into the nose and so on). For various ailments these are essentially remedial methods and do not convey the regular *haṭha yoga* practice. *Haṭhayoga Pradīpikā* specifically says that the *śaṭkriyā* are not for all, but only for those with obesity, phlegmatic disorders or excess of wind or bile. Furthermore, it says everyone including Brahmā, the Creator, prefers *prāṇāyāma* to *kriyā*, and that *prāṇāyāma* can achieve the same results as the *śaṭkriyā* or *śaṭkarma: dhauti, basti, neti, trāṭaka, nauli and kapālabhāti*.

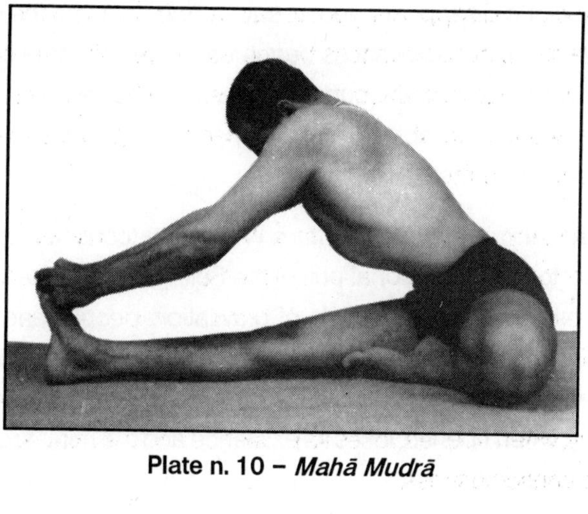

Plate n. 10 – *Mahā Mudrā*

Bandha, mudrā and *kriyā* are the only three additions in *Haṭhayoga Pradīpikā*: why did Patañjali not speak of them? Because he knew that an *āsana* itself has a *bandha*, a lock, and a *mudrā*. That is the beauty of *āsana*. When you do *Sālamba Śīrṣāsana* – headbalance (Plate n. 5) – what do you do? You lock the anus, and the abdominal organs go towards the spine, performing a natural *Uḍḍīyāna bandha*. When you do *Sālamba Sarvāṅgāsana* – shoulderbalance (Plate n. 5) – there is a *Jālandhara Bandha*, or chin lock (Plate n. 20). There is also a contraction of the anal sphincter in *Paśchimottānāsana* (Plate n. 5). *Mahā Mudrā* and *Mahā Bandha* can both be traced in the *āsana*, and that is why Patañjali did not talk about *bandha*.

It is said that there are eighty-four hundreds of thousands of *āsana*, and some say they are countless. In other words, we can make millions and millions of movements in our bodies. We have twenty-two knuckles in the fingers that can move in different directions; we can move the palm or the wrist, forwards, backwards, laterally and so forth. This way there may be eighty-four hundreds of thousands of movements in our body or even more, or as the text says, there may be eight hundred and forty thousand diseases. If you do not use or if you misuse the movements, they get rusted; then they are branded as diseases. Take multiple sclerosis. It affects not just one or two places, but may run all over the body.

In the fourth chapter of the *Yoga Sūtra*, Patañjali speaks of *dharma megha samādhi*. *Dharma megha* conveys that the duty *(dharma)* of the cloud *(megha)* is to rain. This religiousness of the cloud is twofold. It rains or remains just cloudy. Similarly, it is possible that one may experience a partially obscured state of *samādhi* or an enlightened one. *Samādhi* has two sides. It can be partially illumined like the new moon or make one glow like the full.

The moment the cloud disappears, you all say, "let's go out into the sunshine". The sun is the Self. When the *citta* or the consciousness becomes aware of its true condition, it realises that it has no light of its own. Up to now the consciousness had behaved as a subjective organ. Now consciousness realises it is an objective one dependent upon the borrowed light of the Self. At that point, it surrenders to the Self.

Patañjali uses the term *prāgbhāram cittam*. When *citta* (consciousness) realises that it has no life of its own, due to the gravitational pull of the Self, it falls into the lap of the Self. Long before Newton worked out the scientific details of gravitation, people, and certainly Patañjali, were aware of the significance of gravitational attraction. Having practised so many *āsana*, I know exactly where the gravitational forces are in each one. Read *sūtra* I.43, where Patañjali explains how the memory, when ripened, loses its existence and the mind too loses its existence and they dissolve in the consciousness.

There is no doubt in my mind that *haṭha yoga* is equally as important as *pātañjala yoga*, and vice versa. The standard of civilisation in Patañjali's time was high: in Svātmārāma's time it was low, as it is now. Hence, it was important for Svātmārāma to introduce many basic points in his treatise, *Haṭhayoga Pradīpikā*, so that the average intellectual *sādhaka* understands the subject of yoga with ease before jumping to know and understand consciousness. Through Svātmārāma's guidance the *sādhaka* comes to understand first the body and then functions of the organs of action and senses of perception which act as the gates of knowledge to feed the intelligence. The intelligence through practice of *āsana* and *prāṇāyama* understands the difference between the external and the internal body for the *sādhaka* to turn towards the source, the core of Being. This is the meeting point of *haṭha yoga* with *pātañjala yoga*.

Knowledge has no frontier, so let us make full use of the best of *haṭha yoga* or *pātañjala yoga* (or both) without distorting the noble art of yoga.

THE ESSENCE OF *HAṬHA YOGA*

Advances in science and technology have brought an exponential increase in knowledge, but this is sadly accompanied by a tendency to separate and compartmentalise our massive intellectual acquisitions. This process is equally evident in the field of yoga, where *pandits* make nit-picking assertions about the confinement of *haṭha yoga* to the physical realm, and Patañjali's yoga to the spiritual. If the search for knowledge leads us only towards nonsensical division and away from the perception of conjuntion and wholeness, it is tantamount to blasphemy.

MAN AS A TOTAL BEING

Man is a trinity of body, mind and soul. Unless he is affected by physical or mental illness, the life force ebbs and flows evenly in all the three layers, rhythmically and smoothly without any division. No one knows where the body ends and the mind begins and no one knows where the mind ends and soul begins. The body can be divided into three parts, the outer, the inner and the innermost. The outer body is known as *kārya śarīra* (physical body), the abode of action, mind as the *sūkṣma śarīra* (subtle body), the abode of thinking, and finally the soul as *kāraṇa śarīra* (primordial or causal body), the home of ever existing force. For the sake of convenience, the originators of yoga subdivided these three layers of man into five sheaths as the anatomical layer *(annamaya kośa)*, physiological layer *(prāṇamaya kośa)*, mental layer *(manomaya kośa)*, intellectual layer *(vijñānamaya kośa)* and lastly the layer of bliss *(ānandamaya kośa)*. *Kārya śarīra* is composed of *annamaya kośa*, *sūkṣma śarīra* of the *prāṇamaya*, *manomaya* and *vijñānamaya kośa* and *kāraṇa śarīra* is composed of the *ānandamaya kośa*.

This is how the division of man has been outlined in order to explain the functions of his body, his consciousness and self so that he may understand them in detail.

Table n. 4 – *Śarīra and pañcakośa* or five sheaths of human being

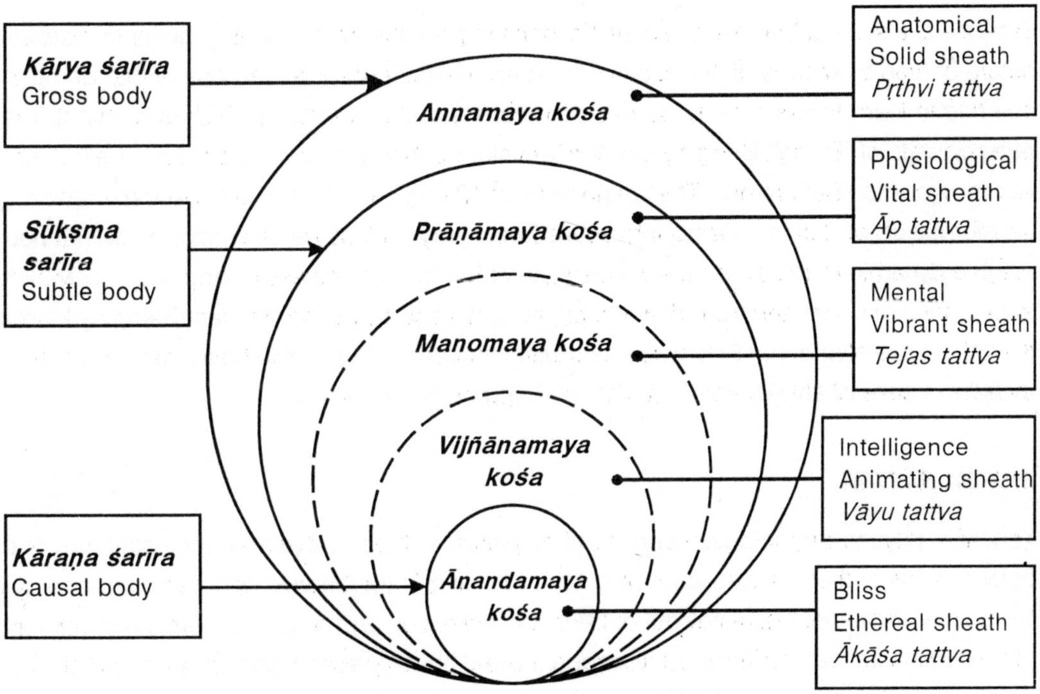

Yoga means integration. Yoga is the art and science which integrates these three bodies with the five sheaths to develop totality of being. We are taught through yoga to develop body, mind and self rhythmically so that the *prāṇa vāhinī* (the river of energy) and the *sva-rasa vāhinī* (the river of consciousness and the essence of the self) flow uninterruptedly without hindrances, bridging all these layers into a single unit. In yogic terminology, this is called *saṁyama*.

PATH IS ONE

God is one but His names are many. Truth is one but is reflected in various facets. Similarly yoga is one yet it is demarcated not only as physical, mental and spiritual yoga but also labelled by different names such as *rāja yoga*, *karma yoga*, *bhakti yoga*, *jñāna yoga*, *haṭha yoga*, *ghaṭa yoga*, *mantra yoga*, *laya yoga*, *trāṭaka yoga*, *kuṇḍalinī yoga*, *śaktipāta yoga*, *anāśakti yoga*, *amṛta yoga*, *tāraka yoga* and so on. There are innumerable paths to take to reach the peak of a mountain. They all lead to the zenith of spirituality. Like a strong tide inundating the land, the minds of people are indoctrinated with the idea that *haṭha yoga* is a purely physical form of yoga. On account of this it is hard for them to see the light of wisdom that dawns on practitioners through the practice of *haṭha yoga*.

BEING AND BECOMING

Essence is a state of being in the core. Essence implies the art of knowing the inner distinctive nature of man by means of this subject. In order to experience the real state of that Being, first one has to learn to Become. In deep sleep, there is a state of Being which is dormant. It is a *tāmasic* state of "Being". Bringing the dormant state of being through a conscious effort into a vibrant state is "Becoming". The attainment of "Being" involves *rajas*. We experience the transformation of dormant Being into active Becoming, so that we can move on still further to live in a dynamic illuminative pure *sāttvic* state of Being. As darkness disappears slowly by the appearance of dawn and from dawn to bright light, yoga helps the dormant Being by kindling the light to live eternally in Self awareness with innocence. This is true being, termed as *kevala avasthā* (a state of absoluteness, a state of Being or aloneness).

MOKṢA ŚĀSTRA

Yoga is a psycho-physiological and psycho-spiritual subject. It deals with the structure of the body, actions of the muscles, current of blood flowing in the arteries and veins, bio-energy or bio-plasma in the nerves, behaviour of the organs of action and senses of perception, influence of mind in ignorance and knowledge, arrogance and humility, sorrow and joy, pain and pleasure, evil and good, bondage and freedom, inspiration and expiration, aspiration and renunciation, and affluence or the abundant wealth of knowledge and resplendence of the Self.

Rāja yoga and *haṭha yoga* are the sciences of freedom *(mokṣa śāstra)*, they are the art of liberating one from the bondages of life and death. They guide man to climb the ladder of spirituality. The only difference between the two is that *haṭha yoga* starts from the body and ends with the soul while *rāja yoga* starts from the consciousness, climbs down to the body and uplifts us again towards the Soul. Both criss-cross each other and reach the destiny of peace, poise and plenitude.

Patañjali enumerates the diseases that come in the way of one's progress towards spiritual realisation (*Y.S.,* I.30). This shows that he deals both with the body and mind and shows also that the eight petals of yoga, (*Y.S.,* II.29), are the ways to free oneself from the shackles of body and mind and guide the *sādhaka* towards Self-realisation and then onwards towards God-realisation.

Svātmārāma, the author of the *Haṭhayoga Pradīpikā,* says that man, being the product of nature, cosmic intelligence, individual mind, intelligence, *ahaṁkāra* ('I'-ness), *mamakāra* (mineness), the five elements and their five qualities, the five senses of perception and five organs of action is susceptible to three types of diseases. He classifies them as *ādhibhautika* (disease due to drought, earthquake, famine, cyclone, tides, bites and so on), *ādhidaivika* (through the influence of planets, which in modern language are termed as genetic diseases and allergy), and *ādhyātmika* (self-made diseases). This *ādhyātmika roga* may be physical or mental or both. As these illnesses come by one's own habits and behaviours, *haṭha yoga* shows the ways of conquering them through one's own efforts.

The *Yoga Sūtra* is divided into four parts as, *Samādhi Pāda*, *Sādhana Pāda*, *Vibhūti Pāda* and *Kaivalya Pāda*. The first chapter explains the *sādhanā* for those who have a balanced mind. The second is meant for those who are raw in body and mind and shows them the way to begin the *sādhanā*. The third speaks of miraculous powers. Though powers are dealt with, Patañjali advises the *sādhaka* to be careful not to get caught in their whirlwind when trying to ride the wind. He cautions that such *siddhi* (powers) may escalate into a tornado of sorrow. The fourth chapter explains in detail the conscious state of the yogi who is in a state of absoluteness or aloneness *(kevala avasthā)*, and how he has to live and act with this state of emancipation.

Svātmārāma divides his book into four chapters. The first deals with *yama* to *āsana* disciplines, the second with *prāṇāyāma*, the third with *mudrā* and *bandha* and the fourth with *samādhi*. Besides these, he has added a few more things, as a curative method with drastic techniques, called *kriyā* or *karma*, for diseases in which the three humours of the body, namely, *vāta*, *pitta* and *śleṣma* are totally vitiated or are in excess. This is the only extra feature in the book. Otherwise his method is almost identical with that of Patañjali's. Hence both are not only complementary to each other but supplementary too.

Patañjali says[1] that the self comes in contact with the objects which are seen and is caught in the web of desires. We forget our true nature and become victims of pain and sorrow. He cautions that one may not be aware of the pain wł.ich may appear in the future (*Y.S.*, II.16) and so he advocates practice *(abhyāsa)* and renunciation *(vairāgya)* (*Y.S.*, I.12)

Svātmārāma says that energy *(prāṇa)* and desire *(vāsanā)* are the two forces which distract the *citta* or the consciousness[2]. Right use of energy is *abhyāsa* and freeing the *citta* from desires which come in the way of practice is *vairāgya*.

---

[1] The association of the seer with the seen is the cause of distress. Avoidance of union between them is the remedy for distress (*Y.S.*, II.17).

[2] The activity of the mind has *vāsanā* and *prāṇa* as the two causes. When one of them becomes inactive, both come to an end (*H.Y.P.*, IV.22).

Practice should be with faith, courage, memory, contemplation and awareness[1], says Patañjali. Svātmārāma uses different terminologies for the same thesis[2]. Practice is that which is done uninterruptedly with devotion and dedication in order to get firmly established in the path of yoga[3]. At the same time to prepare the mind to be free from the things which come in the way of practice is *vairāgya*[4]. Svātmārāma explains *abhyāsa* and *vairāgya* as *ha* and *ṭha*. *Ha* and *ṭha* are *prāṇa* and *apāna* or aspiration *(pravṛtti)* and renunciation *(nivṛtti)*. In the same way as electricity is composed of positive and negative currents, a new dynamic life sets in through *haṭha yoga*. This is known as *ātmajyoti* (light of the soul). According to *Haṭhayoga Pradīpikā*, the body is *tāmasic* (lethargic), the mind is *rājasic* (active) and the soul is *sāttvic* (pure and luminous). *Āsana* practice transforms the body to the level of the mind and then take both body and mind to merge in the seat of the soul[5]. As all rivers join the sea and lose their identities, the vehicles of the Self (the senses, the mind, the intelligence, the ego and the consciousness) lose their identities and live as one integrated being in the sea of the soul. Like a burnt seed which cannot sprout at all, a yogi's actions are free from reactions and from then on he becomes a *jīvanmukta*, a liberated Self in this very life.

Patañjali mentions nowhere that he is speaking of *rāja yoga*. Owing to long-time propaganda, many have the notion that Patañjali's yoga is spiritual and *haṭha yoga* is physical. Most of us are well acquainted with the *Yoga Sūtra* but I am not certain whether all of us are as equally aware of *haṭha yoga* texts.

THE AIM AND ESSENCE

Both the texts, having the same essence, aim at *kaivalya*.

Patañjali explains the essence of yoga in two *sūtra*: "When all the movements and vibrations of the consciousness are stilled and then silenced, the Self stands on its own glory"[6].

---

1 Pursue yogic discipline with faith, vigour, memory, keen intellect and power of absorption to experience the absolute consciousness (*Y.S.*, I.20).

2 Yoga succeeds by six qualities: cheerfulness, adamantine perseverance, courage, intellectual potency, faith and abandoning bad company (*H.Y.P.*, I.16).

3 Residing in such a hut, being free from all worries, the yogi should practise yoga and yoga alone, in the way taught by his guru (*H.Y.P.*, I.14).

4 Yoga fails by over-eating, over-exertion, excessive talk, unsuitable austerity, promiscuous company and unsteadiness (*H.Y.P.*, I.15).

5 *Āsana* make the body and mind firm and steady, make (the practitioner) free from disease and light in the limb (*H.Y.P.*, I.17).

6 *Yogaḥ cittavṛtti nirodhaḥ. Tadā draṣṭuḥ svarūpe avasthānam* (*Y.S.*, I.2 & 3).

Only if the mirror is clean can it reflect an image clearly, whereas in yoga, when the consciousness is silenced at its source, the Self shines forth without the mirror of the mind or the intelligence or the I or Me.

Svātmārāma takes a lot of pains lengthily and lucidly to explain the same thing; how to experience the beauty of this state of Self-reflection *(ātma-darśana).*

Let me quote from the fourth chapter of his text. He says that, *"rājayoga, samādhi, unmanī, manonmanī, śūnyāśūnya, paramapada, amanaskatva, advaita, nirālamba, nirañjana, jīvanmukti, sahaja, turīyā"* are synonymous terms as they imply the same meaning and experience (IV.3&4).

As grains of salt dissolved in water become water (IV.5); as the camphor that merges in the flame becomes flame (IV.59), the body, the mind, the intelligence, the ego and the consciousness merge in the Self and become one.

"The mind is the king of the senses, the king of the mind is *prāṇa*. By sublimating the *prāṇa* through the sound of its flow, both *prāṇa* and *vāsanā* are absorbed". (IV.29 & 30).

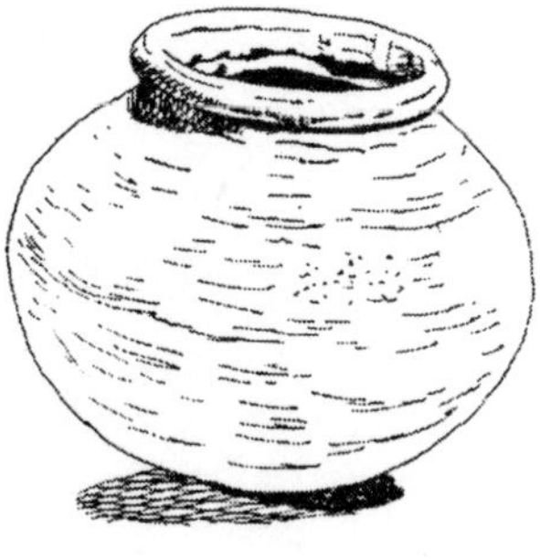

"As an empty earthen pot when exposed to space is empty inside and outside, the yogi is empty inside and empty outside. At the same time, as the pot in the sea is filled inside as well as outside with water, the perfect yogi sees the Self inside and outside" (IV.50).

"Not only does the yogi stop thinking inside and outside, but abandons positively all forces and remains totally silent anywhere and everywhere. Then in that state he experiences the state of *kaivalya* which alone remains" (IV.57 & 62). "In that state he is free from fault, pain, old age, disease, hunger and sleep and becomes a master *(yogeśvara)"* (IV.75 & 77).

"As the fire becomes extinct the moment the wood is extinguished, the *citta* rests in the abode of the Self" (IV.98).

"The yogi blessed with *samādhi* loses all sense of odour, taste, form, touch and sound; he neither knows of himself or others" (IV.109).

"He is neither awake nor asleep, he has neither memory nor forgetfulness, he feels neither heat nor cold, neither pain or pleasure, honour or dishonour but is clear and virtuous" (IV.110, 111 & 112).

The culmination of *haṭha yoga* is when the Self mingles as Self in the rivers of poise, peace, plenty, wisdom and virtue, percolating perennially and freely into the fibres and cells. Then the *haṭha* yogi drinks the essence of yoga.

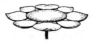

THE YOGA OF LIGHT*

Haṭha yoga is known also as *haṭha vidyā* (the science of *haṭha*). It can be misunderstood and misrepresented as a physical yoga devoid of spiritual light. Hans U. Rieker has done his best to explain the changes taking place in the practitioner's body, mind and Self. The author makes the reader feel the subjective transformation that occurs as he goes on practising, by making the consciousness penetrate the inner body from the skin towards the Self and causing the Self to diffuse outwards towards the skin. He explains that *haṭha yoga* is not just physical gymnastics but an organic and mental science leading towards spiritual evolution.

We are caught up in emotions like lust, anger, greed, infatuation, pride and malice. *Haṭha yoga* helps to overcome these obstacles and hindrances to spiritual development. It is a bio-chemical, psycho-physiological and psycho-spiritual science.

Haṭha yoga, as presented by Svātmārāma, is a science that deals with the moral, physical, physiological, mental, intellectual and spiritual aspects of man. Besides these, it also explains how to purify the nervous system and balance the hormonal system in the body.

Man is known as *mānava* (human) as he is the descendent of Manu, the father of mankind who is said to be the son of Brahmā, the Creator of the world. The word *mana* or *manas*, i.e. mind, originated from the root *man*, meaning to think. Thus one who possesses a mind is man. It also means that one who lives with honour *(māna)* is a *mānava*.

Manas means mind, intellect, thought, design, purpose and will. It is the internal organ for the senses of perception and organs of action, and the outer organ for intelligence, consciousness and the Self. Man is graced with this special organ – the mind – so that he can enjoy the pleasures of the world or seek emancipation and freedom from worldly objects.

---

* Based on the foreword by B.K.S. Iyengar to *Yoga of Light*, Hans-Ulrich Rieker, Harper Collins, London, December 1995.

KNOWLEDGE

Knowledge means acquaintance with facts, truth or principles by study or investigation. As man is ambitious, a mind that is endowed with the faculty of discrimination desires to achieve certain aims and purposes in life.

Knowledge is of two types. The first concerns matters of the world, called *laukika jñāna,* the second is the knowledge of the Self, known as *vaidika jñāna (vaidika* = relating to *Veda* or a religious knowledge, *jñāna* = knowledge). Both are essential for living in the world, as well as for spiritual evolution.

AIMS OF LIFE

The sages of old discovered the means for the betterment of life and called them aims. These are duty *(dharma),* the acquisition of wealth *(artha)* in order to be free from dependence on others, the gratification of desire *(kāma),* and emancipation or final beatitude *(mokṣa).* Beatitude is the deliverance of the Self from its entanglement with material joys, that is freedom from body, senses, vital energy, mind, intellect and consciousness.

Duty *(dharma),* means *(artha)* and passion *(kāma)* are important in matters of worldly life. Duty *(dharma)* and beatitude *(mokṣa)* are to be followed judiciously for Self-realisation. Through yogic practice, both kinds of knowledge encourage the development of a balanced frame of mind in all circumstances.

Even Patañjali, at the end of his treatise, concludes that the practice of yoga makes a yogi free from the aims of life *(dharma, artha, kāma, mokṣa)* and qualities of nature *(sattva, rajas* and *tamas),* so that man can reach the final destination – realisation of himself.

HEALTH AND HARMONY – A PRECONDITION FOR ACQUISITION OF KNOWLEDGE

To acquire either mundane or spiritual knowledge, health of the body, poise of mind and clarity with maturity of intelligence are essential.

Health begets happiness and it ignites and inspires one to further one's knowledge of the world and of the Self. Health means perfect harmony in all our physiological organs and peace of mind. Ill health acts as a hindrance to achieving anything in life. If one does not work to achieve good health and a composed mind, life becomes brutish.

AFFLICTIONS *(TĀPA)*

Afflictions are of three types, physical, mental and spiritual. They are known as *ādhyātmika, ādhidaivika* and *ādhibhautika*. Afflictions arising through self-abuse and self-infliction is *ādhyātmika* torment *(tāpa)*. *Tāpa* means heat, torment, pain, sorrow, affliction and stress. Physical and organic diseases are caused by an imbalance in the required ratio of the five elements in the body, which disturbs the proper functioning of the body. These are called diseases of *ādhibhautika*. Snake bites, scorpion stings and so on are also classified as *ādhibhautika tāpa*. Genetic and allergic diseases or diseases arising from one's past deeds, called fate or destiny, are the diseases of *ādhidaivika*.

HAṬHA YOGA OR *HAṬHA VIDYĀ*

Haṭha means to stick fast, to be devoted and to hold closely or firmly. Yoga means, to associate, to yoke, to join and to unite. It also means zeal, endeavour, fixing the mind on a particular point, keeping the body in a fixed posture, contemplation and meditation; *vidyā* means knowledge, art and science.

Goddess Pārvati, wife of Lord Shiva, approached her Lord – the seed of all knowledge – for guidance to help humanity in their suffering. Out of admiration for His Beloved Pārvati, Lord Shiva explained the greatest of all sciences – the science of *haṭha yoga* which alone, He says, stands high in His esteem for the holistic development of man.

Pārvati, learning this yogic knowledge from Shiva, imparted it to Brahmā, who in turn taught it to his children born of his own will, the sages such as Nārada, Sanaka and Sanatkumāra, and through them to Vasiṣṭa and others.

Svātmārāma Yogīndra, who was also known as Sahajānanda Cintāmaṇi, wrote a treatise entitled *Haṭhayoga Pradīpikā – The Light on Haṭha Yoga*. The author mentions the lineage of yogis before him who practised this noble and majestic art. If we give a thought to this list of names, then we must inevitably conclude that this tradition of yoga is contemporary and supplementary to that of Patañjali.

If Patañjali codified the eight petals of yoga *(aṣṭāṅga yoga)*, Svātmārāma did the same for *haṭha yoga*. If the former is a scholarly exposition with gems of wisdom woven together, the latter is a direct practical and technical handbook. Svātmārāma incorporated ideas from the *Yoga Sūtra*, the *Yoga Upaniṣad*, the *Purāṇa*, the *Bhagavad Gītā* and other works. Because of this, doubts arise in the reader's mind as to its authenticity.

Hans U. Rieker has done very useful work in re-grouping the subject matter so that the reader can understand it more clearly. One should realise that the *Haṭhayoga Pradīpikā* is a major treatise with practical guidelines, including for the raw beginner. It takes the practitioner from the culture of the body towards the sight of the Self.

Patañjali begins his aphorisms with the restraint of the waves of consciousness and Svātmārāma starts with the restraint of cells and sinews *(snāyuvṛtti samādhāna)* and restraint of vital energy *(prāṇavṛtti stambhana)*. Sighting the Self through the restraint of consciousness is *rāja yoga* and when the same is achieved through the restraint of cells and vital energy, it is *haṭha yoga*.

Haṭha means will-power, resoluteness and perseverance, and the path that takes one towards emancipation is *haṭha yoga*. If one breaks *haṭha* into *ha* and *ṭha*, *ha* stands for *puruṣa* (the seer or Self), the sun and the in-breath *(prāṇa)*, while *ṭha* represents *prakṛti* (nature), consciousness, the moon and the out-breath *(apāna)*. Thus, *haṭha yoga* means the union of *puruṣa* with *prakṛti* or consciousness with the Soul, the sun with the moon and *prāṇa* with *apāna*.

The treatise has four chapters *(prakaraṇa)*. The first chapter explains *yama, niyama, āsana* and food; the second, describes *prāṇāyāma* and *kriyā*; the third deals with *mudrā, bandha, nāḍī* and the *kuṇḍalinī* power while the fourth expounds *pratyāhāra, dhāraṇā, dhyāna* and *samādhi*.

Medicine is of two types: oral and surgical. The oral method is followed by a physician and operations are done by a surgeon. *Haṭha yoga* too has two methods to combat diseases; a natural method of *āsana* and *prāṇāyāma* and interventionist means in the form of the *ṣaṭkriyā* and *mudrā* comparable to medical methods like induced vomiting and enema. A caution is given that they should be introduced only if there is an excess of wind, bile and phlegm in the body.

The text contains nearly 390 verses *(śloka)*. Out of these, about forty deal with *āsana*, approximately one hundred and ten with *prāṇāyāma*, one hundred and fifty with *mudrā, bandha* and *kriyā* and the rest with *pratyāhāra, dhāraṇā, dhyāna* and *samādhi*.

ĀSANA

The first chapter begins with *āsana* as the first step in *haṭha yoga*. However, it does not overlook *yama* and *niyama*. Probably at the time of Svātmārāma the ethical disciplines were taken for granted and so the text does not devote much time in explaining them in detail, but only mentions the disciplines of *yama* and *niyama* and goes directly towards *āsana*, as *prathamāṅga* (first step).

Regarding *yama,* he speaks of non-violence, truthfulness, non-covetousness, continence, forbearance, fortitude, compassion, straightforwardness and moderation in food, cleanliness and passion for yoga. For *niyama,* he advises contentment, faith, charity, worship of God, study of spiritual scriptures, modesty, discriminative power of mind, ritual and prayer (I.16).

The ethical disciplines of what to do and what not to do are taught by precept and *āsana, prāṇāyāma, dhāraṇā, bandha, mudrā* and *kriyā* are taught by example so that their effects can be felt subjectively. However, *dhyāna* and *samādhi* cannot be explained, only experienced.

Because the text begins with *āsana,* some people call *haṭha yoga* six-petalled yoga *(ṣaḍāṅga yoga),* and *pātañjala yoga,* which includes *yama* and *niyama* as separate limbs, eight-petalled yoga *(aṣṭāṅga yoga).*

It is said that there are as many *āsana* as living species; the number given is about eighty-four lacs or eighty-four hundreds of thousands. That means the muscles and joints can flex, extend and rotate in several thousand ways. With this huge claim, the text explains only sixteen *āsana.* Similarly, Vyāsa names only eleven *āsana* in his commentary on *Yoga Sūtra.* Probably *yogāsana* practices were a regular daily routine then. They must have thought that it was enough to touch on the subject without going into depth. With only this number of *āsana* in the text, it is ridiculous to claim that *haṭha yoga* is physical yoga.

Yogis were in constant contact with nature and they were searching for natural remedies to combat afflictions. In their search they discovered hundreds of *āsana* to increase and restore the life-giving force to its optimum level.

Āsana is not just physical exercise, but physico-physiological, bio-chemical, psycho-physiological and psycho-spiritual posture. The cells of the body have their own intelligence and memory. Different *āsana* are formed through conscious effort in order to nourish various parts of the body for improved blood circulation and elimination of toxins so that the cells, sinews and nerves are kept at their peak level of condition so that we enjoy robust health in body, mind and self.

If one wishes to know the effect of *āsana,* one should read the commentary of Shri Brahmānanda called *Jyotsnā* on Svātmārāma's *Haṭhayoga Pradīpikā.* He clearly and beautifully sums up the effect of *āsana:* "The body is full of inertia *(tāmasic),* the mind vibrant *(rājasic)* and the Self serene and luminous *(sāttvic).* By perfection in *āsana,* the lazy body is transformed to the level of the vibrant mind and they together are cultured to reach the level of the serenity of the Self". Thus in perfection of *āsana* the intelligence and expressions of body and mind are equal to the purity and serenity of the Self.

According to Patañjali, perfection in *āsana* brings concord between body, mind and self. When *āsana* is performed with the interpenetration of all three bodies (body, mind and self), benevolence in consciousness develops. This puts an end to the pairs of opposites and the indivisible state of existence is experienced.

PRĀṆĀYĀMA

The second chapter is devoted mainly to *prāṇāyāma* and its techniques. *Prāṇāyāma* is often defined as *prāṇavṛtti nirodha* or restraint of the fluctuations of breath, as the breath by nature moves in a zigzag fashion. But in more precise and appropriate terms, *prāṇāyāma* is *prāṇavṛtti stambhana*, or suspension of fluctuations of vital force. According to Svātmārāma, "as the breath flows, so the mind fluctuates, when the breath is stilled, the mind also becomes still and silent" (II.2).

Prāṇāyāma flushes away the toxins and rectifies the disturbances of the humours, wind, bile and phlegm *(vāta, pitta, śleṣma).*

All the yoga texts, including *pātañjala yoga* texts, are emphatic in their view that one has to gain total competence in *āsana* before learning *prāṇāyāma*. This point is overlooked today and many people think that any comfortable sitting *āsana* is good enough for *prāṇāyāma* practice.

Though *āsana* is initially intended for health and lightness of the body, it takes one further towards subtleties like diffusing the consciousness uniformly in the entire region of the body so that the dualities between body, senses, nerves, cells, mind, intelligence, ego and consciousness are eradicated and the whole being acts as one entity. When the nerves, circulatory, respiratory, digestive, endocrine and genito-excretory systems are cleansed through *āsana*, *prāṇa* moves without interruption to the remotest cells and feeds them with copious supply of energy. Through this process, rejuvenation takes place for the instrument of the Self – the body – to reach the goal of Self-realisation. When one begins to interpenetrate the body with effortful means of *āsana*, perfection comes; effort ceases, the gem of joy is experienced. *Ṛtambharā prajñā* surfaces. New light of wisdom dawns.

PRĀṆA

Prāṇa is an auto energising force. The inbreath fans and fuses the two opposing elements of nature, fire and water, so that a new-bio-electrical energy is produced. This energy is called *prāṇa* in yogic terminology. *Prāṇa* neutralises the fluctuations of the mind, and acts as a springboard towards emancipation.

Prāṇāyāma stores *prāṇa* in the seven chambers or *cakra* of the spine so that they can discharge it when necessary to face the upheavals of life.

Patañjali states that "mastery in *prāṇāyāma* removes the veil that covers the flame of intelligence and heralds the dawn of wisdom" (See II.52 and 53).

Though Svātmārāma explains various types of *prāṇāyāma* and their effects, he also cautions the practitioner of *prāṇāyāma* to study the capacity of his lungs and make the brain passive in order to tame the in-coming and out-going breath. If the animal trainer is careless, the animals maim him. In the same way, a wrong practice of *prāṇāyāma* saps the energy of the practitioner.

BANDHA AND *MUDRĀ*

Bandha and *mudrā* are dealt with in the third chapter. *Bandha* means a lock and *mudrā* means a seal. The human system has many apertures or outlets. By locking and sealing these outlets, the divine energy known as *kuṇḍalinī* is awakened and finds its union with *puruṣa* in the *sahasrāra cakra*.

Mudrā and *bandha* act as safety valves in the human system. *Āsana* is also a type of *mudrā* and *bandha*. Hence, *āsana*, *mudrā* and *bandha* help in suspending the fluctuations of the mind, intelligence and ego, so that attention is drawn in towards the Self. The union of the divine force with the divine Self is the essence of the third chapter.

SAMĀDHI

Samādhi being the subjective science of liberation, the fourth chapter is filled with the knowledge of the Self. *Samādhi* is the experience of unalloyed bliss. Before dealing with the path of unalloyed bliss and liberation, Svātmārāma explains about consciousness.

CITTA

Citta is a sprout from the self, and self from the seed (Self or *puruṣa*). *Citta* (consciousness) is permeated by the mind. The concept of mind can be understood by an average intellect, whereas consciousness remains an abstract. Consciousness has many facets and channels which move about in various directions at the same time. The breath cannot move like thought waves. It flows in and out in its own pattern, through a single channel only. Svātmārāma, after watchful study of the mind and breath, says that whether the mind is sleepy, dreamy or awake, the breath moves as in a single channel.

Just as water mixed with milk appears as milk, energy united with consciousness becomes consciousness. So *haṭha yoga* texts emphasise the restraint of energy, as that is easier than the restraint of the fluctuations of the consciousness. A steady and mindful in-breath and out-breath minimises the fluctuations and helps in stabilising the mind. In IV.49, Svātmārāma says that the mind is the king of the senses and energy is the master of the mind. If we learn to make the breath move rhythmically with a sustained steady sound *(nāda)*, the mind becomes calm and the king of the mind shines on its own.

I feel that the majority of commentators must have borrowed the term "king of the senses" from this text and on the basis of this named *pātañjala yoga* as *rāja yoga (rāja* = king*)* though Patañjali himself does not call his work *rāja yoga*.

Svātmārāma says that through *samādhi* the mind dissolves in the consciousness, consciousness in cosmic intelligence, cosmic intelligence in the root of nature and náture in the Universal Self.

The moment the consciousness is quietened, the Self, which is the king of the consciousness, surfaces and shines on its own. According to Svātmārāma, *rājayoga*, absence of mind, conquest of mind, immortal state, absorption, void, non-void, final emancipation, being devoid of intellect or colour, alone, liberated from further birth, in a natural state of disposition, and the Self becoming one with the Universal Self are synonymous words conveying only one meaning, *samādhi*, the sight of the soul (IV.3&4).

In order to get the glimpses of *samādhi*, one should refer to verses, 5, 6, 7, 15, 20, 21, 23, 24, 25, 28, 30, 31, 33, 48, 50, 51, 56, 59, 60, 62, 98, 111 and 112 of chapter IV of *Haṭhayoga Pradīpikā*.

CAUTION

With all these spiritual effects of *haṭha yoga*, in I.69 Svātmārāma cautions that "practice has to be done without thinking of its fruits, but with steadfast attention, living a chaste life and moderation in food". "One should avoid places inhabited by evil minded people, indulging in sex, long walks, early morning cold baths, fasting and exertion" (I.62). Again in I.66, he says, "yoga cannot be experienced by dressing like a holy man nor by reading or speaking about it. Its value is felt and its fragrance tasted by ardent practice alone". Further, he says, "Success comes to those who are zealous, bold, courageous, firm, and who study the spiritual scriptures". Compare this to *Yoga Sūtra* I.20, where Patañjali says that "faith, vigour, sharp memory, absorption and total awareness are the key to success".

Hans Ulrich Rieker has done well to present Indian thought in Western terms so that people can understand them with ease. I am glad to note that he asks his readers to accept the Indian masters' unattached and dispassionate attitudes and their ways of testing the pupils with an open mind. No master accepts a pupil just for the asking. Before he does so he studies the student's capacity for determination and one-pointed devotion. The practice of *haṭha yoga* helps the pupil to keep the body healthy and the mind clean and worthy so that the master can accept him as a fit student to be uplifted towards spiritual emancipation.

Lastly, Rieker's explanation of the mystical terms *nāda*, *bindu* and *kalā* is praiseworthy. *Nāda* means vibration or sound, *bindu* is a dot or a seed and *kalā* means a sprout and to shine or glitter. Here, *bindu* represents the Self, *kalā*, the sprout of the Self, i.e. consciousness and *nāda* the sound of the inner consciousness or the inner voice. A return journey from *nāda* to *kalā* and *kalā* to *bindu* is the ultimate in *haṭha yoga*. Svātmārāma says that if the consciousness is the seed, *haṭha yoga* is the field. He enjoined the student of yoga to water the field with the help of yogic practices and renunciation so that the consciousness becomes stainless and the Self shines forth.

Hans U. Rieker is to be commended for the accuracy of his representation of the original text and I hope his *YOGA OF LIGHT* will be read by yoga aspirants to help them savour the effects of yoga. Then I shall feel proud to have shared in its presentation.

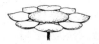

PHILOSOPHY OF *HAṬHA YOGA*

Philosophy is a view of life whereas yoga shows ways to practise the views of philosophy. The aim of *haṭha yoga* is to separate the mind from the contact of the body and then make the mind move closer towards the core of being, for the mind to merge with the Self.

I am deliberately using the term "philosophy of *haṭha yoga*". This subject is wrongly interpreted by present yogis and philosophers as physical yoga, which is far from truth. One should understand that *yama* and *niyama* are in the province of explanations on what to do and what not to do. *Āsana, prāṇāyāma, mudrā, bandha, pratyāhāra* and *dhāraṇā,* are both explanatory, experiential and expressive, while *dhyāna* and *samādhi* are purely experiential states and cannot be taught by instructions. These states are purely subjective. They have to be experienced individually. No words can explain that state though one may view them poetically.

Actually *Haṭhayoga Pradīpikā* is one of the most important technical textbooks on yoga dealing with the growth of the body and cultivation of the mind in order to have the sight of the soul as the final aim. It works in transforming the seeker to become the seer.

In order to understand *haṭha yoga* well, it is advisable to read other texts like *Śiva Saṁhitā, Gheraṇḍa Saṁhitā, Gorakṣa Śataka, Yoga Upaniṣads, Yoga Sūtra* of Patañjali and *Bhagavad Gītā*. Then the reader, whether a practitioner or not, perceives the true nature of *haṭha yoga* as a holistic science, art and philosophy. The text encompasses man as a whole from the gross body to the subtle and causal bodies, comprising anatomical, physiological, mental, intellectual and spiritual layers.

The text begins with the words *haṭha vidyā. Vidyā* means knowledge with discipline and attention; *haṭha* means persistency, determination, to stick fast, to be devoted, to hold closely and firmly, resoluteness, willpower and perseverance. Yoga means union, yoking, to get together, to associate. It also means zeal, endeavour, holding the body in a steady position and contemplation, and fixing the mind to a point.

WHAT REPRESENTS *HAṬHA YOGA*?

Haṭha yoga is a forceful discipline for transforming the inert *(tāmasic)* body to the level of the vibrant *(rājasic)* mind. When body and mind are equally vibrant, both are trained together to reach the serenity of the Self *(ātmā)* so that all three vehicles of man move with rhythm and concord towards illumination and emancipation.

If the word *haṭha* is separated as *ha* and *ṭha*, then *ha* stands for Self, inbreath, sun, seer and practice *(abhyāsa)*; whereas *ṭha* stands for nature, outbreath, moon, seen (consciousness) and renunciation *(vairāgya)*.

Haṭha yoga begins with the body, but it demands consistent physical, ethical, moral, mental and intellectual disciplines. Being a subjective science and philosophy, it builds in the practitioner the knowledge of using the right words, thoughts and deeds.

In *Chāndogya Upaniṣad* (chapter VII), *Bhūmavidyā* or *Brahmavidyā* (knowledge of *Brahma* or *ātma-vidyā)* has been explained in various ways. It begins with all sciences in the name of *Brahma*; "higher than name is speech that is *Brahma*; higher than speech is mind – *Brahma*; higher than mind is will – *Brahma*; higher than will is consciousness – *Brahma*; *dhyāna* is higher than consciousness that is *Brahma*; higher than *dhyāna* is *vijñāna* (discriminative power) – *Brahma*; higher than *vijñāna* is strength that is *Brahma*; higher than strength is food *(anna)* and *anna* is *Brahma*; higher than food is water, so water is *Brahma*; higher than water is fire, hence fire is *Brahma*; higher than fire is ether, that is *Brahma*; higher than ether is memory, this is *Brahma*; higher than memory is aspiration, it is *Brahma*; higher than aspiration or wish is energy *(prāṇa)*. *Prāṇa* is *Brahma* as *prāṇa* is the living self *(jīvātman)*. This is truth and truth is *Brahma*. From truth, one realises the seer, the nectar of life, and this is true bliss and this is *Brahma*".

This quotation from *Chāndogya Upaniṣad* is enough for us to know the importance of *prāṇa* as *Brahma*, since *haṭha yoga's* main emphasis is on *prāṇa*. Its principal aim is the growth of *prāṇa śakti* or the storing of energy from the breath. If the inflow of breath has one gate, the outflow has another; whereas mind has many gates through which it can jump out and wander. As breath has not so many gates, Svātmārāma advises us to control breath.

According to *Praśna Upaniṣad*, energy *(prāṇa)* and awareness *(prajñā)* move together. If consciousness is the rider, *prāṇa* or energy is the horse. Both are dependent upon one another. If one leaves the body, the other follows. Hence the philosophy of *haṭha yoga* is to interpenetrate from the external sheath of man, the body, over the bridge, i.e. energy, so that energy *(prāṇa)* and awareness *(prajñā)* join *jīvātman* or the living core of being. This unity of *prāṇa* and *prajñā* with *ātmā* is the aim of *haṭha yoga*.

ERADICATION OF IMPEDIMENTS

We get tormented with three states of affliction. These may be direct, induced or abetted, tormenting us in mild, middle or intense degree according to our ways of thinking and acting.

Patañjali speaks of afflictions and fluctuations that create not only disharmony between body and mind, but are impediments to spiritual pursuit. Both *haṭha yoga* and *pātañjala yoga* are meant to eradicate such impediments that come in the way of salvation.

All our ways of thinking and acting revolve around the six spokes of the wheel of emotions. These are lust, anger, greed, infatuation, pride and jealousy. They cause the above three types of afflictions and nine types of diseases, namely, physical diseases, langour, doubt, carelessness, physical lethargy, self-indulgence, living in the world of illusions, lack of perseverance and inability to maintain what is achieved.

Haṭha yoga helps one to come out of these emotional upheavals by keeping the body healthy and light and minimising or freeing the consciousness from mental turmoils so that it earns stability, clarity and cleanliness to remain free from intellectual, emotional and instinctive defects.

Svātmārāma says, "Mind is the Lord of senses, energy is the Lord of the mind and the rhythmic vibration in the inner body is the Lord of energy" (*H.Y.P.*, IV.29).

Yoga is one. The essence and principle of yoga remains the same though its titles differ from each other.

Mind is an internal sense of perception organising the functions of the senses of perception and organs of action. These external organs and senses act as windows for attachment and aversion, which feed into the mind, intelligence and consciousness.

Man should have the power of cognisance *(jñāna)* to understand this feedback system of worldly desires, pleasures and freedom from pleasurable objects. This knowledge *(jñāna)* is of two types: one is mundane, pertaining to the material world; the other is of the spiritual world. Both are necessary for life on this planet. Both have to be blended together for one to become a perfect yogi. Without proper understanding of the body, it becomes the temple of pain, pleasure or disease *(bhogamandiram* or *rogamandiram)*. By right use of the temple, auspiciousness and purity *(yogamandiram* or *divyamandiram)* set in.

Therefore *Haṭhayoga* is a powerful structure offering practical guidelines so that the beginner is firmly established in stabilising the body and keeping it healthy with a calm mind, in order to ignite zeal for intellectual aspiration to move towards the sight of the soul. It ends in emancipation.

Even Shri Ādi Shankara, in his work on *Aparokṣānubhūti,* says that *haṭha yoga* is intended for those whose nature requires to be purged from all impurities (see also *Y.S.,* II.28).

Both Patañjali and Svātmārāma explain the aim of yoga as *ātma sākṣātkāra.* If Patañjali's yoga is called *aṣṭāṅga yoga* or "eight-petalled yoga", *haṭha yoga* is known as *ṣaḍāṅga yoga.* Gheraṇḍa, in his treatise *Gheraṇḍa Saṁhitā,* called this yoga *ghaṭa yoga. Ghaṭa* means pot. The body is the pot or vessel of the Self; hence it is known as *ghaṭavidyā).* As an unbaked earthen pot thrown in water dissolves, the body too decays if unattended and not baked in the fire of yoga.

This yoga can be practised by young or old, afflicted, disabled and weak without fear (*H.Y.P.,* I.64). Its only demand is zeal and courage. Its perfection is felt in slimness of the body, brightness in the face, glow in the eyes, a clean and clear tone, stimulating the digestive system with perfect control over the seminal fluid and purity in the nervous system (*H.Y.P.,* II.78).

These results of *haṭha yoga* lead one towards *samādhi.*

Here are some of the quotes from *Haṭhayoga Pradīpikā* in which the spiritual zenith or *samādhi* is dealt with:

a) When salt is disolved in water, the taste is the same at the top, the middle and the bottom. Similarly, through yoga, the body and mind get absorbed by the Self and all appear as Self (IV.59).

b) Silence in breath brings silence in the consciousness (IV.23).

c) When the vessel is empty, it is filled with air and when filled with water, it is full with water. In the same way, body and mind transform to the level of the Self and are illuminated with the flame of the Self (*H.Y.P.,* IV.56).

d) As flame, wick and oil become one when lighted, body, intelligence and consciousness become one when engulfed in the Self.

e) Camphor and flame become one when lighted. So the consciousness and the Self become one with the flame of yoga (IV.59).

f) Like the wood that is consumed by the fire, similarly, when the consciousness is free from desire for objects, attachment and aversion end, and it rests on the lap of the soul.

g) If Self is the seed, yoga is the field and desirelessness the water. By soaking the body with water of desirelessness and sowing the seed of the Self, one frees oneself from actions which entrain afflictions (IV.104).

h) Time and actions do not bind him, and no object of the world influences him (IV.108). This is *haṭha yoga.*

HAṬHA YOGA AND *PĀTAÑJALA YOGA**

Friends and colleagues of yoga,
It is a great honour for me to stand in front of you to exchange views on my practice with your practices, so that you and I can build up a firm foundation in the field of yoga to express that illuminated wisdom that comes through its regular practice. With all the explanations and books available, there is tremendous misunderstanding about me. Many people believe that I am a physical yogi; a yogi who uses props; a yogi who teaches cosmetic yoga. I hear these words wherever I go. It hurts me that one practitioner differentiates and categorises another practitioner of yoga, though you and I, as students of yoga, practise the same art.

Yoga is union. Union of what? Union of me with you. Forget about union with God. If man and man cannot come together, cannot understand each other, why should we think of union with God? In order to clarify that, I wanted to say a few words on *haṭha yoga*. As many of us know, *ha* is a solar energy, *ṭha* is a lunar energy. *Ha* stands for the energy which we call *prāṇa vāhinī*. It is the atmospheric energy which is drawn through the gross air by the practice of *āsana* and *prāṇāyāma*, and converted into bio-energy. *Ṭha* stands for the river of consciousness which is there in the system. Yoga is to unite and integrate together the vital energy and the conscious energy, so that one enjoys the eternal flow of peace and poise, in oneself and with others. This is the goal *(dhyeya)* of *haṭha yoga*. Even from the *Yoga Sūtra* of Patañjali, one can visualise *ha* and *ṭha* in a different way. *Abhyāsa* means positive effort; *vairāgya* means negative touch. It means renunciation. It means to renounce that which obstructs the practice. That which comes in the way of yoga practice should be discarded so that a positive approach in practice is maintained.

Therefore, what is the difference between Patañjali's *Yoga Sūtra* and *haṭha yoga*? Do you know that in the *Haṭhayoga Pradīpikā* not more than fifteen *āsana* are explained? With

---

* Lecture on the 19th May 1984 at the Bharatiya Vidya Bhavan, London, U.K., for the teachers of the British Wheel of Yoga. Reported in *Yoga Today*, vol. 9, no. 7, November 1984.

these fifteen *āsana*, does it become a work on physical yoga? Take the case of Patañjali's *Yoga Sūtra*. Vyāsa, in his commentary, has given eleven *āsana* with names. Then how is it that nobody calls it physical yoga? Only lazy yogis say that sitting in any comfortable posture is enough.

What is a comfortable posture? I put that question to you. If you sit in one position, in a few minutes you would want to change that position for another. When you so how can you say that you were in a comfortable pose? Patañjali's *Yoga Sūtra* says that when the effort of performing the *āsana* is deliberate and that deliberate effort becomes a non-deliberate effort or a state of effortless effort, then one can say that one has mastered the posture. He never says sit in any comfortable pose. When the effort becomes effortless, the firmness in the body and stability in our mind get settled. This is how Patañjali defines an *āsana*.

Sthiratā here refers to the body. *Sukhatā* does not mean that the body enjoys the pleasure of the pose. It is something inside the body that has to say, "Very lovely". That *sukha* according to Patañjali, means grace of the intelligence. So when the intelligence of the body gets firmness and poise, that *āsana* is mastered. Each *āsana* when practised has to reach that state of poise in the self and firmness in the body. Here, he does not refer to one *āsana*. Even the commentators have not said anywhere of sitting in any comfortable pose.

Where do you reach by the practice of *āsana?* The dualities within each individual are vanquished. The dualities between body-mind and self are removed. Though it is a subjective art, they say honour, dishonour, pleasure and pain disappear. These are objective terminologies. What is the subjective one? Subjective is body, mind and self. So, when the dualities between the body, mind and self vanish and these three become one, where is the place for honour and dishonour? Where is the place for heat and cold? When you are in good sleep does honour or dishonour affect you? Does heat and cold affect you? So one has to follow the practice till these dualities are vanquished.

When Patañjali speaks of yoga, he says that unless and until you have acquired perfection in *āsana* you cannot practise *prāṇāyāma* at all. But what are we doing today? Let us look at the characteristics required for the practitioner. *Haṭhayoga Pradīpikā* says: tremendous desire, courage, the hidden force in you are required. Patañjali says: faith, courage, tremendous memory, awareness and absorption in what you are doing are required. I am taking a few *śloka* from *Haṭhayoga Pradīpikā* for you to compare to that of a *sūtra* of *pātñjala yoga* to give you an idea that if you go deep into the texts, you will find absolutely no differences.

Yoga Sūtra has four chapters: *Samādhi Pāda*, *Sādhana Pāda*, *Vibhūti Pāda* and *Kaivalya Pāda* – *kaivalya* means to be alone, free from the body and mind – the seed of all our movements; when you reach that, then you understand what that oneness means, what that aloneness means. *Haṭhayoga Pradīpikā* also has four chapters: the first deals with *āsana*, the second with *prāṇāyāma*, the third with *mudrā*, and the fourth with *samādhi*. See that *Haṭhayoga Pradīpikā* is a textbook which gives the essence of the practice as it appears in the form of *samādhi*.

Haṭha means willpower. Willpower is stronger than the intelligence. You may be tremendously intelligent but if there is no willpower your intelligence has no value; it is rusted. Similarly, *ha* means Self and *ṭha* consciousness, one supplementing and complementing the other. When so many people of today are practising this noble art, let us open a new chapter, let us not divide ourselves by dividing this one word, yoga. Yoga is one; why do people call it by different names, as the aspects of yoga do not vary at all? If some start from the top to understand the bottom, some others may start from the bottom and reach the top. Both convey the same thoughts. Both texts are *mokṣaśāstra*, the science of liberation, freedom and beatitude.

Patañjali starts with the consciousness, because he had already written a book on medicine, or the knowledge of the body. Having written a treatise on the knowledge or wisdom of the body and another on grammar, he started to deal with the functions of mind, intelligence and consciousness. As he was an evolved soul, he started with the development of the mind and consciousness according to the intellectual standard of his day. He speaks of *nirbīja samādhi* in the very first chapter. *Nirbīja* means a state of being alone where words, meaning and expressions come out without any colour of book knowledge or words of the vedas. This state being a seedless state, is known as *nirbīja*. If one reaches this state, then all processes of the intelligence and consciousness sprout directly from the soul that has no other seed at all.

He could have closed the *Yoga Sūtra* there alone, after fifty-one *sūtra*. But one hundred and forty-five more *sūtra* continue afterwards. Perhaps he realised: "I jumped in immediately and spoke about the consciousness, but I have not touched on the body or the mind at all". Hence, he composed the second chapter, known as *Sādhana Pāda*. It is for those who are not initiated. Through this *pāda* he initiates them. I also say that even though you have evolved, remember that still you may get caught in the web of objects of the world, you may by chance fall from grace on account of temptations. He guides us with compassion to practise in order to maintain the development which we have gained.

Then he moves to the third chapter where he explains the effect of meditation and the experiences that the yogi realises through meditation. These are known as *vibhūti* or accomplishments, and not as supernatural powers. This terminology is used by others, and not by Patañjali. Patañjali says that if a real practitioner can continue his practices uninterruptedly, he will come across various experiences, which appear unnatural or supernatural to an average man, but not to the *sādhaka*. Patañjali fears lest those who are caught in such accomplishments forget the path of *samādhi*. He explains about thirty-five various experiences in order to give an impetus to the practitioner so that he can see whether he is on the right path or not. He says that if one of these is experienced, consider that you are on the right path and you must continue without being trapped. If you are caught, retribution may destroy you. These successes are meant only to observe whether your method of practice is right or wrong. Then you have to go ahead, without paying any attention to these successes but to proceed to touch that pure exalted high state of intelligence without any bias.

When that highest state of exalted intelligence is touched, the soul and the intelligence become one; they know the difference between moments and the cycles of moments experienced as movements and they will not be caught in the cycle of *karma* or *karma phala* (fruit of *karma*). He wants the yogi to live only in the moment, and when the moment conjoins like a spur to the next moment, he does not want the yogi to be caught in that next spur but to flow with that exalted intelligence. Then the yogi experiences a state where his action is free from white (good), grey (mixed) and black (bad) actions. This state is beyond the three qualities, which we call *sattva* (luminosity), *rajas* (vibrancy) and *tamas* (inertia). When the yogi goes beyond these three qualities, he reaches an exalted state of intelligence, which is the aim of both *pātañjala yoga* and *haṭha yoga*.

The fourth chapter definitively explains the quality of the evolved self and how he has to serve society and not live in a closed room. Having reached that state of knowledge, how he should work in the world as a *karmin* is explained. Without getting involved in presenting his actions, he works in such a way that his action has no reaction on him. As there are no reactions, he has no fluctuations or afflictions. As he is free from all fluctuations and afflictions, he is considered a man of *dharma*. It means a religious person. The yogi having reached the highest state of *jñāna*, acts through that *jñāna* in the world as a witness without himself becoming afflicted. He remains pure and his pure wisdom flows like torrential rain pouring from the clouds, and he remains in that pristine state. This is the background that I wanted to give you.

I hope after listening we stop our bickerings about which yoga is more important and work together as a unit to build up not only a healthy society but also a sound human race as a whole.

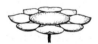

VIṆĀDAṆDA

I am indeed delighted to associate myself with the great living yogi Śri Raghavendra Swamijī of Malladihalli, Chitradurga, Karnataka. He is a true karma yogi who is just living to give all his energies not only to affluent society but also to the lowest and the lost who are more dear to him than the former. His knowledge in yoga is supreme and he willingly imparts this gift of India – yoga – freely to one and all. It is our great good fortune that this sage is ninety years old, but moves like a child of nine. His walk, talk, perfect physical form and mood are an ideal example for anyone to follow, in whatever path one treads.

It is no doubt a fitting tribute to this great sage to bring out the Bṛhad Yoga Darśana to commemorate the silver jubilee function of his centre – Patañjali Yoga Śāstra Śikṣaṇa Kendra – through his teachings, for perfect health of the body, harmony of the mind and reflection of the soul.

It was kind of the editors of Bṛhad Yoga Darśana to ask me to write an article on Vīṇādaṇda (vīṇā = lute) or Merudaṇda (Meru = Gem, name of a mountain), which is commonly known as the spinal column. Though I am not fit for this honour, I, in my own humble way, try to explain the importance of Vīṇādaṇda and seek swamijī's blessings and forgiveness for my shortcomings.

Some say that Lord Ādiśeṣa descended in the shape of a small snake into the palm of Goṇikā. It is said that Goṇikā – the daughter of a sage – prayed to the Sun-God for a son. At once Ananta, the king of the serpents, fell on her palms in the form of a sage. Hence he is named Patañjali.

After intense *sādhanā*, he was blessed with supreme knowledge and wisdom. He wrote three famous treatises namely (a) on grammar, for correct and wise speech, (b) on *āyurveda*, for the purity of the body and (c) on yoga, for control of *citta* – the consciousness.

WHAT IS *DARŚANA?*

Darśana means reflection. When objects are projected on a clean mirror, the mirror reflects the object as it is. Yoga is an art, it acts as a clean mirror which reflects clearly the body, the senses, the mind, the intellect and the self of the *sādhaka* in their true states when its *sādhanā* is perfected. Hence it is called *yoga-darśana*.

BODY – THE *KṢETRA* OR THE FIELD

In order to build a house, pillars are first erected on a firm foundation. The bricks are placed and constructed one above the other systematically, firmly and uniformly so that the inhabitants may dwell in it comfortably and peacefully.

Similarly the various petals of *pātañjala yoga* are to make the dweller *(ātmā)* be at peace in his dwelling place (body). Christ says that the body is the temple of the soul. The yogi goes one step further and says that it is the duty of man to keep the body healthy and pure for its Lord – the *ātman* – to dwell in.

The first five petals of yoga, namely *yama, niyama, āsana, prāṇāyāma* and *pratyāhāra* are very important in any field of science or philosophy. *Yama* cultivates and protects the *karmendriya, niyama* disciplines the *jñānendriya, āsana* keeps the entire human system healthy, *prāṇāyāma* distributes the vital energies to the cells without any interruption, and *pratyāhāra* stills the oscillations of the mind. When these are achieved, then the divine marriage takes place between the *kṣetra* (the field or the body) and the *kṣetrajña* (the knower of the field, or the *ātmā*). This is the *darśana* or reflection of the Self on the body and vice versa.

VĪṆĀDAṆDA

In *Darśanopaniṣad* (IV.6), mention has been made of the spinal column as *vīṇādaṇda* without explaining why it is called so.

While one is practising *āsana, prāṇāyāma* or *dhyāna*, the emphasis is on the spinal column called *merudaṇda* or *vīṇādaṇda*. *Vīṇā* means a lute - an Indian musical instrument with strings. Why there is this special stress on the spinal column is interesting to observe and note.

Vīṇā is the instrument of Goddess Sarasvatī - the Goddess of knowledge. It is a perfect instrument on which one can play any *rāga* without accompaniment by other instruments. *Rāga* is a combination of an orderly sound, harmony, rhythm and melody. *Vīṇā* represents the human spine and brain. The head of the *vīṇā* (the round gourd) is the brain, the sound box is the breathing process. The stem is the spinal column, the knobs are the spinal vertebrae and the strings are the nervous system.

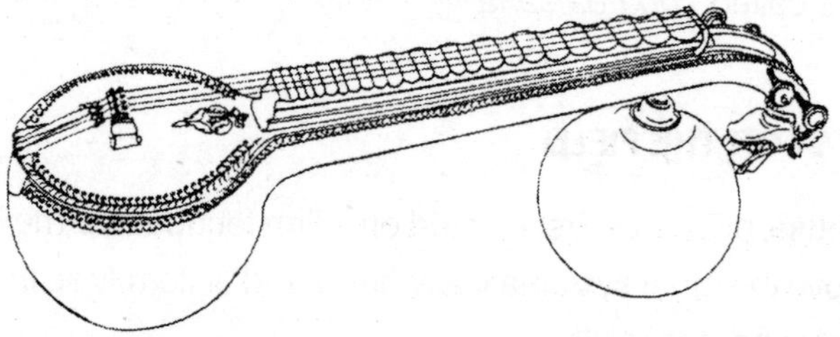

If the gourd is not round and firm with no holes, if the bridge is not rested correctly or the knobs neither tight nor loose, the strings snap or lose their potency and even a master musician cannot produce a sound or play a *rāga* on that *vīṇā*. Our spine can be easily compared to the *vīṇā*. The brain floats on the head of the spine which is the seat of *savitarka* (right logic) and *savicāra* (right reasoning). If the vertebrae of the spine are not kept trim, then the nerves do not get sufficient nourishment and the breathing becomes shallow, affecting the circulatory and digestive systems.

The end part of the *vīṇā* is the *mūlādhāra cakra*. The yogis discovered *āsana* and *prāṇāyāma* in order to carefully exercise the spine, from its base, for the healthy growth of intelligence. When the *vīṇā* is properly tuned, the musician and music become one. By the practice of yoga, the yogi is in tune with the *nāda* of Brahmā and his abode becomes a heaven on earth. If the spine is neglected, then this abode of the *ātmā* becomes the place for *roga* (disease) and leads him to hell on earth.

It is also called *merudaṇḍa*. According to a mythological story, the fabulous mountain Meru is the central point around which the land on Earth exists like islands. The spine is considered the centre of the body to which our physical, physiological, mental, intellectual and spiritual aspects of existence unite. Hence the spine is called *merudaṇḍa*.

We all know the story of Daḍhīci - the great sage who gave away his spine for Lord Indra to make the *vajra* (thunderbolt - the Lord Indra's weapon) to fight the demon Vṛttrāsura. Demon Vṛttrāsura is disease; Daḍhīci stands for happiness and the spine *(vajrāyudha)* which Indra used to fight the demon - the disease *(vṛttrāsura)* - is to be kept healthy.

As each *āsana* has a specific function to play, innumerable *āsanas* were invented to keep the spine strong and healthy. The spine has thirty-three vertebrae. From the spine the nerves get nourishment as the spine is the source of energy supply. It is said that if the entire nervous system of the body is stretched like a single string, it would be about 6,000 to 7,000 miles in length. This suffices to say why so many *āsana* need to be practised and how far and how much they have to be perfected.

The *Varāhopaniṣad* says that the nerves penetrate the body from the crown of the head to the soles of the feet. The body is not merely a bundle of muscles but a vast net of nerves. Yoga texts proclaim 72,000 *nāḍīs* originating from *kandasthāna* (navel area) and each branching off with 72,000 *nāḍīs*. In the same way, 101 *nāḍīs* originate from the seat of *ātmā* (spiritual heart), each having 72,000 branches except one. This one is called the *citrā nāḍī*, which passes through *suṣumṇā* to unite with *brahmarandhra* at the seat of the head.

Cakra are like the flywheels of a gigantic machine. The *vīṇādaṇḍa* has seven *cakra* or chambers. They are *mūlādhāra*, *svādhiṣṭhāna*, *maṇipūraka*, *anāhata*, *viśuddhi*, *ājñā* and *sahasrāra*. As there are *saptasvaras* (seven notes) sa, ri, ga, ma, pa, dha, ni, in music, so also the spinal column has *saptacakra* to climb from *bhūloka* or the terrestrial world *(mūlādhāra)* to *vaikuṇṭha* or the abode of Vishnu *(sahasrāra)*, in order to experience the Infinite and live in that state.

Antennae pick up radio waves and transform them into sounds through radio sets. *Cakra* too pick up the vital energy from the breath we draw in, to be distributed throughout the body for healthy functioning of life in man. When each *cakra* is synchronised and made to function in unison through the disciplines of yoga, the energy of the *ātmā* flows like a river in the *citrā* channel, through the passage of *suṣumṇā*, for the *sādhaka* to merge in the ocean of *sahasrāra*. Then the *sādhaka* is in tune with the brilliance of *ātman* reflecting in his true glory without the vehicles of the *karmendriya*, *jñānendriya*, *manas*, *buddhi* and 'I'-ness.

By keeping the *vīṇādaṇḍa* active and dynamic, the gross and the subtle bodies in us become healthy and mobile and we develop strong willpower with intellectual clarity. The yogi acquires beauty in his words, grace in his action and strength in himself to face life with a calm mind in all situations. Hence yoga *sādhanā*, particularly *āsana* and *prāṇāyāma*, is the fountain for all yogas. By training the *vīṇādaṇḍa*, we keep the *karmendriya* clean for *karma*, *jñānendriya* clear for *jñāna* and the mind and intelligence pure for *bhakti* to surrender ourselves to God or *Paramātmā*.

(1981)

PHYSIOLOGY AND *CAKRA* *

Physiology is a science dealing with the organic processes or functions of living organisms, or their parts in living bodies.

The human body is like a sophisticated machine, but God made. It is an instrument and the apparatus of the soul – the *ātman.* It has three tiers: gross body, subtle body and causal body. These three bodies are demarcated and simplified as sheaths. There are five sheaths known as the anatomical, physiological, psychological, intellectual and the spiritual sheaths[1].

The subtle body is in between the gross or material body and the causal body and hence it is called the middle body. This middle body covers the physiological, mental and intellectual sheaths. This tier being the bridge between the outer and the innermost bodies, becomes the prime factor of thought creation, projection, mutation, fluctuation, modification and modulation. On account of these facets, it becomes the abode of dualities like pain and pleasure, heat and cold and honour and dishonour.

Consequently, all yoga texts advise us to control and sublimate this middle tier of man.

It is the seat of consciousness, which consists of mind, intelligence and 'I'. However, the consciousness *(citta)* acts as the seer *(dṛṣṭā),* seeing, viewing or beholding *(dṛṣṭi)* and as object to be looked at or worth seeing *(dṛśya).* It has the power to evoke, appease, entice and store experiences.

The practice of yoga takes the practitioner beyond mind, intelligence and 'I' to experience that light which never fades. This is the light of the soul or *ātman.*

Wise men discovered and prescribed the ways of practice and renunciation to restrain this middle tier of man and named the ways as the science and philosophy of yoga *(yoga śāstra),* commonly known as *aṣṭāṅga yoga* (the eight petalled yoga).

---

* Talk by B.K.S. Iyengar on his 70th birthday. See also the article entitled *Cakra, Bandha and Kriya.*

1 See Table n. 4

EFFECTS OF YOGA

Practice is an evolutionary path *(pravṛtti mārga)* and renunciation is an involutionary path *(nivṛtti mārga),* though both are evolutionary in one sense. Here, methods to trace the source of consciousness are shown in order to cultivate inner discipline and enjoy unalloyed freedom.

The first four petals of *aṣṭāṅga yoga,* namely *yama, niyama, āsana* and *prāṇāyāma,* are the evolutionary methods as they connect the self to nature. These practices not only give health but purify and sanctify the body, bringing clarity in thought by sharpening the intelligence. The petal of *pratyāhāra* is a bridge between the evolutionary and involutionary practices. The last three petals of yoga, *dhāraṇā, dhyāna* and *samādhi,* are the involutionary or the inward path, a return journey towards God. This latter part of yoga turns man's middle body (the subtle body) towards the causal body, the abode of the soul. Through these various disciplines of yoga, the middle body soon realises the worthlessness of going out to satisfy the gross body.

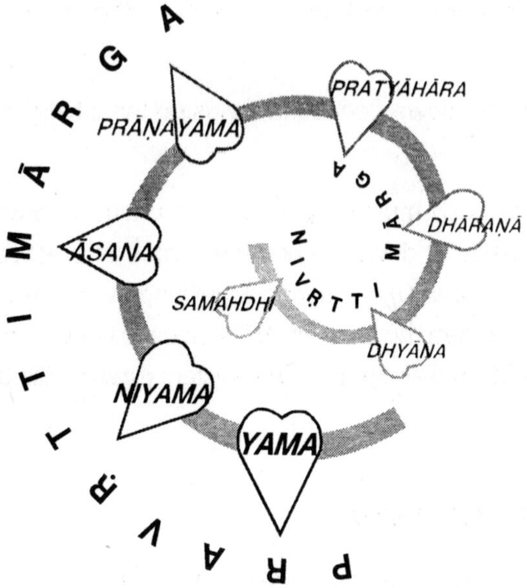

The three tiers of *sādhanā*

Bahiraṅga Sādhanā
yama
niyama
āsana
prāṇāyāma
pratyāhāra

Antaraṅga Sādhanā
dhāraṇā
dhyāna

Antarātma Sādhanā
samādhi

Table n. 5 – *Pravṛtti* and *nivṛtti mārga* in *aṣṭadaḷa yoga*

The first petal of yoga starts from the periphery towards the source with *yama.* It is not only character building but also acts in controling the organs of action. The second petal, *niyama,* helps to discipline the senses of perception. The third petal, *āsana,* cultures the cells of the body; the fourth petal, *prāṇāyāma* stores and evenly distributes energy throughout the body; the fifth petal, *pratyāhāra,* disciplines the mind directly. The sixth petal, *dhāraṇā,* sharpens the intelligence to develop maturity; the seventh petal, *dhyāna,* helps to quieten the consciousness, and the last, the eighth petal, *samādhi,* takes the practitioner towards the source, the sight of the soul *(ātma-darśana).*

We are made up of the respiratory, circulatory, digestive, nervous, glandular and genito-excretory systems. Each one is dependent upon the other for healthy rhythmic functions. The secretions of the hormonal system are considered to be an essential factor for the tranquillity of the mind. The house of all these various systems is the spinal column *(merudaṇḍa).* The spine, its muscles, its nerves and its fluid keep all these systems functioning in concord. The science of yoga was aptly discovered by yogis in order to culture the *merudaṇḍa* or *viṇādaṇḍa* so that the shoots of the spine like the fibres, sinews, cells, nerves, senses, mind, intelligence, ego and consciousness are kept healthy and clear.

Practice and renunciation have to be followed concurrently using the intelligence for analysis and discernment.

By right practice, the sanctity of the body must be built up and maintained and the intelligence sharpened. For earning this quality of development three types of practices are suggested. They are the drying up system *(śoṣana kriyā),* filtering or refining system *(śodhana kriyā)* and appeasing, soothing or quenching system *(śamana kriyā).* These three types of practice are not only in *āyurveda* (vedic system of medicine) and nature cure system *(prakṛti cikitsā kriyā)* but also in yoga *kriyā.*

THE SPINAL COLUMN *(MERUDAṆḌA* OR *VINADAṆḌA)*

The spinal column has different parts such as coccyx, sacral, lumbar, dorsal and cervical regions. Networks of plexuses and ductless glands are situated in contact with the various parts of the spinal column, and they can cause either disturbances in health and poise or help to build up good physical health and mental poise.

Yogis studied the human body in their own ways, particularly the spinal column. Through their intuitive capacity they studied the energy centres within the spinal cord and named them *cakra.* This study gave them experience beyond body and mind.

CAKRA

Cakra means a wheel, a diagram, a cycle or a circle. As the wheel of a gigantic machine is connected to a flywheel, round which the entire machine moves like a chain, similarly the rhythmic discharge of the *cakra* affects the functioning of physical, physiological, mental, mystical and spiritual depressions or elations. *Cakra* is the store house of power; there are seven in number. They are *mūlādhāra, svādhiṣṭhāna, maṇipūraka, anāhata, viśuddhi, ājñā* and *sahasrāra.*

Because of the location of various *cakra* as explained in yoga texts, many authors hold them to represent the plexuses or ductless glands. The *cakra* may or may not be these, though their situation corresponds very closely. If plexuses and glands work on psycho-physiological levels, *cakra* work at the level of spiritual enlightenment. As *cakra* deal with spiritual growth, they are beyond words or expression and hence may remain as mysterious as they are now.

All *cakra* are associated with the five elements of nature and its qualities *(guṇa).* The *cakra* seem to be circular *(maṇḍala)* with different designs like petals *(daḷa).*

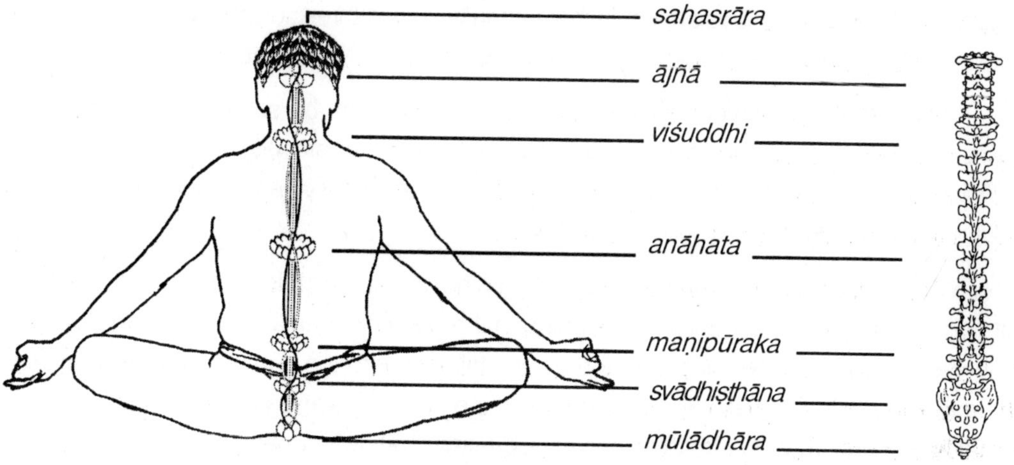

Table n. 6 – *Cakra, pañcabhūta anuguṇa saṁuccaya*

Mūlādhāra cakra belongs to the element of earth *(pṛthvī-tattva)* with four petals and is of *tāmasic* nature. *Svādhiṣṭhāna cakra* belongs to the water element *(āp-tattva)* with six petals and by nature is *tāmasic* also. *Maṇipūraka cakra,* with the element of fire, is *rājasic* and has ten petals. *Anāhata cakra* too is *rājasic* by nature, connected to the element of air *(vāyu-tattva)* and has twelve petals. *Viśuddhi cakra* belongs to the element of ether *(ākāśa-tattva),* has sixteen petals and is *sāttvic* while *ājñā cakra,* which is pure *sāttvic,* has two petals and is connected with the principle of intelligence *(buddhi-tattva).* The last one, *sahasrāra cakra,* is filled with the principle of the *puruṣa,* the Self *(ātma-tattva).* These petals *(daḷa),* represent the fifty letters of the *Sanskṛt* alphabet.

Many are under the impression that Patañjali does not speak of *cakra.* It is far from true. Not only does he but also Sage Vyāsa speak in regard to *cakra* in *sūtra* one of chapter three.

For example, Patañjali mentions *nābhicakra* (*Y.S.,* III.30) for *maṇipūraka cakra; kaṇṭakūpa* (III.31) (well of the throat) for *viśuddhi cakra; mūrdha jyoti* (III.33) for *ājñā cakra* and *hṛdaya* (III.35) for *anāhata cakra.*

Similarly, Sage Vyāsa uses *nābhicakra, hṛdya puṇḍarīka (hṛt* = self; *puṇḍarīka* = white lotus = the seat of God in each individual), *mūrdhani* (forehead), *jyotiṣi* (light, eye, as focal points), *naśikāgra* (tip of the nose), *jihvāgra (viśuddhi)* for concentration and meditation *(dhāraṇā* and *dhyāna).*

NERVOUS SYSTEM

In order to know the functions of the plexuses, glands or *cakra,* one should know something about the nervous system. This system in the human body has three tiers. They are the peripheral nervous system, autonomous nervous system and central nervous system.

The peripheral nervous system gets its feedback from the senses of perception and organs of action. The autonomous nervous system is semi-voluntary as it functions on its own as well as through the volition of the mind. The central nervous system is electrifying, dynamic and functions with the help of judicial intelligence.

The *cakra* are hidden in the core of the spinal canal, which is said to be thinner than a hair and have access to the entire functioning of the body. As mentioned earlier, the *cakra* are within the spinal cord spreading from the base – tailbone – to the apex of the brain – crown of the head. The cord being exactly in the centre of the body, the yogis named it *madhyama nāḍī* or middle nerves. Thus, the middle nerves represent the central nervous system of modern medicine.

We are all aware that with all of the modern scientific equipments, very little is known about this central nervous system. According to the yogis, the energy discharged from the *cakra* is known as life force *(prāṇa śakti* or *jīva śakti),* while the autonomous nervous system is said to be on the right and left sides of the spinal column as an inner part of the nerves *(antaraṅga bhāga);* and peripheral nerves are external *(bahiraṅga bhāga).* Though the functioning of the central nervous system still eludes modern science, it was known and understood by the yogis through their intuition and deep study.

It is said that if the entire nervous system is cut and connected as a single thread it would run to 6,000 miles (9,600 kilometres) while all the blood vessels (arteries, veins and capillaries) if joined run to 60,000 miles (96,000 kilometres). The Indians call even the blood vessels *nāḍīs*. How the Indian sages traced all these systems without sophisticated laboratory equipment is a puzzle to scientists.

The yogis declared that the heart and navel are the centres of the intricate nervous system. They say that 72,000 nerves spring out from the bulb below the navel *(kandasthāna)*, each having 72,000 branches. In the same way 101 nerves originate from the heart centre. Out of these 101 *nāḍīs* only 100 *nāḍīs* emanate with 72,000 branches. But the one *nāḍī* that sprouts from the heart centre has no branch. It is called *citrā nāḍī*, which pierces the *suṣumṇā nāḍī* at *mūlādhāra cakra*. The particularity of *citrā nāḍī* is that it has direct connection from the heart *(hṛdaya)* and to the head *(brahmarandhra)*. Hence, it is considered as a divine *nāḍī (divya nāḍī)* or a sacred *nāḍī (pavitra nāḍī)*.

Yoga texts give various names to *nāḍī*. Amongst them, *iḍā*, *piṅgalā* and *suṣumṇā* are the most important.

Iḍā nāḍī represents the lunar plexus or the parasympathetic nervous system. *Piṅgaḷā* represents the solar plexus or sympathetic nervous system or the autonomous nerves. *Iḍā* controls the emotional centres and *piṅgalā*, the physical and physiological centres. *Suṣumṇā* represents the central nervous system.

Iḍā and *piṅgaḷā* criss-cross each other at each *cakra* and power their energies in the *cakra* for use at times of emergency. When the peripheral and autonomous systems fail, the energy of the central nervous system keeps life going. Similarly, the energy stored in the *cakra* is released as energy at time of need.

KUṆḌALINĪ ŚAKTI (SERPENT POWER)

Kuṇḍalinī is divine energy lying latent or dormant at the *mūlādhāra cakra*. It is called *kuṇḍalinī* as it is coiled three and half times *(kuṇḍalākāra)*. *Kuṇḍala* also means snake. As the snake coils itself at rest, so does this *śakti* or power. The three and a half coils represent the three states, wakeful *(jāgrata)*, dreamy *(svapna)* and sleepy *(suṣupti)*, while the half coil stands for emancipated *(turīyā)* state.

When the *sādhaka* is free from lust, anger, greed, infatuation, pride and malice, the serpent power *(kuṇḍalinī śakti)* rises and flames up through yoga, or by the path of *jñāna*, *karma* or *bhakti*. Otherwise it remains latent or dormant at the base of the spine. The moment the *sādhaka* is free from the above six enemies as well as *triguṇa*, this *kuṇḍalinī* power opens the gate of *mūlādhāra cakra* and ascends chamber after chamber *(cakra* after *cakra)* like fire and reaches the cranium – the *sahasrāra cakra*.

As Lakṣmi is the consort of Lord Vishnu, Pārvati of Lord Shiva, Sarasvatī of Lord Brahmā, *Kuṇḍalinī* is the consort of the *jivātman*.

Kuṇḍalinī has many names. Sage Patañjali terms it *Prakṛti śakti* while others call it *Parameśvari, Bhujañginī, Kuṭilāngī, Īśvarī, Arundhatī, Prāṇa Devatā* and *Bālaraṇḍā (Bāla* = a youth; *raṇḍā* = a widow; *Bālaraṇḍā* = a young pure virgin widow). As the dormant *Kuṇḍalinī* is at the base of the spine, not having united with her lord *(puruṣa* or the Self*)*, it is compared to a young virgin widow. When the *sādhaka* is free from material influences and perseveres in the spiritual path with devotion, this young virgin lady moves at once to unite with her Lord through *brahmarandhra* at *sahasrāra*.

The fluid in the spine acts as a thermometer of the physical, physiological and mental actions and reactions. As temperature runs high, so the mercury rises. Similarly the fluid in the spine ascends or descends according to the activities of the organic and mental bodies. Practice of yoga keeps this fluid of the spine in a steady state without fluctuations.

For example, if we are attentive and observant, we can feel the fluid rising while making an effort to sit erect. Soon it is possible to realise that though we are sitting straight and feeling the fluid low in the base of the spine, we jerk the spine often to keep it erect but do not notice the upward flow of the fluid. When it is so hard to notice this rise and fall of the felt spinal fluid, one can imagine how difficult it would be to observe the ascension of the mystical and spiritual *kuṇḍalinī śakti* at *mūlādhāra*, let alone have the power to maintain or retain it. Often the power may rise to the gate and go back to recoil in its old position.

ĀSANA, *MUDRĀ* AND *BANDHA*

In order to generate the *śakti* of *kuṇḍalinī*, *āsana*, *prāṇāyāma*, *mudrā* and *bandha* were invented and evolved. Their practice pierces the gates of *mūlādhāra* for *suṣumṇā* to receive the energy of *citrā nāḍī* and to allow it to pass through the other *cakra*. By various yogic methods, the cells, nerves, senses, mind, intelligence, ego and consciousness are purified and sanctified for the coiled divine energy to become erect and ascend towards the cranium to meet its Lord.

All the yogic practices help the visual intelligence *(darśana jñāna)* to penetrate inwards and to connect the consciousness *(citta)* with the soul *(ātman)*. Like *āsana* and *prāṇāyāma*, *bandha* and *mudrā* are many. The precise practice of them guides the *sādhaka* to know and understand that the energy oozing out is the same as the energy that oozes in. As common people quickly know the outlets of pleasures, the yogis experience pure delight when energy pours within. We are all aware of various outlets through which energy dissipates from the body. As there are outlets for energy, there are inlets for energy to flow in. These inlets are called *cakra*. If the outlets are blocked through yogic means, energy gets deposited in these various *cakra* creating heat, which stirs the *kuṇḍalinī* to move upwards.

In *Rudrayāmiḷā*, it is said *"mūlādhāre vasati śaktihi sahasrāre sadāśivaḥ"*. It means "*kuṇḍalinī* lives in the abode of *mūlādhāra* and *puruṣa* or *sadāśiva* (Self) at *sahasrāra*".

When *kuṇḍalinī* ascends, the *sādhaka* is chaste in thought, word and deed. He is an *ūrdhvaretan* (one who moves the life force towards *sahasrāra cakra* and lives in chastity). Here, he experiences the fourth state of self *(turīyāvasthā)*.

The three *nāḍī*; *iḍā*, *piṅgalā* and *suṣumṇā* are compared to the three sacred rivers of India, the Ganga, Yamuna and Sarasvatī. They are the sacred rivers in human beings.

As the river Sarasvatī is called *gupta nadi* (concealed river), so *suṣumṇā* is the *gupta nāḍī* (concealed channel of energy) of the human system.

As the subterranean river Sarasvatī is submerged in Ganga and Yamuna, *suṣumṇā* is hidden between *iḍā* and *piṅgalā*. The energy in *suṣumṇā* flows between these two *nāḍī* all over the body. Hence *suṣumṇā* is called the middle nerve or the central nerve.

When energy begins to flow in *suṣumṇā*, the forc e of *iḍā* and *piṅgalā* gets nullified. The energy flowing in *suṣumṇā* is *kuṇḍalinī*. When it flows perennially, the *sādhaka* becomes a yogi, a *jñāni*, a renunciate, a *jīvanmuktan*. This is *dharma megha samādhi* or *nirbīja samādhi*.

CAKRA, BANDHA AND *KRIYĀ*[*]

My prostrations to Lord Patañjali and to the master of all masters, Lord Nārāyaṇa, and to my beloved *Guru*, who enticed me to take this noble path of knowledge with action. I salute and bow to these three *guru*, and pay my respects to them before I begin. You know, the organisers asked me to sit on the platform while speaking. But I have chosen this corner because of my want of knowledge in this subject. In case something happens, I can hide my face in the corner.

This is the most mysterious subject in yoga physiology. You all have heard so much about physiology that I have very little to add to it. The seed is very small, but from it sprouts a gigantic tree. Unfortunately I have not gone beyond that seed and seedling, hence my knowledge of the subject has been of a very slow growth. As the subject, from its seed, has reached the extreme limit of growth, it is most difficult for me to cover.

The inner life force keeps each and every individual dynamically alive and kicking, yet this invisible force being subjective, is very difficult to express in terms of the science of physiology. Before going into the physiological aspect of man, we should know that as human beings we are made up of three elements. Not the elements of nature, but three principles: the body *(śarīra)*, the consciousness *(citta)* and then the seer *(ātman)*. When I speak of consciousness I mean not only the outermost layer or mind *(manas)*, but also the innermost layers like intelligence *(buddhi)* and 'I'-ness *(ahaṁkāra)*, which are very difficult to interpenetrate. Man has these three apparatuses, three instruments, which comprise a *maṇḍala* – body, mind and soul – like a universe mutating within man. Our sages spoke of three bodily frames or *śarīra* enveloping the soul, which are further divided into five sheaths. (Table n. 4).

The first, *kārya śarīra,* is the gross or anatomical body, consisting of one sheath, the sheath of nourishment. The second frame is *sūkṣma śarīra* or subtle body. The third frame, *kāraṇa śarīra* or causal body, is of one sheath, the *ānandamaya kośa* or the sheath of spiritual joy. It is the most interior, the most ethereal of the three bodies. However the second frame is the

---

[*] Lecture given by B.K.S. Iyengar, December 1988, to bring further light on his newly published article, *Physiology of cakra* (also in this volume).

connecting bridge or link between the physical and spiritual bodies. This second, as middle body, contains three sheaths: the physiological sheath (that includes the respiratory, circulatory, digestive, endocrine, excretory and genital systems); the psychological sheath (*manas* or mental) and the intellectual sheath *(buddhi)*, involving awareness, feeling, judgement and subjective experience.

Patañjali attributes tremendous importance to the middle body. As he describes in chapter I, *sūtra* 5 to 11, all actions are created by *vṛtti*. There are five kinds of *vṛtti*, causing mixed pain and pleasure, which may or may not be cognisable. When pleasure is visible, pain is hidden. When the pain is visible, pleasure is hidden. These *vṛtti* trigger this middle body – the physiological, psychological and intellectual sheaths – for the causal body and the gross body to act and react. By this, we see that this middle body is both a troublemaker and a troubleshooter. This middle body has to be brought under control by the life force *(prāṇa)* and the consciousness *(citta)*, as they are interwoven together. Where there is consciousness, there is life force. Where there is life force, there is consciousness. The *prāṇa* and *citta* cannot be separated. Hence, any reactions on these two not only act and react on themselves but also on the outer and inner bodies including facial expressions of dullness or contentment and serenity. Yogic physiology has a tremendous bearing on the psychology of each individual. Patañjali uses the terminology of the physiological functions in the first chapter when he says, *Pracchardana vidhāraṇābhyāṁ vā prāṇasya* (*Y.S.*, I.34). Restrain the outflow of breath, which is the art of releasing tension of the consciousness. When you are in the state of releasing the breath, which is a physiological action, the reaction may be tranquillising and appeasing on the mind. Patañjali wants us to maintain this steady tranquil state by extending and re-adjusting the out-breath with smooth and fine flow as well as pensive retention after the outbreath.

If mutations take place in the consciousness, the reactions are felt immediately in the entire nervous system, the respiratory system, the circulatory system, the digestive system, the glandular system, the excretory system and generative system. They all get boiled up. This reaction or boiling up of these systems affects the causal body. Patañjali says, *Vṛtti sārūpyam itaratra* (*Y.S.*, I.4). The causal body *(kāraṇa* or *ātma śarīra)* gets enmeshed according to the dictates and mutations of the consciousness. So the two *sūtra* of Patañjali cover the entire domain of human development.

As the *vṛtti sārūpyam* (the identification of the seer with the fluctuating consciousness) disturbs the physiological body as well as the psychological body, he wants silence to reign through *abhyāsa* and *vairāgya* (*Y.S.*, I.12-16). *Abhyāsa* is an evolutionary method *(pravṛtti mārga)* and *vairāgya* is the involutionary method *(nivṛtti mārga)*. *Abhyāsa* and *vairāgya* make a *maṇḍala*.

These two unite as two in one, similar to the mind, body and soul which are three in one, trinity in unity. *Abhyāsa* and *vairāgya*, united as one, bring poise and tranquillity. When there is tranquillity, energy is stored in the system. It is not wasted or dissipated at all. So the entire aim of yoga is to develop that *jñāna*, that knowledge which can take us in the right path of *abhyāsa* and *vairāgya* (*pravṛtti mārga* and the *nivṛtti mārga*). *Nivṛtti* means moving from the peripheral areas, from the external body, towards the inner body. The *pravṛtti mārga* means moving from the causal body towards the external body. Understanding inner intricacies and exploring inner channels by external means, conveys what *abhyāsa* and *vairāgya* represent.

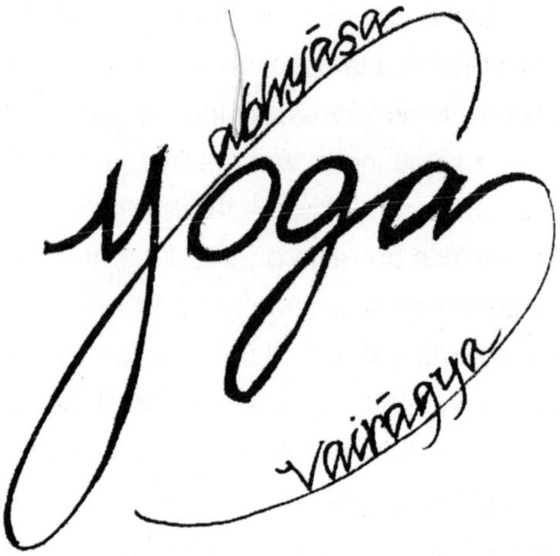

Table n. 7 – *Abhyāsa* and *vairāgya* (paths of evolution and involution)

Abhyāsa and *vairāgya* are both connected to *jñāna*. According to Patañjali, *jñāna* is *savitarkā jñāna*, *savicārā jñāna*, *sānanda jñāna* and *sāsmitā jñāna* known as *samprājñāta jñāna* (*Y.S.*, I.17). It is not just *jñāna*, but *prajñāna*. What is the difference between *jñāna* and *prajñāna? Jñāna* is an acquired knowledge, while *prajñāna* is an experienced knowledge. *Abhyāsa* and *vairāgya* help to develop *prajñāna*. Through acquired knowledge, we find out the pros and cons of objective knowledge in order to come to a final judgement in *savitarkā* and *savicārā*, so that we begin the subjective method in the form of *sānanda* and *sāsmitā*. However, one has to first develop *jñāna* to understand *prajñāna*.

The oscillating intelligence *(buddhivṛtti)* is stopped in *dhāraṇā*. When *buddhivṛtti* is stopped, then comes *cittavṛtti nirodha*. When *jñāna* becomes quiet, then *citta* too becomes quiet. The intelligence *(buddhi)* belongs to the heart while the intellect *(jñāna)*, to the head. In this state neither *jñāna* nor *buddhi* are shaky. *Buddhi* is one *(eka)*, like the *ātman*. This way, yoga takes us from the outer body, step by step, towards the middle body, and from there to the innermost centre, the *ātman*. Hence, *madhyama śarīra* is the right word. Yoga begins with the external sheath, the structural or muscular sheath (the *annamaya kośa* or *sthūla śarīra*). From here one breaks the barriers to enter the *antara śarīra (sūkṣma śarīra)*, which is the organic body or vital areas. The yogis call it *prāṇa śarīra*. After penetrating the physico-physio-psychological body, one penetrates further towards the *vijñānamaya kośa* which western science has never thought of at all. To them, everything is mind. Mind is a gatherer. Mind cannot judge.

The inner instrument of the mind i.e., intelligence alone judges. And that intelligence is *vijñāna*. That is why the yogis – who were scientists in their own way *(vijñāni)* – have used a better terminology for us to tread this path without any confusion. *Jñāna* must be developed into *vijñāna* and *vijñāna* into *prajñāna* and from *prajñāna* one is led towards the *ātman* – the divine source. The science and philosophy of yoga come to an end when an ordinary human being becomes a divine being *(prajñāni)*.

Now we come to *bandha, mudrā, cakra* and *kriyā*. The word *kriyā* is misunderstood in modern times. The *kriyā* of the *haṭha* yoga texts are very different from the *kriyā* of the *pātañjala Yoga Sūtra*. The *ṣaṭkriyā (dhauti, basti, neti, trāṭaka, nauli* and *kapālabhāti)* are on the physiological level, used in yogic texts to keep the vital organs healthy, provided they are not cured by any other means. Hence, they are never used for the growth of spiritual knowledge. They have remedial value to vanquish certain diseases, but should not be brought at all into the picture of *pātañjala kriyā yoga*.

Tapaḥ svādhyāya Īśvarapraṇidhānāni kriyāyogaḥ (*Y.S.*, II.1). Patañjali's *kriyā*, namely *tapas, svādhyāya, Īśvara praṇidhāna*, are practical. *Abhyāsa* and *vairāgya* connect these three *kriyā*. If you do not know the outer body, the middle body and the inner body, is there any way to sanctify and purify the outer, middle or inner, and make them holy? Hence all actions *(kriyā)* are meant to follow *abhyāsa* and *vairāgya* whatever the various terminologies. *Mudrā* means a seal and *bandha* means a lock. Why are these words used? You know today banks have lockers. Why? So that your precious things may be kept safe. All are not allowed to go to the lockers. Only those who have booked the lockers can go to open them. *Mudrā* and *bandha* are like the locks to the doors and windows of the human being. They cannot be opened easily. You cannot open the lockers in the bank without the permission of the manager, can you? He has to come with you to open the main door of the main locker. Then another man comes to open the inner door and then goes away. Then you open your locker yourself. So the *madhya śarīra* and the *antara śarīra* are the agents to unlock before you unlock your door. The doors of the *ātman* have to be opened by your own *ātman*. That is why these lockers have been introduced into the yogic system, as you are the only one who knows the number of the lock in order to unlock it exactly at a right or ripe time.

Why are the locks there? Because there is a precious energy, a precious jewel, hidden in the system known as *kuṇḍalinī*. *Kuṇḍalākāra* means coiled. Why is this energy in a coiled state and not in a stretched state? This energy is given to all of us. It is existing in us as a grace of God. It is in a latent state, therefore coiled. This energy needs to be straightened through yogic practices. *Kuṇḍalinī* is a divine power. Each individual has several divine forces. Even dacoits are known to have shown some restraints of the *guṇa*. Many never molested a woman.

And some only stole from the rich and gave to the poor. There were some very interesting stories about the bright side of these people. We too should look at ourselves, to see what types of dacoitism go on in our own mind, to see where there is violence and thievery, and where there is divine light.

The term *śakti* is used to indicate this divine power. To awaken this *śakti, buddhi-tattva* has to be developed to know the *puruṣa* and character has to be cultivated. But today what is happening? Every Tom, Dick or Harry on the street is going around saying, "My *kuṇḍalinī* has awakened!" You ask anybody, they say, "Oh, the *guru* touched me and my *kuṇḍalinī* was awakened". Only in the fourth chapter does Patañjali speak of *kuṇḍalinī* in the name of *prakṛti.* The original term was *puruṣa prakṛti saṁyogāgni.* The fire which brings union between *puruṣa* and *prakṛti* is *saṁyogāgni.* This divine union of the *puruṣa* with the *prakṛti* makes man divine. An abundant flow of *śakti* runs in him.

Now, what is this union? Lord Vishnu has a consort, Lakṣmi. Lord Shiva has a consort, Pārvati. Lord Brahmā has a consort, Sarasvatī. Similarly, this *jīvātman* has a consort, which is *prakṛti.* So it is nothing new. The science of yoga and the practice of yoga teach us to see how the *puruṣa* can live with his consort, the *prakṛti,* in poise and peace. The *prakṛti* in each individual is in an unpolluted state; and so is the *puruṣa.* But unfortunately the inner (middle) body creates all these problems and pollutes the *prakṛti* and apparently the *puruṣa.* When this middle body becomes clear, then there can be a direct contact of *prakṛti* with *puruṣa* or *puruṣa* with *prakṛti,* without interference. Then there is purity, cleanliness and sanctity, within and without. This is the action of *kuṇḍalinī.*

This latent or dormant energy cannot be awakened by any means except fire. That fire is nothing but the fire of yoga *(yogāgni).* The fire of yoga alone can unlock inside and bring back the inner balance for the *śakti* to rush or to gush to reach its lover, the *puruṣa.* This divine force has different chambers. These chambers are known as the vessels of *śakti.* As electrical energies are stored in power houses, we have power houses in our system. These power houses are known as *śakti kośa* or *cakra.* They are: *mūlādhāra, svādhiṣṭhāna, maṇipūraka, anāhata, viśuddhi* and *ājñā.* From *mūlādhāra, kuṇḍalinī* pierces the five other chambers and moves up towards *sahasrāra* where she reaches the *puruṣa* and remains united with Him. Here ends the polarity between *prakṛti* and *puruṣa.*

The *cakra* possess the principal elements of nature. Each *cakra* has its own shape, its own form or *maṇḍala. Mūlādhāra* has *prithvi-tattva* or the element of earth. It has four petals. You may laugh at these ideas because they are not seen by the naked eye nor by the sophisticated instruments invented by modern scientists. But the yogis had a much deeper awareness than we have today. The heart has four chambers, which we know today. Did they know it had four chambers previously? Only after dissection did they find the four chambers. Similarly, if we go on dissecting the *prakṛti* in us, we may also one day come to the thoughts of the ancients about the various divisions of these different inner chambers, which are natural *(prākṛtic)* but subtle.

The second is the *svādhiṣṭhāna cakra* which has the element water and six petals or six *maṇḍala*. These two have the qualities of the *tamōguṇa*. Why is the energy coiled? Because it is in the *tāmasic* state in these two *cakra*. Then comes the *maṇipūraka*, the third *cakra*, which has the element of fire or *tejas-tattva*, with ten petals. You all know the solar plexus. The *maṇipūraka cakra* has the character of *rajas*. So all mutations take place in this navel area. *Anāhata*, the fourth *cakra*, is of the element air, *vāyu*, with twelve petals. It is both *sāttvic* and *rājasic*. For unenlightened people, *citta* acts in a *rājasic* way as it has to think, act and restrain in order to transform the *sādhaka* towards the *sāttvic* nature. *Viśuddhi*, the fifth, has the *tattva* of ether element, *ākāśa*, with sixteen petals. *Ākāśa-tattva* is full of *sāttvic* nature. The sixth *cakra*, *ājñā*, which is called the third eye, has the *tattva* of *buddhi*. It has two petals, symbolizing the mind functioning in the two regions, *prakṛti* and *puruṣa*. Whereas *sahasrāra* in the head has one thousand petals, hence the name *sahasrāra*[1].

Cakra means a turning wheel. Even in the modern industrial world, all instruments are connected to one wheel or the other. All the multiple wheels are dependent on a central wheel or base wheel. As soon as that wheel begins moving, it triggers the others to start moving as well. *Cakra* makes the energy roll from one to the other through its six chambers. This *prakṛti śakti*, having all the elements of nature, ascends through the *viśuddhi cakra* to become pure in intelligence for the *sādhaka* to experience the state of a *guṇatitan* (free from the qualities of nature). That is why it is called the seat of the third eye. The intuitive eye is the third eye. So when you reach that third eye, you have conquered the *guṇa* of nature. And as the *guṇa* of nature have come to an end, it is *buddhi-tattva* that reaches the culminating area in the *sahasrāra cakra*, the thousand-petalled lotus, or the *cakra* of the thousand *maṇḍala*.

Even people like Vivekananda claimed that the *cakra* had nothing to do with the growth of *rāja yoga*. They all say that it is nothing but a *haṭha yogic, tāntric* method which has nothing to do with yogic method. So I thought that you as students of yoga should know that Sage Patañjali has explained about *cakra* and their locations. *Nābhicakre kāyavyūhajñānam* (*Y.S.*, III.30). What is *nābhicakra?* Navel *cakra*. What is the navel *cakra?* It is the *maṇipūraka cakra* of *Haṭhayoga Pradīpikā*. Though the names differ in the textbooks, the places do not differ at all. Is

---

[1] See Table n. 6.

this not interesting to know that *nābhicakra* of Patañjali is *maṇipūraka cakra* of *Haṭhayoga Pradīpikā?* You may call it one way, I may call it in another way and a third may call it something different. It is just the fancy of the persons giving different names. In *sūtra* III.33, Patañjali refers to another *cakra. Mūrdhajyotiṣi siddhadarśanam. Mūrdhajyoti* refers to the *ājñā cakra*, the third eye (the coronal light under the crown of the head). *Sūtra* III.35 refers to the *anāhata cakra, hṛdaye cittasaṁvit.* Then *kaṇṭhakūpe kṣutpipāsā nivṛttiḥ* (*Y.S.*, III.31). *Kaṇṭhakūpa – kaṇṭha* means neck or throat. According to Patañjali, thirst and hunger are controlled by its restraint. *Viśuddhi cakra* belongs to the element of ether, the subtlest element of nature. You can see the connection to the *ākāśa-tattva.* This means that your *jñāna* has developed to such an extent that you do not thirst for ordinary things. *Kaṇṭha* means the entire portion of the inner throat, the inner part of the neck. *Kūpa* means a well or a vessel to store energy. In our ordinary walk of life we talk and criticise others. We either do this or that. Naturally the well of the throat gets dried up. Hence, the yogis say, "do not dry the well, but keep the vessel of the throat wet". These are the reasons for the introduction of *bandha. Jālandhara Bandha, Uddiyāṇa Bandha* and *Mūla Bandha* are essential to practise in *āsana* and *prāṇāyāma*, so that the energy may not dissipate in wrong ways. When the *sādhaka* gets saturated by energy, his system seeks outlets. Talking is an outlet. Ejection of the semen is an outlet. Excretion is an outlet. When *mudrā* and *bandha* are practised, they act as seals. Remember that in *āsana* there are also seals: *Paśchimottānāsana, Sālamba Sarvāṅgāsana, Sālamba Śīrṣāsana* (Plate n. 5), *Mūlabandhāsana*, act as seals in their own ways. Do not get carried away and think that *bandha* is superior to *āsana.* We have to understand the literal meaning of what a *bandha* is, what a lock is. What is a seal? When you are in *Setu Bandha Sarvāṅgāsana*, what do you do? You seal the entire back portion of the body. When you do *Setu Bandha Sarvāṅgāsana* on the bench, what do you do? Ponder over it. Then you will get lots of ideas.

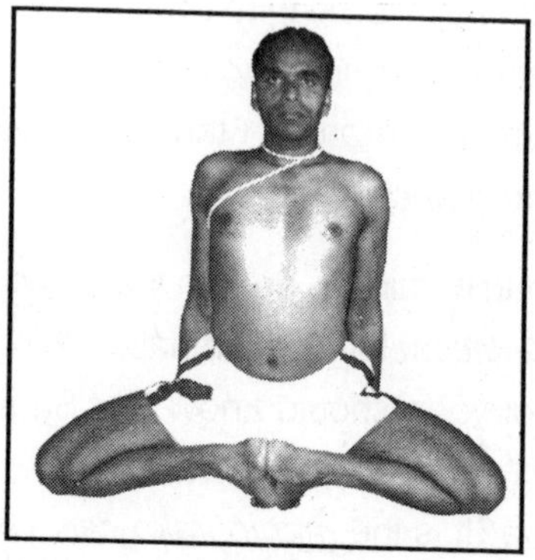

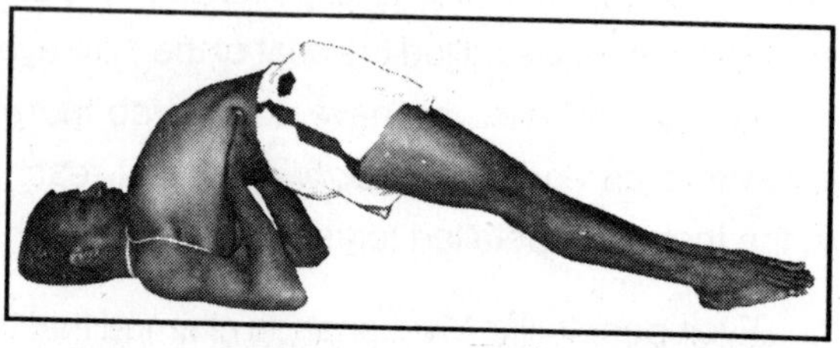

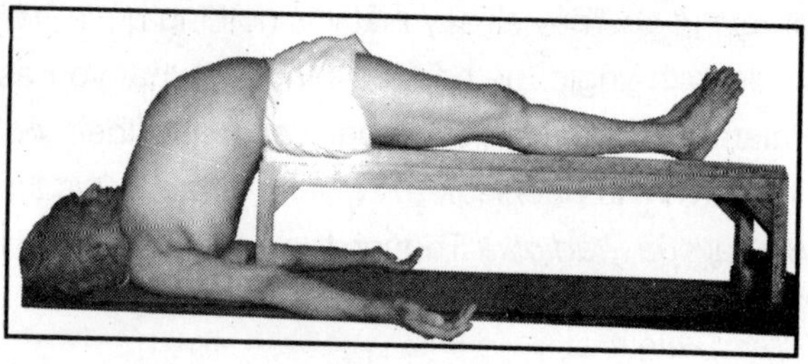

Plate n. 11 – *Mūlabandhāsana, Setu Bandha Sarvāṅgāsana (Uttana Mayūrāsana)* and *Setu Bandha Sarvāṅgāsana* on bench

As yoga practitioners, we do not allow the energy to go out, but find an inlet. As there is an outlet, there must be an inlet too. This is a kind of inlet *(ūrdhvaretas)*. Now you can understand the meaning of *ūrdhvaretas*. The ascension of *kuṇḍalinī* begins from *ūrdhvaretas*, where all the energies are brought together as a single unit. Heat is produced on account of these seals and locks. It cannot escape by any means. It must turn inwards, to the inlet. That inlet is nothing but the *suṣumṇā*. The moment it enters one becomes an *ūrdhvaretan*, a *brahmacārī* in a true sense. The *prakṛti* has moved towards *puruṣa* and he or she is a *brahmacārī* or a *brahmacārīnī*. That is *kuṇḍalinī śakti*.

Now, we come to the most intricate point. We hear about seven plexuses or seven glands and how they correspond to the seven *cakra*. It may be right, or it may be wrong. You are all sitting here. You have all heard of the thermometer, which measures the temperature. The mercury rises and falls as the weather changes. If you have a fever the mercury rises and if you are well, it remains stable at 98.6ºF.

Similarly, there is a thermometer in our system. I am not talking of the hypothalamus, which controls the temperature of the body. You are all seated. Do not disturb yourselves. If you disturb, you will not know what I am saying. You are all sitting here. Be as you are. I will give you a small instance so that you can feel yourselves.

The fluid in your central spine is lower than your spine. You can feel it yourselves. When we are all sitting, the outer spine is slightly warm, but the central spine is not warm. The mercury in your central spine has dropped. Do you feel it, or not?

– [...]

A little louder please! All of you are feeling it?

– Yes, feeling it.

Now stretch your spine. What happened to the fluid? It went up or it went down? When you stretch the spine you should not look into the spine, but look into and feel the fluid. Just try again. Did the outer spine go up, or the fluid go up?

– (Silence...)

What? Nobody knows. Why is everybody quiet? Why are only a few of you replying?

– (Silence...)

Do you understand your *guṇa?* You are dull! That is why Vyāsa was right when he said that "Yoga is not meant for all". But Patañjali being a compassionate man, said let us start somewhere.

Now, you all sat straight, did you not? Some of you are sinking, some of you are yawning. That means the energy has gone down. At least some of you are still sitting straight. Is the fluid remaining at the same height or has it dropped down? Observe the fluid only. The spine is straight. What happened to the fluid? It dropped, did it not?

– Yes, it did.

Understand these things, before you come to me and say, "the *guru* touched me and my *kuṇḍalinī* has awakened". See now. I have awakened your *kuṇḍalinī* but soon it went straight down. Though you are sitting straight, the fluid dipped. If you do not retain, it is as good as sleep. The moment it is awakened, it dips again. What I said is just to show that it happens in the power of *kuṇḍalinī* also. Do you understand why I am bringing this up for you to experience? The medical people can tell you which plexus controls which gland and which glands secrete for what purposes. All these are on the physiological level. *Cakra* have nothing much to do with the physical body or the physiological or psychological bodies. They are connected to the spiritual body. These chambers are hidden inside the spinal cord and hence the yogic method was found to be the key to unlocking these chambers.

The yogis have spoken about *nāḍī*. From the base of the *maṇipūraka cakra* sprout 72,000 *nāḍī*, each one branching off into a further 72,000 *nāḍī*. Besides these, they say 101 nerves sprout from the heart, and except the *citrā nāḍī*, all others further branch into 72,000 *nāḍī*.

This *citrā nāḍī* is unpolluted and virginal. This single *nāḍī* is the bridge that connects *prakṛti* with *puruṣa*. That is why it has no branches. All the others have branches. The other intermediaries do not allow this single *nāḍī* to come in contact with the *puruṣa*. The moment it comes into contact with *puruṣa*, there is *samādhi*.

Modern scientists speak of the influences of drugs and the actions of various drugs on the peripheral nerves and on the autonomous nervous system. The central nervous system solely works on discriminative intelligence. The autonomous nervous system is well dealt with in the *Haṭhayoga Pradīpikā* as *iḍā nāḍī* and *piṅgaḷā nāḍī*. The autonomous nervous system is dependent upon these two. And these 72,000 branches are the peripheral nervous system connecting to the autonomous system, working under the guidance of *iḍā* and *piṅgaḷā*. The word central nervous system means the middle part of the spinal column *(madhyama)*, whereas *cakra* are in the core of the spinal canal. It is said that the fusion of the sympathetic and parasympathetic (parts of the autonomous system) brings electrical fusion. That is *suṣumṇā*. Yogis say that *iḍā* and *piṅgaḷā* control the peripheral and autonomous nerves and feed the *suṣumṇā* to store energy and keep it in reserve. The electrical nerve impulses are in between *iḍā* and *piṅgaḷā*. So all actions and reactions of the peripheral on the autonomous nervous system touch the central nervous system, the *suṣumṇā*. *Suṣumṇā* spreads everywhere, in order to get fed from the autonomous system through the peripheral channels, so that it stores energy.

Yogic practices help to increase or retain that fluid which you felt now, and yet one has to learn with attention to keep it up. Even though it was in the state of ascendance, you felt the fluid start to dip. It wants to be in the *tāmasic* nature, so it dips immediately. Practice of yoga makes this fluid remain in and retain that position, so that it can move up from chamber to chamber. Various *āsana* are prescribed in order to keep this energy active. Tomorrow when you go to practise, whether *Tāḍāsana*, or *Utthita Trikoṇāsana* (Plate n. 8), follow this new lesson when you extend the spine, whether you moved the spine or you moved the fluid of the spine. Similarly, when you do *Ūrdhva Dhanurāsana*, do you extend the spine or do you extend the fluid of the spine? Then you will know what you have learned today.

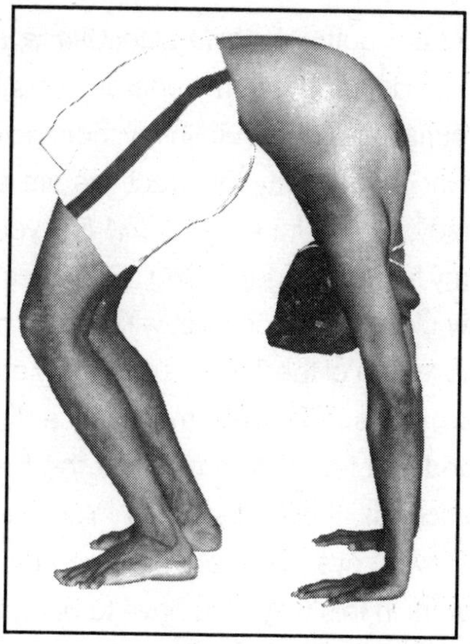

Plate n. 12 – *Ūrdhva Dhanurāsana*

Śakti is a very, very difficult subject to understand. The moment you observe the fluid moving but not the spine, there is no *rajōguṇa* or *tamōguṇa* in your practice. You are in *sāttva guṇa*. The moment you stretch your spine but not the fluid, greed, ambition, pride or anything may come. Your inner qualities, in the form of pride, shine out with ideas of I want to do better, I want to stretch more. If you think like this, *āsana* will remain on the physical level only. When you are ripe in *sādhanā* you come to feel this fluid rising and then learn to maintain it in each *āsana*. When this fluid moves and makes you stretch more, you are a *guṇātīta* at that moment. The moment the fluid falls in an *āsana*, you have come back to the *guṇa*. So, to retain and maintain that rising force of the fluid is known as *bandha* or *mudrā* in *āsana*.

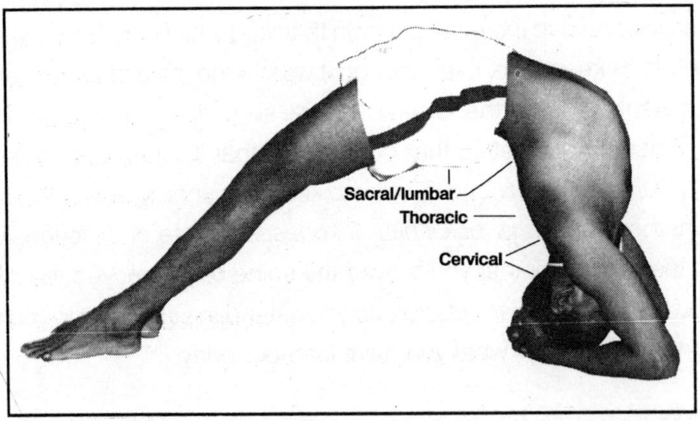

Plate n. 13 - *Dwi Pāda Viparīta Daṇḍāsana* (showing lumbo-sacral and cervical spine)

For example, when you are doing *Viparīta Daṇḍāsana*, the fluids tend to be on your lumbo-sacral and cervical spine. I do not move my energy to fight with the cervical and sacral areas. I say, can I keep the mercurial rise of my fluid in my thoracic dorsal spine without allowing it to hit the cervical or the lumbar? In this way my practices are adjusted inside, all my *āsana* practices are from the inner body, for the inner *sādhanā*. For you they become outer. Stretch your hand. You say, "Oh, I feel my finger has gone long". But when I stretch, I see how much my energy has moved up and how close it is in contact with me. In my stretching, I do not look at the length of my hand, but at the length of the flow of energy. My attention is not on the body, but on the flow of energy. In a sense, this is *vairāgya* in my practice. If you practise like this, you lose the principles of *guṇa-tattva*, and you feel at that moment the fluid of the *prakṛti* intermingling with the *puruṣa*. If the *śakti* descends, the *puruṣa* says, "You are going away from me, come near me". If the *puruṣa* fades, *prakṛti* says, "Where are you, come here. I am here". That is what *āsana* builds up in you, if you work in this way. You have to bring the instruments, the *maṇḍala*, the body, the mind and the self *(sāsmitā)* to be free from the *guṇa*. Due to this feel of experience which continues in my practice, nothing frightens me in my practices and none can shake me away from them. Similarly, you have to cultivate this character by practising yoga so that the inner body, the middle body and the outer body become divine. Then divinity flows in abundance, without the influence of the *guṇa*.

For a *sādhakā*, courage is required. I have given you the background to develop courage on your own. You have to study the *guṇa* of your body, mind and intelligence and the *guṇa* of your nerves all the time. Even you can change your dull body, dull circulation and dull inner frame. Transform them through yoga into vibrancy, and with this vibrancy, illumine them so that each and every cell in the body and consciousness becomes divine, like its indweller, the Self. This unification is *kuṇḍalinī yoga*.

Thank you for your attention.

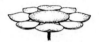

SECTION III

MY VISION OF YOGA

*KṢETRA - KṢETRAJÑA YOGA**

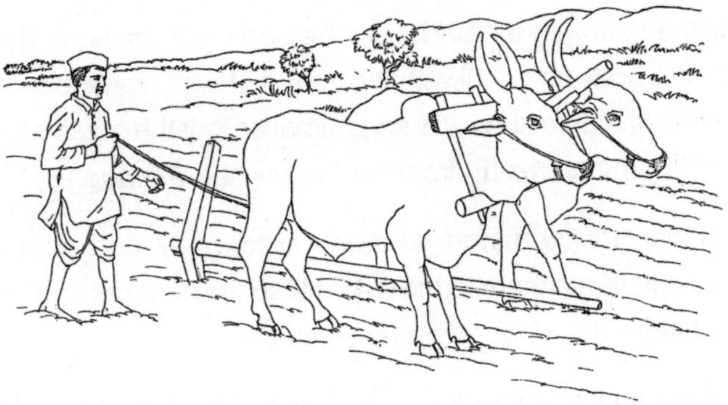

A frequently asked question is, "What is yoga?" The meaning of yoga cannot be conveyed in a few words. It is such a vast and complex subject that it cannot be easily explained or made intelligible in brief. Yoga is a means of coming together. It means to yoke, to join, to unite, to integrate. The question remains, what is to be integrated? What is to be united?

Kṣetra is a *Sanskrit* word which means "field", the "soil". *Kṣetrajña* means "knower of the field", "owner of the field" or "the very cultivator". An owner owns the field to cultivate it. The cultivator is the conscious principle, the Self, the *ātman*. Then what is the field? The body, mind, intelligence, ego and consciousness are the field. The cultivator embraces the whole field. The conscious principle is pervasive and so it pervades the field. The field expresses itself in five prominent composites, namely body, mind, intelligence, ego and consciousness. In fact we are made up of two principles: nature or *prakṛti* and Self or *puruṣa*. These two principles seem to be completely different from each other. The practice of yoga integrates these two principles – nature and Self. The Self is the source whence consciousness flows like a river. As the water of the river wets the field wherever it touches, so too yoga helps the consciousness to flow in the field of the body wetting the inundated elements which are brought to life by the supreme conscious principle, the Self.

The Self is the seed and the principles of nature which grows into a tree from that seed with its trunk, branches and leaves. This is how the *puruṣa* and *prakṛti* express themselves as

* Lecture given by Śri B.K.S. Iyengar on his 73rd birthday, 14th December 1991.

explained in *Bhagavad Gītā* (*B.G.,* XV.1), Lord Krishna says that the Banyan tree has its roots above but its branches are below. Similarly, man too has the root of his intelligence in the brain and it branches its awareness through the mind, senses of perception and organs of action untill it reaches the bottom of the feet, from there it sends back its message to the head (as feed back system), connectiong the entire body's functioning to the root – the brain for further intellectual growth.

Yoga unites the soul with the body and the body with the soul. The practice of yoga is meant to learn to link the body and soul with the thread of consciousness. Yoga is to bring unity in diversity. The evolutes of nature show the separateness, but the percolating conscious energy *(caitanyatā)* flowing in them springs up from the source, the *ātman.*

The field is open for the farmer to reach every nook and corner of it. Similarly, the evolutes of nature in the field are there to make possible the communication with the *ātman.* Let us see how the soul is introduced and communicated.

The *kṣetra* is a vast expanse. Initially, it is made up of five gross elements: earth, water, fire, air and ether. The source energy for the five elements exists in a subtle form. The five subtle elements recognised are: odour, taste, form, touch and sound. These are the *pañcamahābhūta* and the *pañcatanmātra* resting on the first primordial matter, *mahat* of *prakṛti,* which is in the form of *citta* in us.

The field also has five organs of action, called *karmendriya,* and five senses of perception, *jñānendriya.* The mind, intelligence and ego which are the shoot of *mahat,* have their place in the *kṣetra* co-ordinating with the consciousness *(citta).* The source for all these twenty-three evolutes rests finally in *prakṛti,* the twenty-fourth constituent.

This field of evolutes of nature is susceptible to disturbances of disease, sorrow, pain, pleasure, mood and mode. The evolutes get affected and undergo change because of these disturbances. However, discriminative knowledge can check them. The *kṣetra* (field) is encompassed with five sheaths *(pañcakośa):*

1) *Annamaya kośa*	–	physical body
2) *Prāṇamaya kośa*	–	physiological body
3) *Manomaya kośa*	–	mental body
4) *Vijñānamaya kośa*	–	intellectual body
5) *Ānandamaya kośa*	–	blissful body

The five gross elements, the five subtle elements, the five organs of action, the five senses of perception, mind, intelligence, ego and the consciousness, act and interact. Action and interaction are experienced in the form of five *vṛtti* (mental modifications) and five *kleśa* (afflictions), according to the five ranges of consciousness *(śreṇi)*. In short, at each state of consciousness the modifications and afflictions react and interact at different levels.

It is quite interesting to know the five states of consciousness namely:

Pañcaśreṇi citta **(five ranges of consciousness)**

1)	*Mūḍha*	–	dullness or forgetful state
2)	*Kṣipta*	–	distorted state
3)	*Vikṣipta*	–	scattered state
4)	*Ekāgra*	–	state of onepointedness
5)	*Niruddha*	–	state of restraint

Obviously, under the influence of these five states of consciousness, one remains sometimes dull, sometimes intelligent, at times sharp, at times forgetful, at times steady or distracted or full of valour and vigour, silent and dormant, focussed and onepointed or restrained. As the consciousness is governed by these five states, it gets influenced by the afflictions *(kleśa)* as well as by fluctuations and modifications *(vṛtti)* according to its calibre.

Cittavṛtti **(fluctuations and modifications of consciousness)**

1)	*Pramāṇa*	–	right perception, correct knowledge
2)	*Viparyaya*	–	contrary knowledge or wrong perception
3)	*Vikalpa*	–	imagination or wrong conception
4)	*Nidrā*	–	sleep
5)	*Smṛti*	–	memory

The five fluctuations of the consciousness are rooted in the five afflictions:

Pañcakleśa **(five afflictions)**

1)	*Avidyā*	–	lack of spiritual wisdom or perverted knowledge
2)	*Asmitā*	–	egoism, individualism
3)	*Rāga*	–	attachment
4)	*Dveṣa*	–	aversion
5)	*Abhiniveśa*	–	clinging to life passionately

The modifications of *citta* and the afflictions of *citta* work degree-wise according to the five states of *citta*. That is why often a highly Intelligent person seems to be a dullard when his *citta* is in the *mūḍha* plane. One may be in *kṣipta*, *vikṣipta*, *ekāgra* and *niruddha* state, where changes occur too. It is the same with *nidrāvṛtti* (sleep), which is a common experience, different from the other fluctuations. We find our sleep sometimes *tāmasic* and other times *rājasic* or *sāttvic*. These five categories of modifications and afflictions, moods and modes influence the *citta* and affect one, one way or the other but not the same way all the time.

Since the modifications and afflictions are not identical, Patañjali has offered us an eight-petalled yoga to combat these fluctuations and afflictions so that qualitatively they are conquered from their gross manifestation to their subtle manifestation.

Aṣṭadaḷa yoga

1) *Yama*	–	moral restraints
2) *Niyama*	–	fixed practices and observances
3) *Āsana*	–	postures
4) *Prāṇāyāma*	–	regulation of energy, or life force through breath control
5) *Pratyāhāra*	–	withdrawal of senses – quietening of the senses directly by the mind
6) *Dhāraṇā*	–	attention
7) *Dhyāna*	–	meditation or contemplation
8) *Samādhi*	–	absorption

These *aṣṭadaḷa* (eight petals) of yoga are categorised into *bahiraṅga sādhanā*, *antaraṅga sādhanā* and *antarātma sādhanā*. *Sādhanā* is a spiritual endeavour or a journey towards the soul. The means that are used to reach the final destination are recognised as *sādhanā*. Undoubtedly, the *sādhanā* can be on various levels, physical, physiological, psychological, mental, moral, ethical, religious, intellectual and spiritual.

Bahiraṅga sādhanā is composed of *yama*, *niyama*, *āsana* and *prāṇāyāma*. *Pratyāhāra* is the transitory state between *bahiraṅga* and *antaraṅga sādhanā*, whereas *antaraṅga sādhanā* is *dhāraṇā* and *dhyāna*. *Samādhi* is *antarātma sādhanā*.

We know that modern psychology refers to four states of mind, namely, conscious, subconscious, superconscious and unconscious states. If the practice of the eight-petalled yoga that we do in a conscious state cannot penetrate the unconscious state, then that practice remains superficial. We have to pierce the unconscious. Lacking in depth, we can never reach inside. The imprints of practice do not go down, deep into the heart or intelligence of the *ātman*. In this sense, the practice has to undergo transformation to reach the innermost layer of the consciousness. Keeping this aspect in view, the practice of yoga can be put into three categories. Any *āsana* could be first *bahiraṅga*, then *antaraṅga* and finally *antarātma sādhanā*.

In our daily practice, we have to penetrate the peripheral nervous system, autonomous nervous system and central nervous system step by step. The conscious mind is impulsive and can react quickly to the demand of the will. This is not so with the unconscious mind. The *vṛtti* and *kleśa* accumulated in the unconscious mind may remain untouched if you practise yoga without penetration. When you get involved, the *bahiraṅga* practice of yoga silences the impulsive consciousness completely to deal with the subconscious mind. Then the subconscious mind is made to become conscious. This is *antaraṅga sādhanā*. As you proceed and reach the depth of practice, the unconscious mind slowly unfolds. This becomes *antarātma sādhanā*. In this sense, all the eight petals are practised at physical, physiological, psychological, mental, moral, ethical, religious, intellectual and spiritual levels.

The brain functions in tune with the depth of the *sādhanā*. A beginner may remain steady and fast in approach and function physically, but hidden secrets begin to surface if his approach begins from the middle brain and middle body. When the practice becomes intelligent and meaningful, one comes out with firmness and assurance involving the back of the brain.

For the sake of convenience you can say that the frontal brain, which is analytical, is the active brain. The middle brain is the reflective brain, which ponders upon thoughts. The back brain is the meditative brain. Therefore with its discriminating intelligence it reasons on filtered thoughts. The base brain accumulates experiences and deliberates emotionally. However the top brain is the seat of the self, where the bliss is experienced when all thoughts are analysed, filtered, reflected, reasoned and meditated upon. This brain concludes the truth and experiences only the truth.

Even if you think of yogic practice at the body level, it has its own depth in approach. The *karmendriya* are brought under control by *yama* and *jñānendriya* are controlled by *niyama* first at the physical and then at the mental and spiritual levels. A beginner practises *āsana* at the physical level, then gradually connects his practice to the inner body and then to the innermost body. The objective of practice is to tame, control, channel, recharge, transform and finally transcend all the twenty-four elements of nature.

Know that *yama* and *niyama* are present in all the other petals of yoga. A *sādhaka* cannot achieve anything without practising all the petals of yoga.

The deep-seated afflictions *(kleśa)* and mental modifications *(vṛtti)* penetrate the five sheaths of man and the practice of *aṣṭāṅga yoga* is meant to penetrate these five sheaths for a *sādhaka* to become a qualitative *sādhaka (lakṣaṇa puruṣa)*.

This penetration is two-fold:

a) the different depths which are reached in the practice of each petal of yoga, as explained in the previous paragraphs,

b) the different depths which are reached by the different petals of *aṣṭadaḷa yoga*. Let me explain this in detail.

Table n. 8 – *Aṣṭadaḷa yoga* and *prakṛti jaya (viśeṣa, aviśeṣa, liṅga, aliṅga)*

Aṣṭadaḷa	Meaning	Range of conquest	Conquest of stages *(parvajaya)*	
1) *Yama*	Social discipline	Understanding of *karmendriya* (five organs of action) and conquest of *karmendriya*, which are mainly of five elements *(bhūta)*	*Bhūtajaya*	*Viśeṣa*
2) *Niyama*	Individual discipline	Understanding of *jñānendriya* (five senses of perception) and conquest of *jñānendriya*	*Bhūtajaya*	*Viśeṣa*
3) *Āsana*	Postures	Conquest of elemental body (gross, subtle) and mind		
4) *Prāṇāyāma*	Discipline of breath	Control and conquest of vital energy	*Bhūtajaya*	*Viśesa Aviśeṣa*
5) *Pratyāhāra*	Withdrawal of the *indriyas* and mind	Control of the inner mind and conquest of the outer mind		
6) *Dhāraṇā*	Concentration	Conquest of intelligence *(buddhi)*	*Buddhi*	*Aviśeṣa* and
7) *Dhyāna*	Meditation	Understanding of *tanmātra* and conquest of ego or *ahaṁkāra*	*Ahaṁkāra*	*Liṅgamātra*
8) *Samādhi*	Total absorption	Conquest of conscious-ness *(citta)*, *guṇa*. (*Y.S.*, I.19). After this, *kaivalya* – *puruṣa khyāti* (*Y.S.*, II.23)	*Citta*	*Aliṅga*

If *yama* and *niyama* are meant to conquer the *karmendriya* and *jñānendriya*, *āsana* is intended to purify the *pañcabhautika* and *pañcatanmātrika* body. *Prāṇāyāma* is for control of the five vital energies *(pañcaprāṇa)*. *Pratyāhāra* is for the quietness of mind. *Dhāraṇā*, for the clarity of intelligence *(buddhi)*. *Dhyāna* is for sublimating the *ahaṁkāra* or the ego, while *samādhi* transforms the *citta* with crystal clarity for the *ātman* to shine. This is how *aṣṭāṅga yoga* helps the *sādhaka* to reach the ultimate. Hence, I have given the graph of this *aṣṭadaḷa* for you to recollect and remember.

Āsana is to purify each and every cell of the body. The cellular body changes totally with the *āsana saṁskāra*. Do not entertain the idea that *āsana* is a mere physical exercise. It is a physico-psycho-ethical and ethico-spiritual practice. The practice of *āsana*, without the ethical background of *yama* and *niyama*, is merely physical. The five gross and five subtle elements of the body have to be purified and sanctified by *āsana* by incorporating *yama* and *niyama* in them. This has to be remembered and followed by each practitioner. *Yama* and *niyama* are like the foundation on which the six-storied building of yoga is raised. One has to learn to incorporate *yama* and *niyama* in each limb of yoga. This can be explained only practically and not by theory.

Āsana deals with *annamaya kośa* and *prāṇāyāma kośa*, whereas *prāṇāyāma* deals with *prāṇāmaya kośa* and *manomaya kośa*. The physiological body consists of respiratory, circulatory, digestive, urinary and glandular systems, and the vital organs like heart, kidney, liver, spleen, pancreas and intestines. All these comprise the physiological territory. In *prāṇāyāma* the cells are vitalised, the living content of the bioplasma is stored, the bioenergy is added and balanced. Every tissue is invigorated. With *prāṇāyāma* practice, the doer learns to utilise, discharge and recharge the energy. Perfect physiological harmony is established by *prāṇāyāmic* practices for the mind to work healthily.

Then come the facets of *manomaya kośa*. *Pratyāhāra* means withdrawal of the senses from objects. The mind is the king of the organs of action and perception. The mind can lead the organs either towards pleasure or towards auspiciousness. *Pratyāhāra* leads the mind from pleasantness to auspiciousness, from *bhoga* to yoga. The mind, which would continue in its undisciplined movement, is made to function in a disciplined way for the outer mind to move in, towards the inner mind.

Let us come to *vijñānamaya kośa*. *Vijñānamaya kośa* is complexly fabricated by the interplay of mind, intelligence, ego and consciousness, and needs taming. This job is done by *dhāraṇā*. *Dhāraṇā* tunes the mind that is scattered in various directions. A scattered mind is brittle. *Dhāraṇā* unites the energy of the mind and holds it. The outgoing and expressive ego is reversed and reduced or purified and made to focus well on the *kṣetrajña*. The *kṣetra* has various divisions *(vibhāga)* and hence *dhāraṇā* could be on the different regions of the body *(kṣetra)* or on the soul *(kṣetrajña)*. However, in *dhāraṇā* the focussing of consciousness is objective, whether it is *kṣetra* or *kṣetrajña*. The scope of *vijñānamaya kośa* is quite expansive. Therefore, the states of *dhāraṇā, dhyāna* and *samādhi* are not vivid. The consciousness tends to oscillate from *dhāraṇā* to *dhyāna* and from *dhyāna* to *dhāraṇā*. It is only after the penetration of *ānandamaya kośa* that the state becomes vivid.

When *dhāraṇā, dhyāna* and *samādhi* are fused with vividness and clarity, that state is *saṁyama*. The intelligence is purified by the constant practice of *dhyāna* so that the tinge of 'I'-ness does not remain in it. Thus, the purified intelligence is digested in order to be assimilated in *samādhi*. *Citta* or the consciousness, which remained in the manifested *(vyakta)* state, begins to become unmanifested *(avyakta)* by dissolving in the *ātman*, which is eternal, ever present, never decays and has no beginning and no end. When this is felt, the *ātman* that remained in unmanifested form manifests as daylight. Then the field in its pure state merges in the cultivator. The field and the field-holder become one. The knower of the field is known as *puruṣa*. The divine union of *prakṛti* and *puruṣa* occurs only in the sheath of *ānandamaya kośa* or the sheath of ether.

To reach this hidden *puruṣa* in the space of ether *(cidākāśa)*, *prakṛti* has to travel penetrating the *pañcakośa* through *aṣṭāṅga yoga*. As we saw in *sādhanā* how it gets transformed from *bahiraṅga* to *antaraṅga* and from *antaraṅga* to *antarātma*, it is interesting to see how the means of restraint are applied, how the embellishment of consciousness is brought about.

Patañjali says, *Śraddhā vīrya smṛti samādhi prajñā pūrvaka itareṣām* (*Y.S.*, I.20). Pursue yogic discipline with faith, vigour, memory, keen intellect and power of absorption to experience the absolute consciousness. While dealing with *prakṛti*, you should understand that it can cheat by taking you to a wrong destination rather than towards the *ātman*. Here the *sādhaka* is likely to stagnate rather than be liberated. To move from stagnation towards emancipation, Patañjali advises us to redouble the efforts of practice with five aids namely, faith *(śraddhā)*, vigour *(vīrya)*, memory *(smṛti)*, total absorption *(samādhi)* or supreme wisdom *(prajñā)* with a single pointed attention *(ekāgra)*. While penetrating each *kośa* in order to filter the *vṛtti* and *kleśa*, the restraints listed above are essential.

Do not think that one can burn the afflictions or restrain the mental modifications by applying the above five aids directly. Effective and intensive application of these means is not that easy. The consciousness does not permit us effectively to utilise these means intensely and directly. It tries to create obstructions. Therefore, Patañjali has given a method to tame and train the consciousness, in order to smooth the way towards realisation.

The method of cleansing, culturing and embellishing the consciousness is *citta prasādanam.* The *citta prasādanam* is developed by the consciousness only through the practice of *aṣṭāṅga yoga.*

Patañjali stresses that we should develop friendliness towards the happy, compassion towards the miserable, joy towards the virtuous and indifference towards the malicious. He offers other alternatives, like control over breath, or engaging the mind to be engrossed in a chosen object, to contemplate on the sorrowless luminous effulgent light, or to follow the desireless mind of enlightened men, or to concentrate on dreamy or sleepy and wakeful states, or to contemplate on a thing which is conducive and pleasing to bring about steadiness. All these alternative methods are the subtle forms of the *aṣṭadala* of yoga, while many attribute these to meditation techniques and processes and not to *aṣṭāṅga yoga.*

Patañjali, while explaining various types of *samādhi prajñā,* mentions that the yoga *sādhaka* reaches a state where *prakṛti* takes him to the state of dissolution of the consciousness with, or the state of merging in, the elements of nature *(prakṛti laya)* or a bodiless state *(videha)* state – *Bhavapratyayaḥ videha prakṛtilayānām* (*Y.S.,* I.19) – which should not be mistaken for *kaivalya* as this state explains the function of *prakṛti.*

Patañjali clearly explains the divisional functions of *prakrti.* The evolution of *prakṛti* takes place in four stages – noumenal *(aliṅga),* phenomenal *(liṅgamātra),* non-distinguishable *(aviśeṣa)* and distinguishable *(viśeṣa).* He explains it in *sūtra* II.19, *Viśeṣa aviśeṣa liṅgamātra aliṅgāni guṇaparvāṇi. Prakṛti* is primeval and springs up as the first evolute *(mahat), pañcatanmātra* and *ahaṁkāra* are *aviśeṣa* (non-distinguishable) and *pañcabhūta, karmendriya, jñānendriya* and *manas* are *viśeṣa* (distinguishable).

The practice of yoga begins from the evolved gross stage of *prakṛti* and progresses towards dissolution in *prakṛti.* It is a journey from evolution to involution. The evolutes of *prakṛti* are reinvested in their source in order to be dissolved. This return journey is from distinguishable to non-distinguishable. The elemental body, along with the organs of action, senses of perception and mind, dissolves in the five subtle elements and ego. The five subtle elements and ego return to *mahat,* the phenomenal stage *(liṅgamātra)* and finally *mahat* into the noumenal. That is what Patañjali explains in *Sūkṣmaviṣayatvaṁ ca aliṅga paryavasānam* (*Y.S.,* I.45). The subtlest component of nature is consciousness. When it dissolves on its own in the seat of the Self, it is free from stain. He explains the merging of the gross body and elements, the subtle body *(ahaṁkāra)* and *pañcatanmātra* in *mahat,* and *mahat* in *prakṛti.* Thus, *sūtra* II.19 and I.45 help to understand *sūtra* I.19 clearly.

It is also interesting to note that Svātmārāma explains four stages of *sādhanā* as *ārambhāvasthā* – for understanding the *viśeṣa* of *prakṛti*, as *ghaṭāvasthā* for acquiring *aviśeṣa jñāna* of *prakṛti*, then *paricayāvasthā* to go to the root of the first evolute *(liṅga* or *mahat)*, then *niṣpattyāvasthā (aliṅga to prakṛtilaya)*: *Ārambhaśca ghaṭavaścaiva tatha paricayō'pi ca / niṣpattiḥ sarvayogeṣu syādavasthācatuṣṭayam //* (*H.Y.P.*, IV.69). In all the yogic practices there are four stages; viz., *ārambha, ghaṭa, paricaya* and *niṣpattī*.

The state beyond *aliṅga (prakṛti)* is the state of emancipation *(kaivalya)*. The seer dwells in his own true splendour. Hence, Patañjali wants the *sādhaka* to go in a methodical way. He does not accept the chance way of achievement. In this sense Patañjali is very close to Lord Krishna. Lord Krishna calls it *kṣetra kṣetrajña yoga* (*B.G.*, chapter XIII). For Patañjali the aim is to bring about the union between *kṣetra* and *kṣetrajña* at the highest plane. He is not happy at a little bit of achievement and attainment, coming through *kṣetra*. He unequivocally states it in two *sūtra:*

Sattva puruṣayoh śuddhi sāmye kaivalyam iti (*Y.S.*, III.56). This exalted intelligence being equal to the purity of the seer, he has reached perfection in yoga, and *Puruṣārtha śūnyānāṁ guṇānām pratiprasavaḥkaivalyaṁ svarūpapratiṣṭhā vā citiśaktiḥ iti* (*Y.S.*, IV.34). From now on, the yogi is devoid of all aims of life. He is free from the qualities of nature and lives in the state of emancipation.

These two *sūtra* clinch my thoughts on the issue. The intelligence which shines in consciousness in a state of exaltation, drops the mind and ego and becomes as pure as the seed. At this stage the seer and the seen both are in a pure state.

The yogi in such a state is devoid of all aims and ambitions. No modifications or afflictions touch or bother him. All the evolutes of nature in their pure and pristine form reach the very source and dissolve for the seer to shine. The *puruṣa* presents himself in his original state. The *kṣetra* and *kṣetrajña*, in this sense, become one in a flawless purity.

This is Divine Union – Divine Yoga.

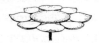

YOGĀSANA: A SEARCH OF THE INFINITE IN THE FINITE BODY*

Our six systems of philosophy are known as *darśana* (mirror or direct spiritual perceptions of the Ultimate, the Real). They are based on the firm foundation of experience. Unfortunately, this great and glorious tradition moored to experience has been forgotten. Hair-splitting textual scholarship and logical skills of intellectual debate have made it an armchair philosophy. Yoga is one of the six systems, but it is more practical and experiential than theoretical. Being a practical discipline par excellence, it needs matured experience to explain it.

Though Patañjali accords an important place for *yogāsana* in his treatise, denigration of *yogāsana* as physical has created doubts in many practitioners who are seeking the Supreme. According to Patañjali, mastery of *āsana* is a precondition for *prāṇāyāma*. In the *Sādhana Pāda*, Patañjali devotes three *sūtra* to *āsana* and in *Vibhūti Pāda*, abundant references to the wealth of the body *(kāya saṁpat)* and physical attainments *(siddhi)* are made.

Many yogic texts emphasise meditative postures. It is also equally true that yogic texts like *Śiva Saṁhitā* speak of 84,00,000 *āsana*, revealing that there are as many *āsana* as species on this planet.

It is rather hard to describe *āsana* at one stretch. Each *āsana* has many complex, subtle and fine adjustments, not only in the limbs of the body but on the very fabric of the intelligence and consciousness. One has to train and tone the body to have strength, flexibility, endurance, poise and integration sufficient to sit comfortably and correctly for a considerable length of time even in a meditative posture.

The value of *āsana* as *tapas* has been explained by Patañjali in *Y.S.* II.43, wherein he says that one has to burn out the impurities of the body, senses and mind for the soul to rekindle the spark of divinity which is hidden within. Hence, I feel that *āsana* is a form of *tapas* demanding rigorous discipline.

---

* From *Yoga Rahasya*, vol. 2, no. 1 (an excerpt of this article is published as "How to perform *yogāsanas*").

Today, this rigorous discipline has been transformed into soft instant yoga. This soft casual practice has lost the critical, scientific, experimental and experiential exposition of *āsana,* but abundant stereotyped facile writings on the subject are available.

Though *āsana* has been accepted as an alternative method of medicine owing to health consciousness in people, let us not forget the holistic nature of the body as each *āsana* is filled with profound scientific know-how of the body and mind, starting from the gross body and then piercing the various inner layers of the body to reach the inner ruler – the *ātman.*

Āsana, as a science, deals with health and perfection of the body. It helps to uncover the differences between the body and the mind in order to keep the Self in a crystal pure state.

Āsana sublimates the senses of perception and organs of action and develops harmony in the functioning of the body, keeping the entire nervous system free from blockages. We cannot forget that the body is the only instrument to be used for worldly as well as spiritual pursuits.

Let us start to learn from the known, a visible object like the body, before exploring the unknown, in order to move towards the subtlest of the subtle, and the finest of the fine – the Self.

Āsana play a major role in correcting the defects of matter and energy so that these two are educated to move towards the refinement of intelligence and consciousness.

The structure of an *āsana* cannot change, as each *āsana* is an art of holiness in itself. But when the *sādhaka* performs, he does his best at it. One has to study the structure of each *āsana,* arithmetically and geometrically. As arithmetic is based on addition, subtraction, multiplication and division, one has to add proper action in order to have proper adjustments; minus the unwanted, unnecessary and wrong actions by avoiding underdoing or overdoing; multiply the intensity of awareness and divide and distribute the energy evenly. In order to adjust geometrically, we have to measure the dimensions of *āsana* so that we fit properly into it. Each *āsana* in its methodology has certain measurements of its height, length, width and girth. Again there is a direction to the movement and action of the body which has to be followed properly. One has to analyse and realise the real shape and form of each *āsana* so that it is expressed and presented properly.

Āsana may be angular or triangular, straight or oblique, circular or semi-circular, round or oval shaped, upright or inverted. One has to note all these points in each *āsana* by observation and study and then act in the field – the body – for the knower of the field – the Self – to perform in its pristine glory. It means total involvement of the whole body with senses, mind, intelligence, consciousness and self. One has to be careful not to create room for emptiness and forgetfulness in the known and the unknown bodies. One has to use the weapon of ego or 'I'-consciousness carefully so that it neither gets inflated nor loses its will. This way it becomes submissive at the right moment.

It is not right to perform *āsana* according to one's pliability and mobility. One has to mould the body to the *āsana* and not the *āsana* to fit into the body. It is not ethical to do the *āsana* to one's individual convenience. Constant study and trial is needed to educate and mould the limbs of the body to fit into the right frame of each posture.

Know the structure, process and functions of an *āsana* and how it interfaces with body, mind and self. In each *āsana* one has to feel the flow of intelligence and consciousness from the periphery of the body towards the centre – the *ātman* – and from the *ātman* towards the periphery. *Āsana* is not a posture where one mindlessly and mechanically scrambles in and out.

First, one has to figure the structure of an *āsana* and realise the basic or fundamental points by conatively spacing the structural or anatomical body through adjustment and arrangement of the limbs for placement in the movements; then one has to mould the body to fit into the structure of the *āsana*. Resistance and movement should move in concord. Distribution of weight should be even in the muscles, bones, joints, mind and intelligence.

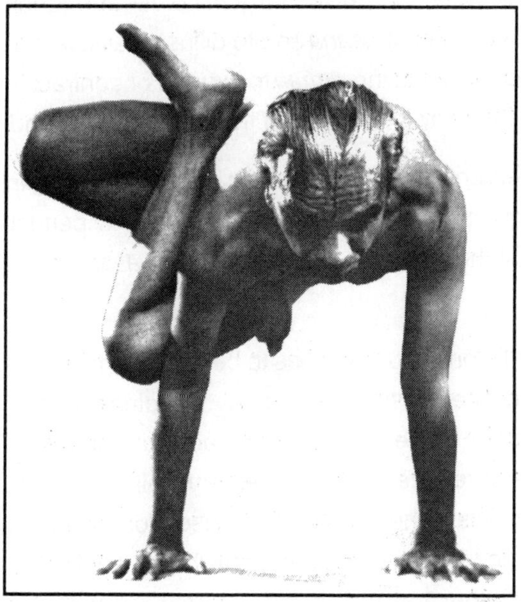

Plate n. 14 – Harmony and balance, equipoise and serenity in *Pārśva Kukkuṭāsana*.

Trim the jewel of the body like a well-cut diamond by creating space in joints, muscles and skin so that the fine network of the body fits into the *āsana*. This helps the senses of perception to cognise the conative action. This conjunction between organs of action and senses of perception brings about reflection in thought and subjective understanding begins to prompt re-adjustment. Then one begins to act, react, reflect, readjust, correct and perform the best in a conscious way.

One can go further towards finer actions and feelings for further growth of sensitivity in intelligence and consciousness, so that the body with the mind and consciousness come closer to the self. The life force then moves in the entire system of man, introducing a new light of discrimination so that evolution of the Self and involution of matter may converge and unite. Then harmony and balance, equipoise and serenity set in. The doer, the body and the *āsana* become one.

From here the *sādhaka* uses the body as a bow, and *āsana* as arrows to hit the target – the *ātman*.

Yoga is practised in four stages, viz., *āraṁbhāvasthā, ghaṭāvasthā, parichayāvasthā* and *niṣpattyāvasthā*. In the *āraṁbhāvasthā, āsana* are done objectively and mechanically. In the *ghaṭāvasthā* one performs with a series of adjustments. Then one tries to acquaint the mind and intelligence with the *āsana*. This is *parichayāvasthā*. Then one does a perfect *āsana* with absolute consciousness where the divisions vanish and the *āsana*, the body and the soul are blended together. This is *niṣpattyāvasthā*.

Performance of *āsana* can also be studied and understood in terms of the five elements: earth, water, fire, air and ether, and their counterparts, namely odour, taste, shape, touch and sound (as vibration), to gain rich insights into the structure, process and functions of each *āsana*.

Earth and odour represent the anatomical sheath and physical health, water and taste represent the physiological sheath giving organic health. Fire and shape characterise mental health by burning out the toxins and bringing coolness and poise in the mind. Air and touch help the intelligence to discriminate and discern the effect of *āsana* and to diffuse it all over the body, the mind and the self. This contact and touch enlivens the *ātman* to expand or contract in the ethereal sheath listening to the language of the body in the form of the vibration of sound.

Each practitioner has to feel these five elements with their dynamic qualities working in unison in each *āsana* or in each flow of energy in *prāṇāyāma*. Then the *āsana* is perfect, comfortable and stable according to Patañjali. Till then it is not a perfect state of *āsana* but a process towards performance of it.

In the final stage of perfection, the ego or 'I'-consciousness has to become humble and drop down like a ripe juicy fruit falling from the tree. Observe and study the placement of muscles, joints, tissues and cells at the starting point: in the *āsana*, feel the adjustment, reflect, readjust and reshape. While releasing from *āsana*, retrace all the movements, all the points, step by step, and come back to the starting point. This is the right key to be used for mastering an *āsana*. One has to see that no jerks or jolts occur in the body and mind. The intellectual flame and energy neither fade nor brighten. Neither the ego nor the vanity pervade the consciousness. This is how *āsana sādhanā* has to be done.

Conscious and regular practice not only keeps the cells of the body healthy but develops clear and pure intelligence and memory in them, creating purity in thought for one to move closer towards the *ātman*. The practice of *āsana* with reflective and meditative attention leads the *sādhaka* to move with the right attitude, right poise and stability bringing about loveliness, liveliness and dynamism. This method of practising *āsana* carries one from the bank of sorrow towards the bank of freedom.

Tataḥ dvandvaḥ anabhighatahaḥ (Y.S., II.48), i.e., From then on the *sādhaka* is undisturbed by dualities and experiences the infinite Self in the finite body.

PRACTISE YOGA WITH ATTENTIVE EYES*

What these two eyes can see, see well! If they cannot see, then you have to use the inner conscious intelligent eye to activise the physical eyes to be attentive to see.

ഇരു

We use our intelligence to see external things, but we do not know how to use the intelligence to penetrate internally. This internal movement of the intelligence begins through the practice of yoga and it travels from the body to the mind, mind to intelligence, intelligence to consciousness and consciousness to the self, so that you are drawn towards the core of Being – the Self.

ഇരു

Believing that "Iyengar Yoga" is meant only for physical fitness is a misconception. Those who make a separation between body and mind as well as mind and Self, do not understand the depth of yoga.

I use the body as an instrument to reach the Self. It is essential to transform the mind, the seeker, into a seer for physical, mental and spiritual well being. I use the body as a temple for the in-dweller to glow in life. As such, my emphasis on *āsana* is to bring total attention, so that the peripheral mind is transformed into the deep mind to be closer to the Self. This is my way of teaching and uplifting the students.

ഇരു

When I started practising I tried to remove all the weeds which grew in the body creating all sorts of cloudy feelings. As yoga is a factual subject, it should be judiciously practised so that it is accepted by the body, mind and consciousness. Unity of the body and mind is the keypoint of yoga. I want each of you to experience

---

* Excerpts from a lecture-demonstration at Harvard University, Cambridge, Massachusetts, August 20th, 1987.

this unity. When I practise, I study and compare the physiology of anatomy of that *āsana* to the physiology of the anatomy of the body for adjustment. I had to work and plan how to mould and build the body as required by each *āsana* and not make the *āsana* fit into my body's flexibility or stiffness. This way, the object and the instrument used reach unity, so that divisions disappear. I want you all to work to reach this state. I am sure that when this happens you will all experience a feeling of timelessness.

Pleasures are not permanent, whereas emancipation is permanent. Yoga brings that permanent freedom.

"THE ULTIMATE FREEDOM"*
BRING THE UNKNOWN INTO THE SPHERE OF THE KNOWN

Unless and until each and every part of our body, each and every limb of our body, the gross body, is released completely from tension, the subtle body, which is composed of the mind, intelligence, ego and consciousness, cannot be known, cannot be felt, cannot be understood. Unless and until freedom is gained in the body, freedom of the mind is a far-fetched idea. However, the gross body is cognised in two stages. What we call the "known body" also has a hidden layer of the unknown. Therefore, *āsana* is meant to conquer first the known, cognisable body in order to go towards the unknown body and to cognise it further. Later, the cognised body takes us closer towards the unknown inner body – the intelligence, ego and consciousness – so that both dissolve on their own in the seat of the Soul. The practice of *āsana* is meant to bring the unknown into the sphere of the known.

When I am in an *āsana*, I not only attend to the extension of each and every portion of my body, which moves in various directions, but I contact the intelligence and consciousness and connect them in unity, in order to be with myself.

FREEDOM OF BODY AND MIND

Each and every joint of my body has its own freedom and hence, I know what freedom is. Because for me my body is not one bulk or one piece, the space within is so great that it can be articulated piece by piece. Therefore my mind is free. It is not caught in the bulk of the body. My mind moves freely within. However, for an average person, the body is in one piece and the mind is in pieces.

The art of yoga is not only meant to keep oneself healthy but to keep the body light, which is why yogis have given several *āsana* to lighten the weight of the body.

---

* Demonstration at YMCA, Ann Arbor, 1976.

Each and every *āsana*, if perfected, is as comfortable as sitting on a chair. As the sculptor uses the chisel, the painter uses the brush and colour, or a musician uses his instrument, the yogi uses his own body to refine his inner intelligence. *Āsana* have to be practised in such a way that a sensitive refinement takes place in the body.

FREEDOM OF THE SPINE

In this modern technological world we have lost the resonance of the spine, which is why today the majority of people, due to the limited movements of the spine, are suffering from scoliosis, slipped discs and other spinal problems.

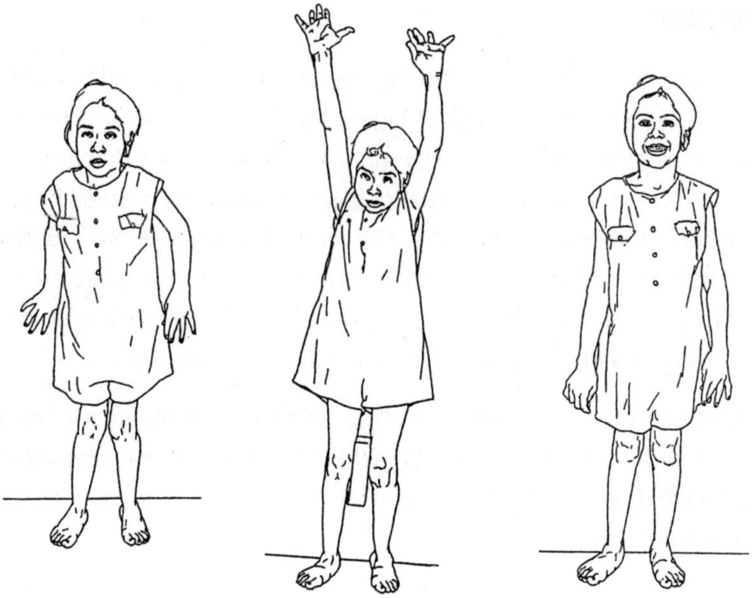

You must have seen people when they are not stable. They cannot stand steadily. Therefore, postures like the standing *āsana* help people who have defects in their legs or who are physically and mentally challenged. These postures strengthen the legs, so that they begin to stand firmly and see clearly. If the eyes are steady, the brain gains stability. If one knows the art of balancing the feet correctly, the brain floats in the fluid of the spine accurately and then it is centred. If the standing position is wrong, the brain cannot float exactly in the centre. These *āsana* are meant for the brain to float exactly in its position so that there is harmony in the brain and mind.

REMOVAL OF OBSTRUCTIONS

In the practice of *āsana* each and every pore of the skin, each and every part of the body, each and every ray of the intelligence is made to work to the optimum level penetrating from the extreme end of the foot to the top of the skull. The intelligence penetrates without obstruction. The practice of *āsana* removes obstructions and makes the energy and intelligence flow everywhere, in every nook and corner of the body. The practitioner no more remains caught in the web of the body. He goes beyond the body. For me, it is not merely the elasticity of the muscles and joints, it is not merely the freedom in the movement. Rather it is an ultimate freedom since I am not caught in the shackles of body-consciousness.

SĀLAMBA ŚĪRṢĀSANA

One needs to stand on one's head correctly. The fluid between skull and brain should not get compressed and should remain undisturbed. Liquid finds its own level. Similarly the fluid in the brain finds its own level. When you stand on your head correctly, then due to gravity the blood is pumped to the brain cells without any strain or injury because the arteries have elastic walls which contract and expand. So head balance *(Sālamba Śīrṣāsana* - Plate n. 5) does not make the blood pressure shoot up. Rather it oxygenates the brain. The brain needs one fourth of our oxygenated blood. Here the brain cells bathe in pure blood. The freshness of the brain brings clarity in thinking. Thoughts are filtered. Unwanted thoughts are expunged.

We all stand on our feet for hours each day. The venous return becomes poor at the end of the day. If we stand on our head for at least ten to fifteen minutes, the venous blood will return to the heart easily to be oxygenated. We will not only be free from varicose veins but save the heart from stress and strain.

SĀLAMBA SARVĀṄGĀSANA

In *Sālamba Sarvāṅgāsana* (Plate n. 5), the thyroid gland bathes in blood so secretion improves, whereas in *Sālamba Śīrṣāsana* (Plate n. 5) the pineal and pituitary glands bathe in blood. The advantage of the practice of *yogāsana* is that they regulate overworking glands and activate the underworking ones.

As the farmer ploughs the field and makes the soil soft, the yogi ploughs his nerves and organs by performing these *āsanas*, so that the body becomes a more fertile ground to produce vital energy for a better, healthy life.

These two *āsana* generate abundant energy – the life force – and make one free from mental and psychological tensions. The mind is freed from its enemies such as anger, desire and malice.

ŚAVĀSANA

Śavāsana (Plate n. 3) does not mean just dropping the body on to the floor and saying: "I am relaxing". The body, the mind and the self have to be kept in a state of equipoise. It is not merely either stillness or silence. It is the discipline of the body, senses and mind without feeling the stress of the discipline. It is a state where the fluctuations of the mind and intellect cease, the ego is subdued and finally disappears.

ULTIMATE FREEDOM

When the physical and physiological systems are kept completely healthy, the mind is free from the conflicts of the body; man is free from physical and physiological diseases and develops a clear and stable intellect. When the body is released from the shackles of diseases, then one experiences freedom. When the mind is free from the shackles of fears, then the intellect becomes ever alert and active. And in that activity there is creativity and in that creativity there is freedom. In freedom there is precision and in that precision alone there is God – God is Truth.

This practice of *āsana* leads one to experience the Inner Invisible Truth. Ultimate Truth means wisdom, which can never be shaken, which has no oscillations, which has no doubts. So when all the *āsana* are perfectly done, then the *sādhaka* is taken to that extreme subtle peace which we all call eternal truth, eternal poise, bliss and freedom from sorrow.

INTENSITY IS INTERPENETRATION*

In July 1989 a group from the U.K. (and a few others) had the good fortune to attend an intensive course in Pune taught by Gurujī. This was unexpected, as Gurujī was teaching only because of his son Prashant's recent accident.

The group contained a mixture of teachers and students some of whom were beginners. Many were visiting Pune for the first time.

Prior to the course Gurujī had said, "I am an old man now. I will give the best I can, but it may not be up to your expectation. Do not expect wonders. The course will be basic and consolidative."

On arrival at the Institute he warned us, "I do not know if you will be able to stand the pace!"

In fact he excelled himself. The class was made to exert physically and mentally to their maximum and new ideas and insights were explained each day. Even so, Gurujī told us, "Do not think this exhausts my knowledge. I am giving only thirty per-cent of what I know".

He explained the purpose of the intensive course from his point of view:

Intensity is interpenetration. We must intensify our intelligence to internalise and interpenetrate the body, mind, 'I'-consciousness and intelligence. The stretches or extensions are not limited only to the muscles of the body, but reach the consciousness so that it can expand.

My actions and words synchronise exactly in this sense. They do not vary at all. There is oneness. Interpenetration is devotedness. Though one has to penetrate inwards as well as outwards, it is an inner journey. You need to balance the inner intelligence with the peripheral intelligence of body in order to know the body and its wisdom. It is simultaneously balancing the intensity of action with the intensity of intelligence. The intensity of intelligence has to grasp the intensity of action. For this the brain should be completely pensive, calm and cool.

---

* from *Dipika Supplements*, nº 4, May 1990.

Before proceeding, please know that I am of average intellect; that is why I help others through my experiences. I am not selfish so I cannot keep what I know for myself. What little I know and have experienced, I want to give to you all. That is why I am happy.

I do not keep you in confusion. If you are in confusion, I am with you to remove that confusion. Often I read confusion on your face. If you are confused and do not admit that you are confused, I lose my temper. If you do not get it, then it is confusion which stops you from finding clarity. Therefore do not cover yourself under a cloak of confusion or ignorance. Know that this temper is genuinely to burn out your ignorance. It is meant to constructively build up, it is not a destructive apparatus.

You may not like my weapon of anger which is meant to build up and improve you. Where is your chance to improve, when I am gone? We should always try to understand what we do not understand. We have to study our habitual cultivated defects by looking microscopically at the action of the skin, then the spine, the buttocks, the thighs, the lower legs, in fact, each area of the body, and afterwards learn to adjust through discrimination in all the postures.

As a prisoner is put in a cell, the flesh is imprisoned by the skin which does not allow the expansion or contraction of the flesh. Prisoners are rehabilitated in the prison in order to restore them to normalcy. They are given freedom within the compound of the prison to improve themselves. Similarly, you have to create freedom to stretch and to move into vastness within its boundary or frontier. Sometimes the skin has to touch the flesh; sometimes the flesh has to touch the skin; sometimes there should be the creation of space between the flesh and the skin and vice versa.

We should be aware of each and every area of the body; where resistance should be, where co-operation should be, what the density should be; what the girth should be; how the movement should be and so on. This is called inner freedom.

For instance see *Tāḍāsana* and *Naṭarājāsana* (Plate n. 15). This is the first *āsana* and that is the last one. But is not the behaviour of the legs the same? See the parallel in these two different *āsana*. See how the parallelity is maintained though one is a standing pose and the other is a backward extension.

That is discretion: how is the outer side leg, or how does the socket of the hip function; is the resistance of the muscles and joints the same inside and outside the legs? This understanding of action in *āsana* comes only when there is a depth in the penetration. The similarity, or unity in diversity (two different *āsana*) is seen because of the intensity in interpenetration. For this reason you need to go back from the peripheral body to the inner body, then from the inner body to the outer body. The Self has to balance both on the inner body as well as on the outer body. Experience the intensity of the touch of intelligence and consciousness.

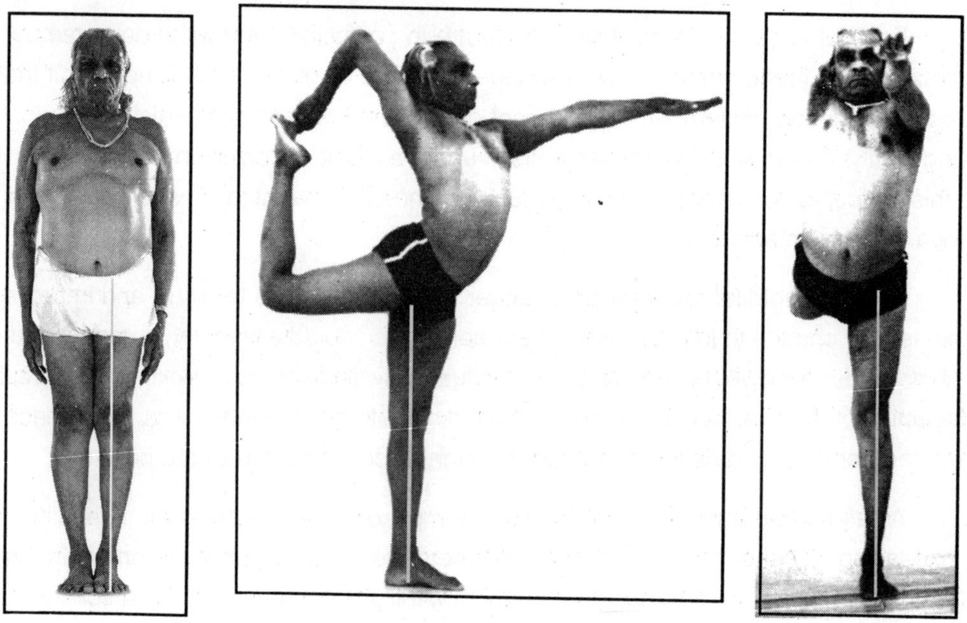

Plate n. 15 – *Tāḍāsana* and *Naṭarājāsana*

When one does *āsana* with intelligent awareness one gets the real light from the right performance of *āsana*. Observe the intelligent light flashing more and more. If it does not, there is darkness and stalemate in the body as well as in mind.

Devotedness means to soak all parts of the body from the outer skin, the inner skin and the flesh in the intelligence. It is the distribution of intelligence and energy in the body that is important in the presentation of the *āsana*. The moment the distribution takes place, the flesh is free from its prison.

In the *Bhagavad Gītā* it is said that one out of a million is devoted to any art, that is, they do it for its own sake. The rest do it with a motive. I am giving these points so that I can make millions develop the same inner awakening of intelligence *(prajñā)*.

If attention is intelligence, know that awareness is consciousness. Awareness is *citta*. What is the difference between *prajñā* and *citta? Prajñā* is the intelligent character of *citta*. If there is no *citta*, it is a dead body. In the first chapter, Patañjali uses the word *saṁprajñāta* (self awareness). He says, *saṁprajñāta citta* is full awareness of the *citta* which comes with *sabīja*

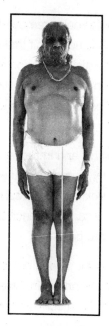

samādhi. It is untinged transformation of the consciousness. It is true that it takes a long time to transform the *citta* since it is tainted with so many thoughts. But if you remember your *Sālamba Śīrṣāsana* (Plate n. 5) of the first day, you will know that when you stood on your head, your mind was totally engrossed in *Sālamba Śīrṣāsana*. You could not think of anything else. Did you noticed the quality of *citta* at that time which was fully aware of only *Sālamba Śīrṣāsana* and nothing else? The *citta* remained fully charged with awareness. In a sense it was *samprajñāta* state wherein the *citta* was charged with self awareness even though it was time-bound. You learnt a new level of your own *citta*. When this *prajñā* or attention and awareness was lost, you fell down. In fact one has to learn the quality of *citta*, replete with *prajñā* in those few minutes which help you to understand the *samprajñāta citta* of *samādhi* state.

You need to be intense in your practice and very fast in your observations. Use your intelligence and awareness to adjust when or where you go wrong so that you spend no time dwelling in a wrong *āsana*. The misunderstanding and confusion only vanish when your approach is correct.

The mind is like a dog's tail. As long as you are straightening it, it remains straight. The moment you remove your hand, the tail immediately goes back to its old shape. So be careful and see that your intelligence does not curl back but maintains its extension, expansion and freedom.

I have given you a very sound base. It is a healthy approach. You cannot jump and miss anything. I have taught the ways to feel the right movement and wrong movement. Even if you practise for ten minutes a day with a reflective state, you build up a sharp intelligence. The moment the fragrance of intelligence is lost in an *āsana*, do not continue. Better that you go to the next *āsana*, so that you revitalise and renew your intelligence.

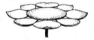

YOGĀSANA – TO YOKE THE BODY-MIND TO THE SELF*

As healthy plants and trees yield good flowers and fruits, so does the healthy body. It is the means for man to reach the goal of life, which is the realisation of the Self.

As a result of one's *karma,* a chain of reactions is generated. This chain makes one succumb to the dual afflictions of pleasure and pain. Pleasure is an affliction, as it increases desires and wants; these in turn lead to unhappiness if one fails to achieve them. Even if one has all the pleasures within one's reach, for one reason or the other one will not be able to enjoy them. For example, ill health can stand in the way of enjoyment.

The afflictions that affect man can be classified as *adhyātmika, ādhidaivika* and *ādhibhautika*[1]; they appear in the form of physical, mental and spiritual disorders. *Ādhidaivika* and *ādhibhautika* diseases affect man as a result of external influences, whereas *ādhyātmika* disease is a result of one's own deliberate deeds.

Most people are affected by physical, mental and spiritual afflictions, which are of their own making, thinking and acting. *Yogāsana* can change man's vision and help him to develop right thinking and right action so that he can put a stop to the accumulation of physical and mental disorders.

Āsana deals with the health of the body, harmony of the mind and clarity of the intelligence. *Āsana* acts as a bridge to unite the body with the mind and the mind with the Self. If the Self is the core, the body is its envelope. If the envelope is strong and well glued together, it carries the letter safely. The content is preserved. Hence it is wrong for spiritual seekers to treat *āsana* as if it is inferior and untouchable. It shows that they are dull in their thinking and behaviour. Actually *āsana* is the stepping stone towards a spiritual life. Those who treat the body as a separate entity and a hindrance to spiritual life are ignorant of its value.

---

* From *Bhavan's Journal,* August 1, 1981 - also *Dipika,* Spring 1981 and *Dipika,* Spring 1982.

1 *Adhyātmika* means pertaining to the self, *ādhidaivika,* pertaining to the divine sphere; and *ādhibhautika,* pertaining to worldly phenomena.

Āsana helps one to know the known fully and realise it. When the known – the body – is fully understood, then this known, which is finite, guides one to move beyond the known, towards the infinite, the Self. Then the True Self is expressed through actions. At this time there is neither known nor unknown, subject or object. Both become one and that is the essence of *yogāsana* and that is the reason for its daily practice.

As the body is the shrine of the soul, it has to be kept healthy, clean and pure – as a heaven on earth. If it is neglected, it becomes a hell for the person possessing it.

Regular and perfect practice of *āsana* cleanses the senses of perception and organs of action, controls and sublimates them for the Self to shine forth.

While performing *āsana*, certain things must be observed in each state of the *āsana*: an even stretch on either side of the body and even attention all over the body is non-violence in *āsana*. Its truthful presentation is in its essence. To do less than one's capacity towards perfection is false practice. It is dishonesty. The co-ordination of body and mind without losing the contact with the self has to be maintained. One should not be in *āsana* just physically. Then it becomes a physical performance. Rather there should be a total absorption and involvement when one is in *āsana*. As the *āsana* should be pure and faultless, the body and mind too should be clean and sacred. One should not feel contented, just because the posture is good and comfortable. The contentment is in the perfection of the *āsana*, where the body is firm and the intelligence is steady. When these are achieved, the very performance of *āsana* leads the performer towards Self-realisation.

Each movement begins from the seat of the heart. The seat of the heart is known as the knower of the field (the body). The field and the knower of the field should be divinely wedded while performing *āsana*[1]. Then one becomes a light unto oneself.

The practice of *yogāsana* transforms man totally. His views and aims change for better purpose. It makes him sacrifice the desires of the world in order to reach the goal of complete surrender of himself to The Almighty – *Īśvara praṇidhāna*.

If *yogāsana* is done without bringing the body and the Self together, then the practice becomes *ajñāna yoga*, the yoga of ignorance or foolish yoga. When *yogāsana* is done thoroughly and thoughtfully, then that practice becomes *prajñāna yoga* or yoga with full knowledge.

---

1 See *Kṣetra-kṣetrajña*, pp. 197.

YOGA – MUSIC FOR THE BODY AND SOUL*

Yoga is the talented presentation or the balancing of the various regions or frontiers of the body, the mind, the consciousness, the ego and the very Being. Water is even on the surface of a lake though there are many dents at the bottom. The body, like a lake, has several dents and in spite of these dents, it is possible to spread the flow of consciousness evenly. And that is what yoga guides us to learn.

All yogic postures – *yogāsana* – ventilate the entire human system through two ventilators, namely the respiratory and the circulatory systems. They function harmoniously, keeping the other systems in balance. They bring understanding and intercommunication between each other. Each cell of the body communicates with the others and appears as a true Self for the practitioner. They have their own voiceless language.

The practice of *āsana* helps to increase the calibre of intelligence by destroying the impurities of the body and mind so that the crown of wisdom radiates in each individual making him friendly and compassionate towards himself, to his neighbour and to his society. That is what the art of yoga teaches mankind.

Yoga is music for the body and the soul. The best of all music is silence. Silence has got its own rhythm and melody. Peace with silence brings harmony in the music of the soul.

The vibration of breath without any movement is known as silence in stillness. This silence is not found only in the body but also in the mind. This stillness and silence of the mind bring one into the present moment. As long as one lives witnessing the movement without getting involved in it, moment to moment, one experiences the music of the divine.

An unhealthy body cannot hear or experience the music of the divine.

---

* Lecture – demonstration at Davies Hall, San Francisco, July 1984.

The most important key for health is the art of using the respiratory system through *prāṇāyāma* in order to derive the maximum benefit from the bio-nuclear energy that is in the atmospheric air, so that each and every cell in our system is fed with nuclear energy. The nerve-fibres which are nothing but strings of this instrument – the body – then vibrate rhythmically and melodiously to produce divine music.

The interior decorator decorates the house in order to beautify it. Similarly, each *āsana* and *prāṇāyāma* decorates the entire system from within. Thus the Lord of the house, the *ātman*, enjoys free movement in any direction. He finds chamber after chamber opening for him to observe their beauty.

However, due to our limited capacity we are able to perceive our body only partially. The front of the body is the visible body, whereas the back portion of the body is unperceived. The senses of perception perceive the front body. We see the entire front body through the eyes, whereas we can conceive the back body only through feeling. Sensitivity alone can make us feel. Feeling the back or posterior body involves drawing the energy, intelligence and senses of perception inwards. This is a kind of *pratyāhāra*. Such sensitivity is developed only through *pratyāhāra*. *Pratyāhāra* inhibits the known sensitivity and brings the unknown sensitivity to the surface. Thus, in *pratyāhāra* one learns how to change the conscious into the unconscious, and the unconscious into conscious states. The balance of consciousness with the unconscious is learnt. Then there are no subconscious, unconscious or conscious divisions. They all are one. When they all become one, some call it a superconscious state. This is how *pratyāhāra* accompanies the performance of *āsana*.

The practices of *āsana* and *prāṇāyāma* are done at two levels. A beginner just performs, acts and does. But at a certain stage he begins to reflect on what he does. The action is *karma* whereas the reflection is *jñāna*. When *karma* and *jñāna*, action and reflection, go together, spiritual *sādhanā* begins. Undoubtedly *sādhanā* (practice), unites the physical body and the spiritual body. But one has to cross the bridge of the consciousness (the mind, the intelligence and ego). If one end of the bridge is bondage, the other end is emancipation. Patañjali calls it *kaivalyam*. *Kaivalya* or emancipation is the absolute state of aloneness. It is certainly not loneliness. This aloneness has to be felt in each individual cell. When each cell works individually and lives in freedom, the Self too is free. This is *kaivalya*.

Many a time, people think that the performing of *āsana* is something like a violent action. One who acts at the physical level only will have violence and aggressiveness. But when one performs by co-ordinating the action and reflection, then there is no aggressiveness. There is neither non-violence, nor violence. When non-violence and violence move together, there is yoga. Patañjali says, *Vitarkabādhane pratipakṣabhāvanam* (*Y.S.,* II.33). Please read the commentaries on this *sūtra* in the *Light on the Yoga Sūtra of Patañjali* [1]. Do not stick to the theory, "If you're angry, think of non-anger". That is what others have said, but I do not think it is Patañjali's idea. He says, go with the anger and analyse it. When there is a certain pain in a certain part of the body and there is no pain on the other identical part, analyse the part where there is no pain, analyse the part where there is pain. How do you analyse? Do the movement several times to find out how the pain comes and how it does not come and exchange *(pratipakṣa)* by reversing the process. Adjust the position on the bad side or the afflicted side to that of the good side, then both the feelings of good and bad disappear. This is the melody that has to be felt in our practice. Similarly, when one goes deep into anger and studies it, then anger and non-anger, violence or non-violence, disappear. The practitioner begins to get clarity in his judgement. The action may seem to start from aggressiveness, but reflection leads one towards non-aggression. The practice of *āsana* and *prāṇāyāma* teach each individual cell to be non-violent *(ahiṁsaka).*

Patañjali says: "Do not covet!" While in *āsana* you may stretch, extend or create the space on one side of the body or one part of the body forgetting or neglecting the other side or other parts. This is called covetousness *(parigraha).* In that case, the vibration will be rough and crude. Obviously the sound will be harsh. It ends up in greed, as you are neglecting many things in that covetousness. You create a barrier for your intelligence and energy. You don't release it to flow everywhere evenly. So learn to tune your attention on the side which is neglected. Try to feel the rhythmic vibration (*nāda)* where there is no overstretching. This way, if you observe both sides of the body and adjust and tune evenly, then the truth reveals itself so that the grossness and roughness disappear. Otherwise one side sings the truth because that side has depth, while the other side rambles because that side cannot reflect right vibration in action. When all things are put together in presentation of the *āsana,* we experience oneness in the melody of vibration in the body.

You all know that *brahmacarya* means celibacy. You do not know how the state of celibacy is experienced in the *āsana.* When both right and left sides of the body, anterior and posterior body as well as outer and inner body are tuned in unison, your mind is raised above the body. You remain non-attached to your body and forget it. The mind is tuned to flow with the self. You find within you a divine tune – a divine music. The reverse flow of your *(prāṇic)* bio-energy, mind, intelligence and consciousness from outwards towards inwards is called *brahmacarya.*

---

[1] See the Author's *Light on the Yoga Sūtras of Patañjali,* Harper Collins, London

Unless and until the *āsana* and *prāṇāyāma* are well-performed, well-managed and well-balanced, know well that you have already put the seed of imbalance, incoherence and non-co-ordination in the nervous system, circulatory system, digestive system. This way it goes on creating various disturbing sounds in body and mind. There is neither toning nor tuning. While in *āsana* one learns to extend the inner structure in the interior space of the body to its capacity in order to allow it to stretch fully, without strain or tension. By this you learn the way to surrender the body and mind. If there is any restlessness, the eyes indicate it immediately. Then know that you are doing something wrong. Restfulness brings equipoise in the cells and mind and helps one to be receptive. This receptive passivity with alertness helps one to surrender to the practice. This surrender is *bhakti* in the *āsana*. When the pose is fully performed, surrender of oneself to that *āsana* is as good as *Īśvara praṇidhāna* (surrendering to God who is within).

What is anger? It is a kind of hyperextension. You go red when you are angry. You get hyper-tensed. Your face and temples become tense. Your eyes get puffed. All these are the symptoms of hypertension. Hyperextension of the muscles in *āsana* too is, in a way, an anger of the muscles. You have to check and stop the hyperextensions in *āsana*. The hyperextension of the muscles not only damages the muscles but also the nerves. Similarly, a hypertensed person not only invites high blood pressure but indirectly damages his nerves. Anger damages and dries up the nerves. As the strings of musical instruments break when overstretched, so also the nerves, due to hyperextension, get over-burdened and result in nervous breakdown. Therefore the practitioners need to have an eye on such hyperextensions, overdoing. You have to check your over-enthusiasm.

When the physical body fuses with the physiological body, the physical and physiological bodies come in contact with the mind. The mind sends the message to the intelligence: "This cell is telling me something, please, listen to that." The *āsana* needs to be adjusted on a cellular level. Each *āsana* will have its own direction in which to extend and turn. Each cell has to be placed in its location. Then, from the cell the self is connected, and from the self the cell is connected by the *sādhaka* like the musician with his instrument and music.

While practising *āsana* you have to do the dual part, moving the intelligence from the self towards the extremities of the body and the intelligence of the extremities towards the self. Energy moving from the self towards the body is the outgoing energy and the energy that moves from the body towards the self is the incoming energy. This ascending and descending movement of energy between body, mind and self is the music of the Soul. Uniting these two energies is the essence of performing *āsana*.

Patañjali has said: *Prayatna śaithilya ananta samāpattibhyām* (II.47). When the effortful effort transfers itself into an effortless effort, you have touched the subtle sound of that *āsana*. Similarly, you have to get this effortless effort in all *āsana*. When you have conquered an *āsana*, at that time the dualities between the joints, the muscles, the systems, disappear. The disparity between the body and mind dissolves, and then you live not as a single individual, but alone as universal personality. If I am struggling to get the *āsana*, I am an individual, but the moment effortlessness sets in, there is no individuality, no struggle and there is no 'I', there is no 'me', there is no 'you', but *nāda*, the music alone.

Anatomists know the limited range of movements in the joints. The yogis of yore found the way to go beyond. They were courageous and cheerful to advance in order to find out the new, unknown and hidden movements in joints and muscles. That is why they could visualise, perform and practise innumerable *āsana*. If I show more *āsanas*, the anatomists brand me as a contortionist. It is an underestimation of the intelligence of the body's functions or the body-wisdom. They do not understand that if one human being can do it, another can also do it. If the ankle is sprained, you are in plaster: you are kept for twenty days with support, but the yogis know how to curve in, how to move the ankle, how to move the inner ankle out or the outer ankle in to minimise the pain and at the sametime to rest this part. In this way, *āsana* teaches various movements, bringing out the hidden intelligence of the body for the adjustment of the fluids of the body. This is the beauty of *yogāsana*. It is a very difficult and sensitive art, which does not mean that it should be abandoned and forgotten. Today, people have the *jñāna* (knowledge) of the body but not its *prajñā* (subjective awareness).

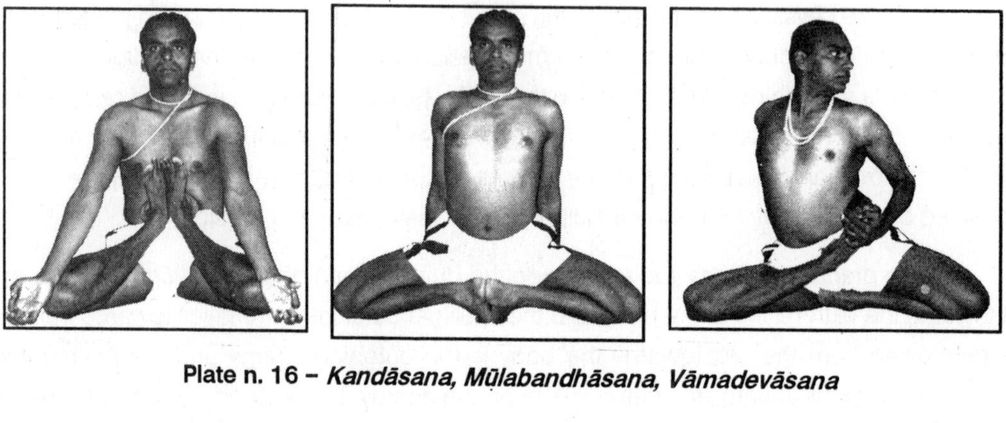

Plate n. 16 – *Kandāsana, Mūlabandhāsana, Vāmadevāsana*

I am presenting the postures not to show my ego or my greatness, but to fasten your attention deliberately, so that you may not do false movements. False movements are a waste of energy. Hitting the *āsana* ten times and collapsing is not practice. Music is never practised

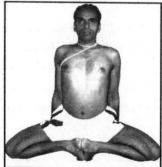

like this. If it does not come, stop it, what does it matter? Have patience, be soft, as all motions need softness and not hardness. Motion is like using the accelerator and the hardness is like a brake. How could they move together? This results in injury. So you have to give room for each muscle which moves like a wheel. Each muscle, each cell, is a wheel of this human system. It needs to be charged with *prāṇa* and *prajñā*.

The practice of yoga should be filled with *śauca, santoṣa, tapaḥ, svādhyāya* and *Īśvarapraṇidhānā*. *Śauca* means cleanliness. If you do your *āsana* just a little here and a little there, it is as good as doing nothing. It is a waste of time. "Warming up" is not the right word. If I want to warm this finger, knuckle, I have to only stretch for the blood to circulate. Touch the thing directly to feel the movement directly! This is *śauca*.

One requires a tremendous awareness in the practice of yoga: *Vivekakyātiḥ aviplavā hānopāyaḥ* (*Y.S.*, II.26). Awareness should run uninterruptedly when the *abhyāsa* is getting complicated. Similarly, while practising *āsana, prāṇāyāma* or *dhyāna*, if that uninterrupted awareness is slightly lost, you are in the dark. You are in suspense and you do not know what to do. What happens to you when the light suddenly goes off, your nervous system may go into a sort of suspense inside which may not come to the surface for days or months or years. That is why especially the practice of *āsana* has to be done with tremendous awareness and not with greed of ambition in mind that "I want to do it". You love backbends, but is your body prepared to do backbends or not? One should know that. You want to do the balances. Are your hands and your shoulders strong? Practitioners do not put these questions to themselves. If I show the *āsana* on a platform, some of you may stupidly go and try. Remember I have done yoga with sanity for fifty years. You should have in your mind that I did not get these *āsana* in a day. How did I manage to get that rhythm from years of practice is unknown to you all? And you are fortunate as you have at least a person who helps to remove the weeds from your practices. Learn to remove the weeds first, so that the plant of *āsana* may grow well in you. That needs a healthy mind and a clear intelligence. This is *śauca;* I have cleansed the body, I have cleansed the nerves. In that cleanliness, what do I get? – "Rhythm, and that is contentment". Because of a good circulation, a healthy feeling has been felt in those parts. Health may come, but cleanliness has to be present. From this health and cleanliness the real yoga commences. From *śauca* and *santoṣa,* the real hard work commences in the form of *tapas, svādhyāya* and *Īśvara praṇidhāna*.

Patañjali does not say: "Have the delight, have the pleasures," but, "go beyond pleasures and delight." He wants us to develop a tremendous inner urge and aspiration to penetrate further in the form of *tapas*. In that search comes the knowledge of the body, knowledge of the muscles, knowledge of the organs, knowledge of the nerves and knowledge of the mind. This is *svādhyāya*. From this aspiration you develop the discipline to study yourself, which you all call: "Know thyself". To know thyself there should be an aspiration. Here *santoṣa* does not mean just the pleasure of contentment but also aspiration. *Śauca* does not mean just taking a bath and keeping the body clean. Taking a bath does not keep your blood clean, but it may keep the pores of the skin clean. The question remains, how to keep the cells clean, how to keep the organs clean? It is possible only by *santoṣa*. Each organ has to live and love itself, and smile. The stomach has to smile, the intestines have to smile. When that is learnt, then: "Know thyself" comes, because your interest in the art increases. As the interest increases, the search for the Self begins. In that searching you have to become one within yourself through the *āsana*.

When I am performing the *āsana*, the *āsana* is an object, I am a subject. I am seeking through that *āsana*. When I have searched out everything in that *āsana*, which is an object, then I enter into that object, I lose my identity, the object becomes the subject and I become the object. I become the witness. This is *Īśvara praṇidhāna*. My self is witnessing this universal, cosmic structure in each *āsana*. This is the real, spiritual, yogic practice. When the raw, false yoga ends, the real yoga commences. Confining oneself to the health aspect is raw yoga. After gaining health, what one has to do becomes real yoga. Real yoga is a science of liberation, a science of freedom. So one cannot stop at the point of health and happiness, which is common to all. One has to go still further to perform carefully, watching each and every cell to see that it co-operates with one's willpower. When the will of the mind unites with the will of the self, it is *haṭha yoga*.

Ha is also compared to consciousness and *ṭha* to energy. How to make the energy of the breath mingle with intelligence and consciousness, so that they are communicating with and understanding each other, is also *haṭha yoga*. Lazy yogis who do not practise, who cannot stand straight, who cannot walk, who need a support, say: "*Haṭha yoga* is a physical yoga", because they cannot do it. Three-fourths of my life have gone in the practice of yoga and I am very near the grave. So I want to reach that grave with benevolent friendliness. This is why I am practising. Those who are afraid of practising *āsana* and *prāṇāyāma* take shelter under the cover that they are teaching spiritual yoga. What is spiritual yoga? To say *mantra* you have to use your mouth, do you not? *Auṁ Namo Nārāyanāya*, "I am thinking of God". Which part of your body is used? Is the self saying it, or are your lips and your mouth saying it? If I say: "*Auṁ, Auṁ, Auṁ, Auṁ*, I am doing *japa yoga*", and if I move my hand, I learn whether my intelligence can reach there or not. Is it then a "physical" yoga? The discriminative faculty in you cannot help you if you do not test these so called yogis and *swamis!* Ask them to stand erect: they want a chair. If *swamis* come with robes you give them a chair to sit. And for me you offer nothing because I am not in that robe. I stand and am still standing. And they say: "My young pupil will be performing for you." Because they cannot stand, they are using someone. Their limbs are rusted. But my limbs are not rusted, I am living everywhere, that is the meaning of "know yourself" – "know yourself" because "I know myself". This is the music of the body, mind and Soul.

Age makes one nervous. People are afraid of old age, believing that age stops one from doing *āsana* and *prāṇāyāma*. Remember, soul has no age. Old age comes through the mind, old age does not come to the Self. Often these questions are put to me: How can *āsana* be done in old age? Will it not be harmful? When sex life (desire) has no age, why should there be a fear to do good things in the world, when there is so much room for evil deeds? To do good practices in the world, why should there be doubts? Why should one question? Do not be nervous. If you can abuse evil things like drinking, smoking, sex and what not, why do you not also abuse the good things in life a little more? If you abuse the good things more, you will have more good effect; by abusing the bad things you get illnesses. Then you have to leave off smoking, you have to leave off drinking. By doing good, there is nothing to leave, as nothing bad happens. That advantage is there forever.

I beg my pupils to protect their pupils more than themselves when they are teaching. Do not say as a teacher that you are protecting yourself so that you can help your students more tomorrow.

Let this ancient knowledge flow like the sound of music from one generation to another. Art is infinite but we are bound in finite time. The *riṣi* of yore were right to tell us to pass on our knowledge to the next generation. We may not live but art remains alive and vital for ever.

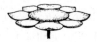

THE GRACE OF CONSCIOUSNESS IN *ĀSANA**

Before we begin today's special course, I would like you all to know that this will not be an intensive work. I believe that it will be inspiring work. It will not be a session of hard work where you all perspire. As intelligence is universal these are going to be judiciously intellectual sessions where the universality, or the feel of oneness in our teaching may be experienced by all so that all will carry the message of yoga uniformly from now on.

In *Sanskṛt* there are words like *cintana* and *manana*. *Cintana* means analysis and *manana* means that which is analysed and synthesised through action. These two words hold a beauty for us to make use of in the path of yoga. Where analysis and synthesis meet, skill in intelligence emerges, which is why yoga is called skill in action *(karmasu kauśalam)*[1]. Skill in performance is the true *karma mārga* of yoga. When skill in analysis and synthesis meet, you are in a state of meditation. Suppose you reach that state where action is reflected, then from there you begin to readjust accurately and you reach the final state of the *āsana*. I want to show and teach this as well as guide you. That is what I have in mind. However, the base and essence of what I say has to be taken within yourselves from the very first word and presentation. In the limited time of these sessions it is impossible for me to teach the essence of all the two hundred *āsana* to everyone. Then we may have to work for months together. Therefore I have decided to give you the base, and from this base you will have to practise to experience the essence of the *āsana*. Once you know the base, then you are able to introduce the pattern in various other *āsana*. It is important that you digest what you learn here before you share it with your students. You need to learn and practise with a subtle sensitivity of intelligence.

In the first chapter of the *Yoga Sūtra,* Patañjali uses the term *citta prasādanam*. *Prasādanam* means grace. It is not just awareness, but also the grace of the consciousness. As you go to the temple or to the church and ask for the Lord's blessing and grace on you, similarly, as yogis, you would like to have the grace of consciousness on the body, mind and intelligence,

---

* Introductory talk given at a course held in Panchgani, India, 29th November 1993.
1 See *Bhagavad Gītā* II.50

in your practices. When consciousness graces you, then it is possible to have *ātma-prasādanam* – the grace of the Self. Then you experience the totality of yourselves and live in each and every part of your body, every part of your expression and in every part of your feelings. Therefore, from *citta prasādanam* (gracefulness of the consciousness), leap or go ahead to earn the gracefulness of the seer. Patañjali uses the term *citta prasādanam* first since *ātma-prasạdanam* has to follow. He does not use the term *ātma-prasādanam*, knowing very well that people cannot see or visualise the seer. So he makes us aware of our consciousness, which we can know and grasp. Then he uses the consciousness to work as a bridge to unite the intelligence and the seer. You awaken the hidden essence and bring it to awareness and so you have been awakened. The moment you have been awakened, from that point on it is the job of the seer to see using the consciousness as his instrument. Your job now is to awaken and alert the consciousness. After that, allow the seer within you to see if consciousness is alerted in each and every part of your body. Then the seer engulfs the body and uses it as his instrument, along with the mind, intelligence, ego and consciousness, co-ordinating them with him, and they all become one and divine. Here both the seen and the seer unite and become divine. I hope with this background of understanding you begin to practise *āsana*.

No other path except *aṣṭāṅga yoga* brings out this hidden quality of attention. The need for practice with attention and awareness is essential in order to follow the paths of *jñāna, bhakti or karma*. This attention and awareness definitely flowers through *āsana* and *prāṇāyāma*.

Āsana is a path of *jñāna mārga,* where you develop the knowledge of yourself, your body, your mind and your consciousness, through action *(karma)*, while in *prāṇāyāma* you learn the path of devotion. These two petals of *aṣṭāṅga yoga,* as instructed by Patañjali, come to my mind as *jñāna* cum *karma mārga* and *bhakti* cum *jñāna* and *karma mārga*. The practice of *yama* and *niyama* helps one to follow *karma mārga*. True *karma* (right action) cannot come without the acquisition of knowledge *(jñāna)* and devotion *(bhakti)*. Without mastery in *āsana*, *jñāna* does not develop, and without *prāṇāyāma*, dedication and devotion do not come. Without *jñāna* and *bhakti*, right action does not rise.

Actually the culmination of *jñāna* and *bhakti* or even *samādhi* is nothing but actions that have no reactions. Therefore no fruit of those actions touch the *sādhaka*. Many people acquire knowledge but only do so with a certain motivation. However, knowledge without motivation is developed through *āsana*, and dedication and devotion through *prāṇāyāma*. These non-motivated actions are beyond black (evil), grey (mixture of good and evil) and white (good) actions. So these two aspects of yoga are the guides for us to reach ripeness in our spiritual development. This is the reason why through this session I am trying to show to you what it may be possible to achieve through *āsana* and *prāṇāyāma*. In the case that it is not possible, then we must accept our limited intellectual condition, but in the meantime let us make a serious and attentive effort. In these sessions I will try to present you with this aspiration, so that you may understand and feel what you can experience without prejudice or conditions.

First you have to study *āsana* correctly and then understand the homogenous movements in various parts of the body that are involved. Without a correct understanding of the *āsana*, a rhythm and homogeneity in doing it, as well as a tranquil feeling, will not come. So first learn not to speak out before you feel the sense of poise and calm and how it is happening. You cannot feel this unless you give your ears to understanding exactly what is said.

ĀSANA AND THE ELEMENTS

Our body is a combination and co-ordination of five elements: earth, water, fire, air and ether, with five qualities like odour, taste, form, touch and sound. You can call these the atomic structures of the above five elements. All these elements with their qualities are in our body. Through the organs of action and the senses of perception, we can feel these elements and the qualities of the elements. While practising *āsana* you begin to control the elements so that they function in unison, and through the practice of *prāṇāyāma* the same with the atomic structures of the elements. This means that through *āsana* and *prāṇāyāma* practices you learn to recognise and control the ten elements and qualities of nature in you. At the next level comes *citta,* comprised of mind, intelligence and ego, which are to be co-ordinated attentively with the organs of action and senses of perception in order to make all facets of nature function healthily.

The first evolute of *prakṛti* (nature) is the cosmic consciousness, known as *mahat.* In man this cosmic consciousness *(mahat)* transforms into individual consciousness *(citta).* When you are practising *āsana,* this individual consciousness has to be transformed into cosmic consciousness in the entire body so that the individual and the cosmic come together to become one. The *cidākāṣa* and *mahadākāṣa* unite. Then the differences or the separation between the two exist no more. When this state is reached, the twenty-four principles of nature in the body are brought under control for the seer – the twenty-fifth principle – to see and guide directly thereafter. This is what *āsana* and *prāṇāyāma* teach and it is what you and I have to work for.

I am glad to tell you that to some extent I have reached this state. I have experienced it. I want you also to learn how, by the practice of *āsana* and *prāṇāyāma,* these vehicles of nature are understood and trained, so that the seer uses them to see how this drama that is each of us is enacted. As God uses the world as a playground for Him to play, treat this body as the playground for the seer to play. I play well in this playground of myself, using all parts of my body, my consciousness, awareness and intelligence, through the performance of hundreds of *āsana* and *prāṇāyāma.*

Each of us may have different facets to our intellect, but factual intelligence should not vary at all. Though the intellect varies, experiential knowledge is of one piece. At the end it is matured intelligence that codifies, synthesises and unifies all varying points for right understanding and homogeneity in action. The intellect earns the knowledge *(vidyā),* whereas the intelligence experiences, filters and feels the knowledge *(buddhi),* that leads one towards wisdom. *Vidyā* is knowledge earned through intellect, and *buddhi* – the intelligence – cleanses the knowledge.

The filtered intelligence – *buddhi* – does not vary. But you have to learn how to spread the filtered intelligence in its abode of the body. You can experience this while performing *āsana* along with reflective observation. When correct placement of intelligence with awareness is learnt, then rhythmic, smooth movement of energy is made to flow throughout the body. When you proceed further you find that the *āsana* helps the consciousness to spread and engulf all the sheaths of the body. With this total awareness, you can tap your intelligence *(buddhi)* and consciousness *(citta)* to move towards the level of the intelligence of the seer and view at once the entire frame of the physical, physiological, mental, intellectual and conscious sheaths, part by part and as a whole. It is this message of the uniformity of the feeling of experience that I want to give you in these sessions.

Each teacher thinks that what he or she teaches is according to his or her study or to the condition of the students. I try to break this illusion as far as possible. Only then may it be possible for you all to compare and decide whether it is the teacher's mental condition or the student's mental condition that you are dealing with. Afterwards, before you convey the essence of yoga, you have to share your experiences with your colleagues, to find out whether they too felt the same feeling as you experienced. Hence, we are all here to feel that oneness of the essence that is tested and tasted while performing each *āsana,* so that the work in this session makes each one of you experience the same sensitive feeling. When I make you taste the same experience, then you can go back and begin teaching with this new taste. This is the aim of us all being here.

On your return, you can transmit this new dimension to those whose destiny has not brought them to attend these classes. Please be humble; you need not be devoted to me, but please be devoted to the art you practise. Know that without devotional practice, no development comes. *Āsana* and *prāṇāyāma* are the two aspects in the field of yoga where knowledge needs to be developed. Remember that no one teaches and no one tells you this requirement as their minds get blocked owing to their limitations or dogmatism. We are here to study that *āsana* is not just a physical performance, but that there is something further hidden in it, i.e., the flow of intelligence. *Āsana* sponsors the intelligence in each of us to become a powerful helping hand for the understanding of ourselves as well as of others. *Āsana* helps us to bring to the surface this latent quality of attention and awareness, which we all have, but we do not tap.

The subduing and conquest of nature by *āsana* and *prāṇāyāma* is to make the seer establish Himself so that He dictates terms for nature to follow Him. As long as you are not practising *āsana* and *prāṇāyāma* with this aim, then it is the other way around: nature plays supreme and the seer acts in servitude to nature. By the judicious practice of *āsana* and *prāṇāyāma* that state is reversed and you become your own master and remain master of nature. The five elements with their atomic nuclei, the mind, the intelligence, ego and the consciousness are under your command.

Āsana and *prāṇāyāma* teach you to go beyond the vehicles of nature so that the seer and all his vehicles become a single unit. Then the *puruṣa* graces your body (*puri* - fort or city - *śete* - dwells in - *iti puruṣaḥ* = since He dwells in His abode, everywhere He is the Lord of the fort or Lord of the body).

I want to convey to you this grace of the seer or *puruṣa* throughout this session. I hope you have grasped something of what I said about the principles behind *āsana* and *prāṇāyāma* so that you play well in the yogic field. Good luck and better understanding of yoga from now on. May God's grace be on you all.

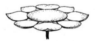

ĀSANA – COSMIC AND NOT COSMETIC*

Friends,

I am grateful to the organisers of the International Yoga Teachers Association, for having invited me to present something on my practice of yoga.

I know that you are all eager to watch my performance. I am not sure whether I can enthuse you towards the subject after finishing my demonstration.

I know many of you are more devoted than I. There is a truth in this. The only difference is that I cannot call myself a devotee of yoga, because yoga is running in my bloodstream. Therefore I do not know what I have to call myself, but I say I am just a student of yoga. The student of yoga should know that yoga alone is the master, and no one who practises it has the right to call himself or herself a Master of Yoga. After all, art is God and hence art alone, and not its practitioner, can be the Master. The more you know, the more you realise that the unknown is far beyond the known. As such, art is the master, not you or I.

Amazingly, in this world everything is moving in triune – creation, continuity and destruction. One calls this movement the work of God. This work of God is expressed by the word *AUṀ*. To pronounce *AUṀ* you have to open your mouth, roll the tongue for continuity and then close it to listen to the silence. *A* stands for opening of the mouth, *u* for continuity and *ṁ* for silence. As communication is dependent on the organs of speech, the syllable *AUṀ* becomes significant and important in this sense. If you take the qualities of nature *(guṇa)*, they are triune; *sattva*, *rajas* and *tamas*. If you take the humours of the body *(dośa)*, they are three, *vāta*, *pitta* and *śleṣma*. The human being has three components, *śarīra*, *manas* and *ātma*. The power of humans is again hidden in triune, *icchā* (will), *kriyā* (action) and *jñāna* (knowledge). Knowledge *(jñāna)* is gained only by triune *śravaṇa* (listening), *manana* (mental reflection) and *nidhidyāsana* (engrossment). Even our lives have three divisions: childhood, youth and old age. Take our states of living, it is wakefulness *(jñāna)*, sleep *(nidrā)* and dream *(svapna)*. Take recitation of

---

* International Yoga Teachers Association convention, Maseru, Lesotho, South Africa, 1978.

mantra, it is *japa*, *artha* and *bhāvana*. Take *sādhanā*, it is *bahiraṅga*, *antaraṅga* and *antarātmā* – the external quest, internal quest, innermost quest. Take *prāṇāyāma*, it is composed of *pūraka*, *recaka* and *kuṁbhaka* – inhalation, exhalation and retention. Again it is practised on three levels, gross, subtle and fine. The practitioner of *prāṇāyāma* may be an *adhama*, *madhyama* and *uttama*. The intelligence also is *mṛdu*, *madhyama* and *adhimātra*. Music has *mandrā*, – low octave, *madhya* – middle octave, and *tāra* – top octave. In many ways the qualities of nature in us and the way we practise yoga have this triune as an underlying structure.

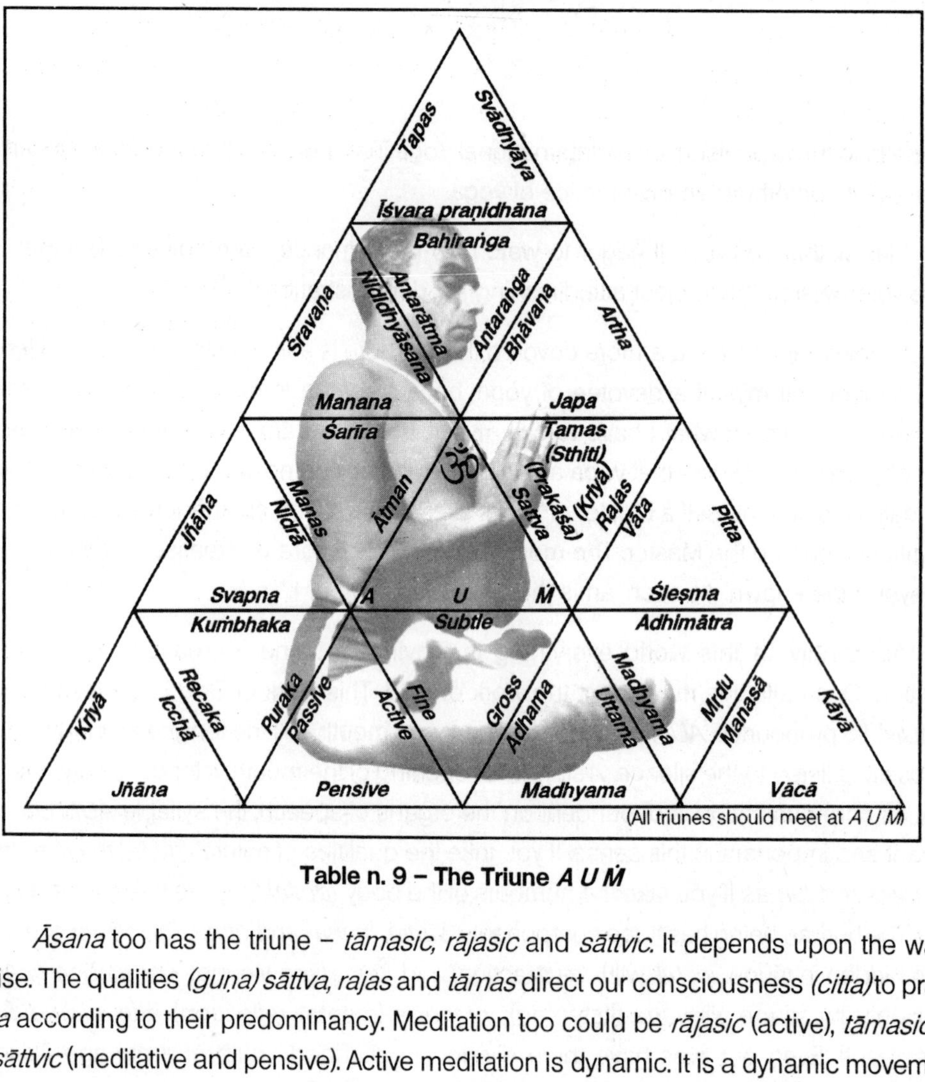

Table n. 9 – The Triune *A U Ṁ*

Āsana too has the triune – *tāmasic*, *rājasic* and *sāttvic*. It depends upon the way we practise. The qualities *(guṇa) sāttva*, *rajas* and *tāmas* direct our consciousness *(citta)* to practise *āsana* according to their predominancy. Meditation too could be *rājasic* (active), *tāmasic* (dull) and *sāttvic* (meditative and pensive). Active meditation is dynamic. It is a dynamic movement in the body that involves mind and self. When a person completely integrates himself, without a difference between body, mind and self, that becomes active meditation. In pensive meditation he tries to penetrate the space within himself. As one sees with open eyes the outer space, so the observation of the inner space *(ātmā)* in the place (body) is penetration. When the *sādhaka* penetrates inwards to measure the source of his consciousness, it is known as reflective or pensive meditation. Dull passive practice makes one live without the experience of knowledge or illumination.

You must have read in the *Rāmāyaṇa* about three brothers, Rāvaṇa, Kumbhakarṇa and Vibhīṣaṇa. Rāvaṇa had Kailasa in his hand. Kumbhakarṇa had Brahmā in his hand, and Vibhīṣaṇa had Rāma in his hand. All the three worlds had been conquered by Rāvaṇa. Rāvaṇa, having Lord Shiva in his hand, could not control the greed, the infatuation he had towards Sīta, and hence his meditation was *rājasic* due to his passion. Kumbhakarṇa had the Creator Brahmā in his hand, but was sleeping six months at a stretch, in a year. He was not to be disturbed, as his strength would fail if awakened. When Rāvaṇa woke him up to fight, he saw his downfall approaching. His meditation was of *tamō guṇa*. Vibhīṣaṇa's was a *sāttvic* meditation; it was he who advised both his brothers about morality. Vibhīṣaṇa came very close to the Lord, because of his *sāttvic* meditation, whereas the other brothers drifted away. We have to look carefully within ourselves in what way we are meditating, whether we are meditating in the *sāttvic, rājasic* or *tāmasic* way.

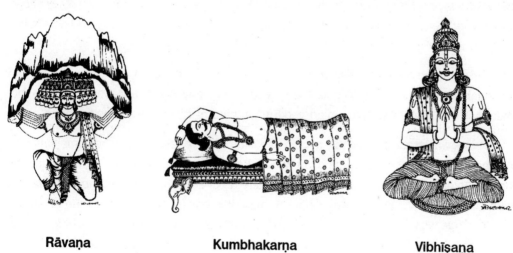

Rāvaṇa

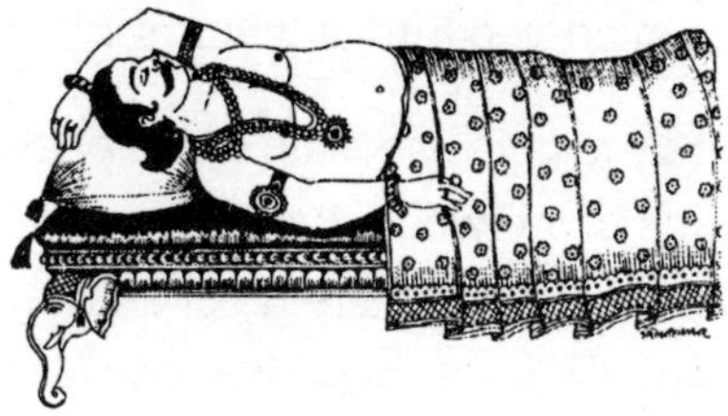

Kumbhakarṇa

Vibhīṣaṇa

We had three great men in India whom we have heard of and many of us have seen. One was Ramana Maharshi, another was Sri Aurobindo, and the third was Mahatma Gandhi. Ramana Maharshi, a *jñāna* yogi, was completely static in relation to the external world, but he was thoroughly dynamic within himself. He never moved the physical body, but his mind and his Self were ever alert. He was completely dynamic within. He wanted each one of us to find out who we are. It is interesting to know that this happened even in past times. Indra and Virocana went and asked Brahmā for knowledge. One of them said, "I can see", the other said, "I did not see". When Ramana said, "Find out who you are", people started interpreting in different ways. Like Virocana and Indra, each one said, "I have seen Brahmā". But only the man, Ramana, realised the dynamic self within himself.

Then comes a man of dynamic action and the dynamic vibration of the Self – Mahatma Gandhi. He was a great *karma yogin.* He never said, "I stay alone". Though he had communed with the Lord, he looked after the interest of common people. He never said, "I know my Self", nor asked people to go to him, but he went out to people to spread his experiences through expression. He was physically, intellectually and spiritually vibrant and dynamic.

Many of us have not seen, but heard of Sri Aurobindo. Sri Aurobindo was a *bhaktan,* completely quiet to the external world but also dynamic within. Not many could meet him, but only through his books could one know him and his knowledge on Self and Mother. Ramana and Mahatma Gandhi gave direct knowledge of the value of life and how one could develop a spiritual way of living while facing the turmoils of the world. One could know Sri Aurobindo through his books, his experiences and the value of his life. These three great men are examples of *jñāna, karma* and *bhakti.* Though all had expert knowledge of all the three paths, they chose their paths for the good of man according to their study of human psychology and needs. We have to understand this triune of their life within ourselves.

These three great men showed us that we have to be perfect in our body, in our mind and in our heart. Mahatma Gandhi's *karma* represents the body. Ramana Maharshi's represents tremendous clarity of *jñāna* in the mind and Sri Aurobindo's *bhakti* represents the heart.

Yoga was practised not only to gain liberation within oneself, but at the same time with mind control to enjoy the pleasures of the world. *Vairāgya* means having the potency and yet living the life of a renunciate. What use would there be of a talk given by an impotent man on *brahmacarya?* We, living in this world, have to dip within ourselves and sample the objects of the world. Yoga was presented to us to live in the world and at the same time show us how to be aloof from it. Yoga (auspicious living) enables one to have the *bhoga* (sensual pleasures) and to be free from *roga* or diseases. Practice of yoga first attracts one towards pleasures *(bhoga).* If one is attracted towards pleasures excessively, then it leads to *roga.* Today, people do yoga not for the sake of yoga, but to get rid of *roga* (diseases). They come with zeal to learn yoga, but their interest is to relieve themselves from their sufferance.

The yoga that I am going to demonstrate is based on the triune of *karma, jñāna* and *bhakti* (path). Patañjali advocates the practice of *śauca, santoṣa, tapas, svādhyāya, Īśvara praṇidhāna. Śauca* means internal and external purification. *Santoṣa* is a word that conveys the whole meaning of Patañjali's *maitrī, karuṇā, muditā, upekṣā* (friendliness, compassion, gladness and indifference). What is *tapas*? *Kāyendriya siddhiḥ aśuddhikṣyāt tapasaḥ* (*Y.S.*, II.43). *Tapas* is not merely an austerity. It is a self-discipline in order to burn away the impurities of the body, *jñānendriya* (senses of perception) and *karmendriya* (organs of action). When the impurities are burnt, the sensitivity is also refined. Our sensitivity is unclear because of impurities. It is tainted. Taintless sensitivity can lead one towards higher sensitivity. I am writing a book on *prāṇāyāma*. The publishers wanted some chapters of it, which I sent. I had mentioned in it that: "When you are doing *prāṇāyāma*, you have to differentiate the movements between the skin, the nerve endings and the inner organ"[1]. I got the reply: "This is nonsense". It is acceptable if I tell you about the *kośa*, the sheaths of our body. If I speak about the skin and the nerve endings, it becomes nonsense. The skin is the envelope of the body. You write a letter and put it in an envelope. Similarly the whole sheet of your body is covered in the envelope – the skin. If this envelope and its content are kept well clean, the entire body will be sensitive, attentive and intelligent. If the envelope is the external intelligence of the body, the one that is kept inside is the internal intelligence of the Self. If one understands and communicates between the skin, which is the external intelligence, and the Self, which is the internal intelligence, whether one does *āsana* or *prāṇāyāma* one experiences a quiet state in body and mind which is as real as meditation. If this communication is there, then one can experience harmony, balance and alignment. This communication from the skin, through nerve endings towards the intelligence to feel the felt experiences in order to carry that feeling to the Self cannot be a "non-sense" but "super-sense" knowledge.

Tapas has to be practised carefully to understand the *kārya* or *sthūla śarīra* (the body) and *sūkṣma śarīra* (the mind) as instruments that acquire knowledge. *Vidyā* is acquired knowledge, which is put into practice to experience *prajñā* (awareness). In *tapas*, the five layers of the body have to be kept perfectly clean, pure and serene. Hence, *tapas* is action. So it comes under *karma mārga*.

The fourth aspect of *niyama* is *svādhyāya* – *sva* and *adhyāya*. It means to study our own self. To know who you are, you should know what you are. To know what you are, you have to know all the five sheaths and the three bodies, namely, *kārya (sthūla) śarīra, sūkṣma śarīra* and *kāraṇa śarīra*. These three put together become the knowledge of a total man. This knowledge comes under *jñāna mārga*.

---

1 See the Author's *Light on Prāṇāyāma*, Harper Collins, London

The fifth part of *niyama* is *Īśvara praṇidhāna*. *Īśvara praṇidhāna* begins when the body and the mind are free from impurities. Acquiring this subjective purification is *svādhyāya*. We call it *buddhi* and not *vidyā*, because *vidyā* belongs to *manomaya kośa* and *buddhi* belongs to *vijñānamaya kośa*. With a clean *citta* only *Īśvara praṇidhāna* (the surrender of the Self unto that Universal Soul) begins. This is *bhakti mārga*.

Knowledge is predominant in *jñāna mārga*, action is predominant in *karma mārga*, whereas surrendering devotionally is predominant in *bhakti mārga*. But whatever the path *(mārga)* one follows, the others co-exist without a doubt. In order to reach any of these paths, one has to follow the principles of *niyama*. As long as one does not follow the principles of *niyama*, one cannot be a *bhaktan*, one cannot be a *jñānin* and one cannot be a *karmin*. Yoga was developed in order to acquire stability to follow these three paths by keeping man free from the contact of the objects of the world that create disturbing impressions on the mind. The mind sends these impressions as a message to *buddhi*. The *buddhi* receives and studies the message and guides the mind how to act or react. Like the light of a star, which may take millions of years to reach us, the imprint on one's movement of consciousness may take a long time to surface on the mind and to make the senses act. This is an ongoing process, known as *kāla cakra* (the wheel of time). The people who make pots use a wheel called *kulāla cakra*. The pot is made only when the *kulāla cakra* (rotating wheel) moves in the *kāla cakra* (time). With the help of the *kāla cakra* (wheel of time) and the *kulāla cakra* (potter's wheel), the three *guṇa (sattva, rajas, tamas)* manifest in man according to the mutations of the consciousness on these wheels. When we are born, we are born pure, then we come in contact with the objects of the world and our minds and our characters get influenced and start changing. So we have to re-think and re-change our values to come to that original pure state.

Undoubtedly *ātmā* is pure, but that *ātmā* gets tainted as it is influenced by the other sheaths, namely *annamaya, prāṇamaya, manomaya* and *vijñānamaya*. So if the sun is shining brightly, and if the clouds are there, where is the brightness of that sun? Though the sun is bright, how can the rays touch the earth if there are clouds in the middle? Similarly, our minds, our senses, our intelligence come in between like clouds and block the Self. Therefore the *ātmā* does not shine. Yoga has been given for us to see that these blocks of the Self are to be moved away in order to generate brightness in our senses, mind, intelligence and self, so that the Self shines brilliantly, like the sun that irradiates the earth when the clouds are not there. That is why this subject was given as a fountainhead of *abhyāsa*. The practice of *āsana* and *prāṇāyāma* are meant to remove these clouds.

In this convention before my talk, you heard *swamijī* who was saying that he heard from someone that Iyengar teaches cosmetic yoga. Is it fair for a holy man like him to bring this issue here? By quoting words of hearsay does not his word become unholy? In what way did *swamijī* see the truth of this statement? How can he differentiate, when this art was given to the whole of humanity for the good of spiritual health and unalloyed bliss? Please know that I cosmetise the inner body through *āsana* and *prāṇāyāma* practices to experience the cosmic state of oneself. Let us learn to see the cosmic purity in these paths and not take advantage of gossip.

Gheraṇḍa Saṁhitā speaks of *ghaṭa yoga*. *Ghaṭa* means pot, i.e. the body as the vessel of the Self. But this does not mean that *Gheraṇḍa Saṁhitā* is about cosmetic yoga. The body, which is the temple of the soul, was never ever neglected by yogis of yore. As Patañjali demands the purity of body and mind, the other texts such as *Haṭhayoga Pradīpika, Gheraṇḍa Saṁhitā* and *Śiva Saṁhitā* followed it. *Haṭhayoga Pradīpikā* concludes in the second chapter the effect of the practice of *āsana* and *prāṇāyāma:* they make the body slim and light, bring lustre on the face, the voice becomes clear, the eyes become clean and bright, the body remains free from disease, the senses of perception and mind come under control, the gastric fire is stimulated and the nerves are purified.

Pandit Shiv Sharma (an authority on *āyurveda*) recently wrote a book called *Yoga and Sex*, which was well read and well received. I told him that a man of his calibre should not have written such a book. A person of great calibre like him should always think and present ideal views in writings. He said, "People wanted it, so I wrote it". So how can such a highly intelligent man write on yoga as if it is only for sensual experiences? Friends, I have spoken much, but I have spoken with feeling. To be short, I have done this practice for forty-five years and I have met the cream of the world, I have taught yoga to the geniuses of the world and I have also taught the people who sweep the streets and those who were sex obsessed. So I know the psychological development of the human being, from the lowest level to the highest. It is my good fortune that this art, just labelled as cosmetic yoga, is enjoying a considerable revival.

I came across a word the other day in one of the *Upaniṣads*, *viṣamāsana*. It means "a wrong, uneven, unequal or odd pose". I was pleased to see the *Upaniṣads* mentioning that even a pose done wrongly is an obstacle to progress in yoga. Today in meditation the holy men say, "Sit in any position which is comfortable or as you like". This is known as *viṣamāsana* according to the *Upaniṣads*.

Friends, do not treat the *āsana* aspect as a physical thing. Know its importance and the vital role it plays in *sādhanā*. You have seen a tree. Yoga is like a tree. The tree has got the root, trunk, branches, leaves, bark, sap, flowers and fruit. The tree has eight limbs. Yoga too has eight limbs. They are *yama, niyama, āsana, prāṇāyāma, pratyāhāra, dhāraṇā, dhyāna* and *samādhi*. The root of the tree is *yama*. The trunk is *niyama*. If the root and the trunk are not strong, the tree decays. A fall is certain if your practice is not supported by the pillars of *yama* and *niyama*. The base has to be firm. The branches are *āsana*. The leaves are the *prāṇāyāma* which feed the bark. The bark is *pratyāhāra*. The sap that flows within the bark is *dhāraṇā*. The flower blossoms as *dhyāna*, and the fruit as *samādhi*. The spiritual ascent of the tree is the fruit. The tree does not hanker after flowers, or fruit. They are a natural growth of the development of a tree. Integrity, advertance and sincerity are the only source. When you are doing this yoga with an advertent, sincere mind and with a surrendering approach, you come out – like the spiritual ascent of the tree with a fruit – as a divine man. When you practise *āsana, yama, niyama* or *prāṇāyāma*, do not think that you are in a lower state of *sādhanā*. They are all together, like a tree. As you cannot separate the tree, you cannot separate the eight petals of yoga. Those who separate it do not know yoga in depth. Words can be spoken very cleverly. But the facts that are felt cannot be spoken cleverly, they can be spoken only with clarity. So clarity comes with practice. Cleverness comes only by articulating words. It is my wish that, instead of articulating words and reading books, you acquire knowledge through experience. Conviction, clarity, courage and compassion are the seed for this experiential knowledge.

Droṇa said to his *śiṣya* (disciple) Arjuna, that he would only train him and no one else. A hunter called Ekalavya went to Droṇa and requested to be taught in the art of archery. Droṇa denied this opportunity to Ekalavya since his lineage was of a hunter class. Ekalavya went back to his forest and made an image of Droṇa. He started prostrating to that image of his *guru* before practising and mastered the art of archery *(dhanur vidyā)*.

My life story too is somewhat analogous to the above story. I also have my *guru*, whom some of you might have heard about. He told me, "You are not born for yoga, what little I gave is all you need, and not beyond". I am carrying that blessing still. Even today my *guru* does not know what I am doing. I meet him, I talk to him, and we discuss, but not about yoga. After all he is my brother-in-law (my sister's husband). So, I practised yoga like Ekalavya. Something from inside forced me to learn this art.

I request you now to pay attention to my presentation of this cosmic and divine art.

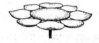

*VINYĀSA YOGA**

Yoga is one. So is *āsana* but people give it different names and forms. Nothing like *vinyāsa yoga* existed for *aṣṭāṅga yoga* and it is unfair to name yoga as *vinyāsa yoga*. I am sorry for the doubts that have risen in the mind of the students of yoga. Do not make yoga a cheap product for sale under various names and brands. All the yogic texts proclaim that the means and aims of yoga are the same. They were the same in the past; they are same in the present and will remain the same in the future also. To reach the ultimate state of the *āsana* may be termed as *vinyāsa* only. Even the eight aspects of yoga, namely, *yama, niyama, āsana, prāṇāyāma, pratyāhāra, dhāraṇā, dhyāna* and *samādhi* are a *vinyāsa krama* sequentially arranged by Patañjali.

I, being a pupil of my guru, learnt yoga as did his other pupils. He never referred to the *vinyāsa* practice as *vinyāsa yoga*. He never said that he was teaching *aṣṭāṅga yoga*. He always referred to the very practice as *pātañjala yoga*.

While doing *āsana, prāṇāyāma* or *dhyāna*, the body, mind and intelligence need to be trained, toned and tuned so that they pick up a rhythmic vibration and correct modulation like an antenna which receives the news and, when tuned, emits it also. They have their own modus operandi and we, as *sādhaka,* need to recognise them. The word *vinyāsa* has two parts – *vi* and *nyāsa*. *Vi* means separating or disjuncting. *Nyāsa* means placing or putting down. *Vinyāsa* means separating and putting down or placing in a sequential order. It is a way of arrangement or a method of proper disposition. In order to practise *āsana, prāṇāyāma* or *dhyāna,* one has to conceive an idea of the work involved that is to be done, and then, a kind of disposition, articulation and delivery has to take place. Through *vinyāsa* one finds an organised practical approach from the start in each stage, in each step and in each station.

In the 1930s and 40s my *Gurujī* taught the means to achieve the *āsana* in a *vinyāsa* way, in the *yogaśālā* as well as outside the *śālā*. When he was sent on "yoga tours" by the patron of the *Śri yogaśālā,* the *Maharaja* of Mysore, he was then young and we too were young. He taught us to do the *āsana* linking them with those which are popularly known as

* An excerpt from an answer to a letter published in *News,* a magazine of the Oxford Iyengar Yoga Institute, Summer 1996.

Sūryanamaskār. But actually *Sūryanamaskār* are all *āsana. Āsana* such as *Ūrdhva Hastāsana, Uttānāsana, Chaturanga Daṇḍāsana, Ūrdhva Mukha Śvānāsana* and *Adho Mukha Śvānāsana* **(1)** (Plate n. 17) were linked in various ways so as to go towards the main *āsana* that was aimed at. For instance, in order to go to *Paśchimottānāsana,* he used to ask us to do *Samasthiti, Ūrdhva Hastāsana, Uttānāsana, Chaturanga Daṇḍāsana, Ūrdhva Mukha Śvānāsana, Chaturanga Daṇḍāsana, Adho Mukha Śvānāsana, Lolāsana, Daṇḍāsana, Paśchimottānāsana,* and return back to *Samasthiti* reversing the sequence. Today this method of sequencing the *āsana* or *vinyāsa krama* is popularly known as "jumpings" **(2)** (Plate n. 17). When I was in Pune in 1937, I had to teach this way in various educational institutions. I continued this method up to 60s and 70s.

Children and youngsters do like this method and thoroughly enjoy it since it gives them quickness, agility, speed and variety. In the late 40s, *Gurujī* abandoned it. In my case, as I had to teach in schools, colleges, as well as the cadets of the National Defence Academy, I followed it wherever and whenever it was appropriate. In the Institute even now we do continue to teach this method in children's classes and once in a while in other classes too. But they are not done as a permanent feature. In children's classes, I often teach with *vinyāsa krama.* If I have to take them into the depth of the *āsana,* I preserve their energies from "jumpings" and make them concentrate on parts of the body that are needed for the *āsana* and use their minds to penetrate their bodies with study in depth.

I was teaching this type of so called *vinyāsa yoga* for many years as my young pupils wanted power, strength and endurance. When the very same students reached thirty-five to forty years of age, they were getting exhausted by this method and began dropping out. On account of this drop out rate, I had to change my way of doing and teach from a pure physical standard to a higher level of yoga.

In those days Pune was the temple of physical activities and it was a known place for bringing out wrestlers. Even the mall-khāmb was popular. Mall-khāmb is a form of exercise in which a wooden pole and ropes are used. Various *āsana* are performed while balancing on the pole. Having a toned body, practitioners were unhappy about doing yoga with *vinyāsa* as it only worked on their peripheral body and did not penetrate the mind or intelligence. It was a challenge for me at that age and I had to work the ways for myself and search the means to feel that inter-penetration of how to reach the unknown inner depth of the body.

By *vinyāsa krama,* people with diabetes, blood pressure, back-aches, restlessness, nervous breakdown and whiplash felt hotness in their eyes and ears. Then I thought that if I insist on jumpings, this yoga may not flourish at all. So I stopped introducing *vinyāsa* for them so that they did not get tired or breathless or add to their existing problems.

Instead of the *vinyāsa* movements, I started to explore the inner invisible hidden body and began explaining to my students the art of inner observation and penetration. This ignited interest and gathered momentum for yoga and it gained respect. In the early days, even in performances all over the world, I was performing with *vinyāsa krama* to show the external expressions and dynamism. It did attract the viewers. Then I began to demonstrate a few *āsana* by jumpings and then moved on to explain the inner action. The audiences started to admire these hitherto unheard of explanations. Since then, I started demonstrating and explaining more and more of the mind, intelligence and consciousness and how they percolate throughout the body in various presentations of the *āsana*. I would certainly admit that I first attracted them towards this subject and then intelligised them to know the real depth of the subject that added respect to this art.

So my view is that the sequential jumpings in *āsana* end up only on the physical or peripheral level of the body and *vinyāsa* is a sequence to reach the ultimate or final state of the *āsana*. Whoever does jumpings, gets stuck there only, because his mind will be on jumpings and motions and not on aligning the intelligence or the exploration of the dark caves in the body. For me alignment is stability and entering the dark caves of the body is enlightenment.

Even in this penetration of approach, *vinyāsa krama* is there but it is applied in different mental and intellectual ways and attitudes. By this approach the mind and intelligence, along with energy *(prāṇa)* and conscious awareness *(prajñā)*, are built up within the system in different aspects of human beings sequentially and gradually.

Similarly *vinyāsa krama* is not necessarily fast movements with the *Sūryanamaskār* jumpings. It could be with slow movements too. For instance, in order to do *Sālamba Śīrṣāsana*, one can prepare oneself for the inverted position by following the sequence of *Adho Mukha Śvānāsana, Uttānāsana, Prasārita Pādottānāsana, Jānu Śīrṣāsana, Paśchimottānāsana, Adho Mukha Vīrāsana.* After staying in *Sālamba Śīrṣāsana,* one can come down and follow the sequence in reverse. This kind of *vinyāsa* prepares one to go to *Sālamba Śīrṣāsana* (Plate n. 5) physically, mentally, intellectually and consciously. The return journey helps to maintain a soothing and quietening sensation. Apart from this, it helps those who are physically weak, or those suffering from high blood pressure and those who have defects in the eyes. On the other hand, *Adho Mukha Vṛkṣāsana, Pīncha Mayūrāsana,* enliven us prior to *Sālamba Śīrṣāsana* **(5)** (Plate n. 17). When the main *āsana* is encased with *vinyāsa krama,* it is called as *sampuṭana kriyā* – the action of encasement **(3)** (Plate n. 17).

The opposite to *vinyāsa* is called *viṣamanyāsa*. *Viṣamanyāsa* means placing in an odd or irregular manner. Certainly it is not done in a disorderly way. Rather it is a method of challenge.

In this method, *āsana* from different categories are linked together without breaking the flow of the movements. For instance, *Eka Pāda Śīrṣāsana* and the variations in an *āsana* are *grathana sthiti* (body knotting). This category works as follows: *Eka Pāda Śīrṣāsana* from sitting *(Upaviṣṭha Sthiti), Skandāsana* (forward extension or *Paścima pratana sthiti), Bhairavāsana* (supine or *Supta sthiti), Kāla Bhairavāsana* or *Chakorāsana* (arm-balance or *Bhujatolāsana sthiti), Dūrvāsāsana* (standing – *Uttiṣṭha sthiti), Richikāsana (Uttiṣṭha paśchima pratana sthiti)* and so on **(4)** (Plate n. 17).

A mixed group of *āsana* is also known as *viṣamanyāsa*. For instance, *Tāḍāsana, Uttānāsana, Adho Mukha Śvānāsana, Paripūrṇa Nāvāsana, Utkaṭāsana, Uṣṭrāsana, Kapotāsana, Adho Mukha Vīrāsana* and so on **(6)** (Plate n. 17). Because of a flexible body, children enjoy practising this way since the changes are challenging ones. My *guru* used to ask me to do any *āsana* in this way. He would ask me to do *Sālamba Śīrṣāsana* and suddenly jump over to *Naṭarājāsana*.

Vinyāsa and *viṣamanyāsa* is again classified as *viloma, anuloma* and *pratiloma*. *Viloma vinyāsa* means linking with regular interruption. In *viloma vinyāsa, āsana* belonging to the same classification are linked each time with one single chosen *āsana* such as *Jānu Śīrṣāsana – Paśchimottānāsana, Trieng Mukhaikapāda Paśchimottānāsana – Paśchimottānāsana, Ardha Baddha Padma Paśchimottānāsana – Paśchimottānāsana, Upaviṣṭha Koṇāsana – Paśchimottānāsana,* and so forth **(7)** (Plate n. 17).

In *viloma viṣamanyāsa*, the *āsana* forming separate or opposite classifications are linked with one single chosen *āsana*. That means practising one forward extension and one backward extension *(Paścima pratana sthiti* and *pūrva pratana sthiti)* such as *Paśchimottānāsana – Ūrdhva Dhanurāsana, Paśchimottānāsana – Uṣṭrāsana, Paśchimottānāsana – Dwi Pāda Viparīta Daṇḍāsana* **(8)** (Plate n. 17)

Earlier I explained the sequence of *āsana* leading up to, and returning from, *Sālamba Śīrṣāsana*. In that method, there is *pratiloma vinyāsa* and *anuloma vinyāsa*. The journey from *Adho Mukha Śvānāsana* to *Sālamba Śīrṣāsana* is *pratiloma vinyāsa* (going against the current). It is an ascending or unnatural order, whereas from *Sālamba Śīrṣāsana* to *Adho Mukha Śvānāsana* is *anuloma vinyāsa* (going with the current) or natural order. In *pratiloma vinyāsa* the practice proceeds in an ascending order and in *anuloma vinyāsa* it proceeds with a descending order. In order to go to any advanced *āsana*, you go from simple to complicated *āsana*. This way of charging the body, vital energy, mind, senses of perception, and igniting the intelligence and 'I'-consciousness (ego) is called *pratiloma vinyāsa;* whereas returning from complicated to simple *āsana* and pacifying the complete system of body and consciousness is called *anuloma vinyāsa*. This way the alertness of activity and passivity in the body are increased or decreased, which helps to open the horizon of the mind. Often in the regular classes and in regular practice you all might have noted that the beginning is done in such a way that from simple to complicated *āsana* you proceed *(pratiloma)* and come back *(anuloma)* from complicated to simple *āsana*.

Prāṇāyāma practice is also done in this way. *Ujjāyi* is done with an alternate normal breathing cycle or *Viloma prāṇāyāma* is done with an alternate *Ujjāyi* cycle.

Even in *dhyāna*, whenever a shift or a drift of consciousness occurs, recharge of the consciousness is required. Patañjali reminds us of *mantra japa*, the sacred syllable *Auṁ*. He asks us to know the meaning and to feel it. *Citta prasādanam* or favourable disposition and deliberation of the consciousness during meditation *(dhyāna)* has to be done as *vinyāsa* alone. However, in *dhyāna vinyāsa* is refined and very subtly adjusted. It cannot be done on a gross level.

As pupils of yoga, remember that *vinyāsa* is not merely a fast mobile movement in *āsana*. It is a procedure of building oneself. A fast and gross movement is enchanting to youngsters who get carried away by them. If the practitioner of yoga is satisfied at a gross level by scratching the external body and not penetrating, then that kind of practice helps but at a certain point it becomes a yoga of pleasure *(preyas yoga)*. What I teach and practise is to explore the subtlety and firmness in each *āsana*. Therefore it is auspicious yoga *(śreyas yoga)*. Let us not be carried away by motion, but static dynamism in action.

We all learnt this method from our *guru* and there is no division. The former method is for youngsters to stimulate their interest and build up their valour and the second is the art of sublimating the ego and a road towards intellectual progression.

Plate n. 17 – *Vinyāsa Krama*
(1) *Sūryanamaskār*

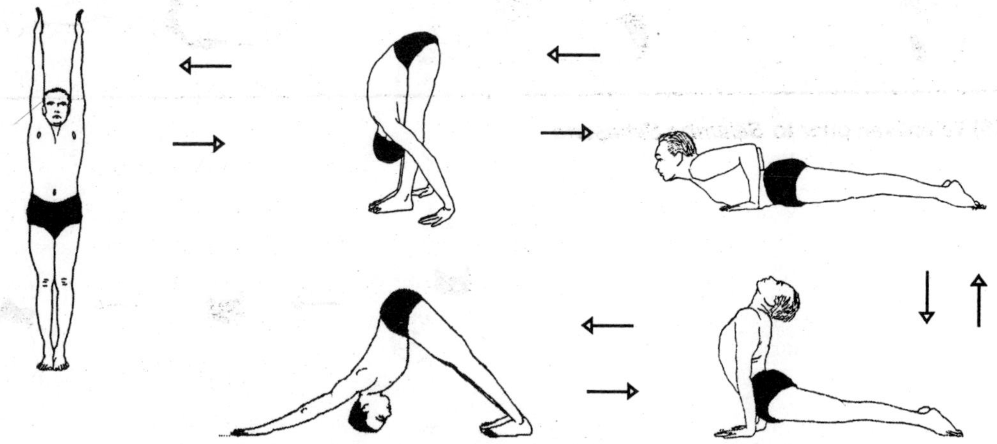

(2) *Vinyāsa krama* – jumpings (as taught at the *Yogaśālā*, Mysore in the 30's and 40's)

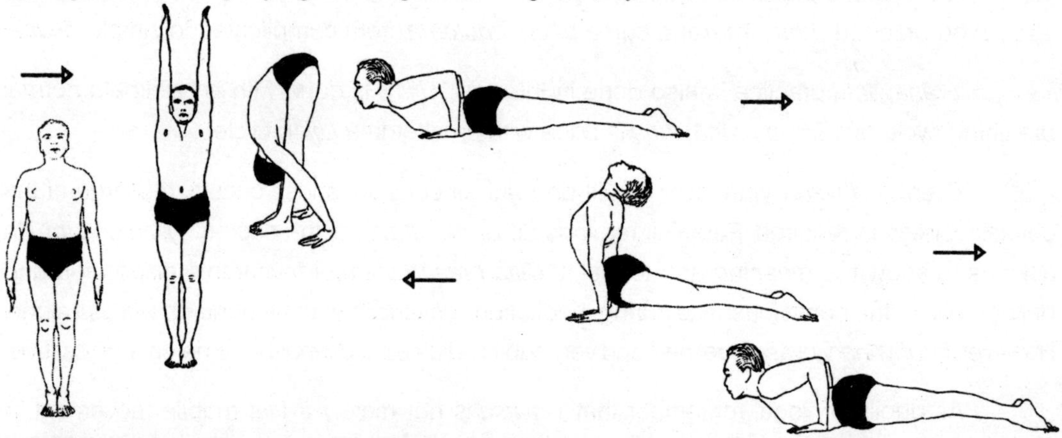

(3) *Saṁpuṭana kriyā* – action of encasement

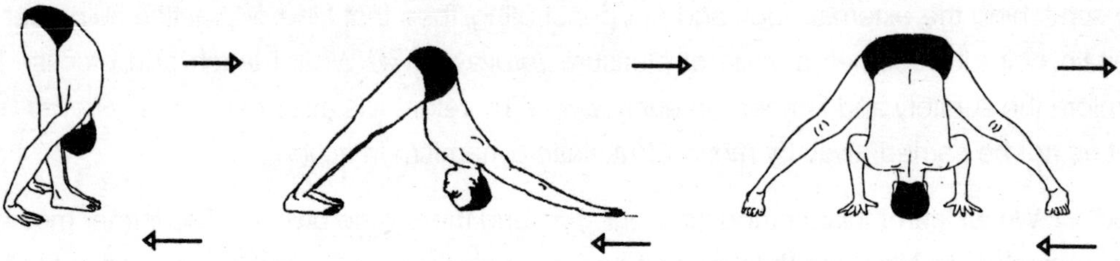

(4) *Viṣamanyāsa krama – grathana sthiti*

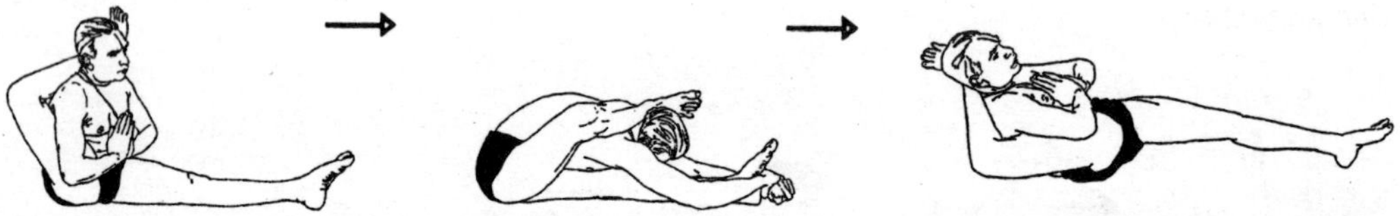

(5) To enliven prior to *Sālamba Śīrṣāsana*

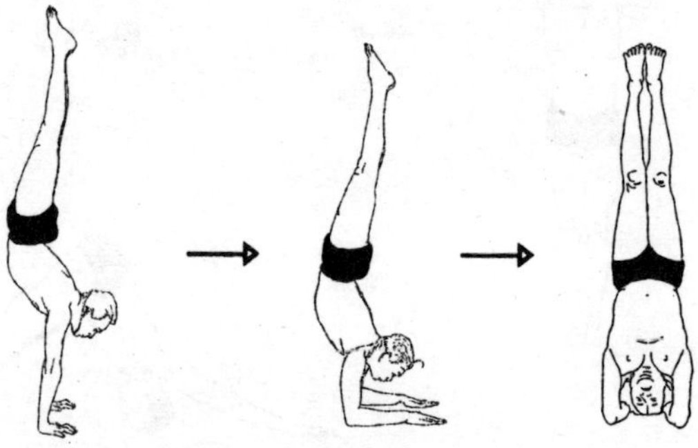

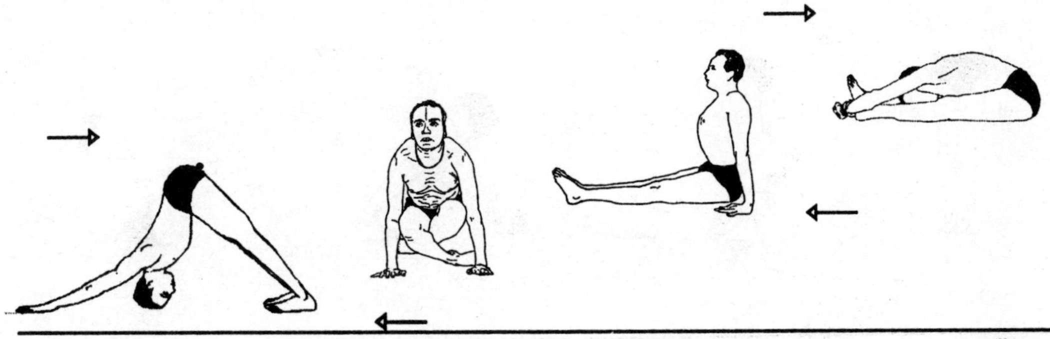

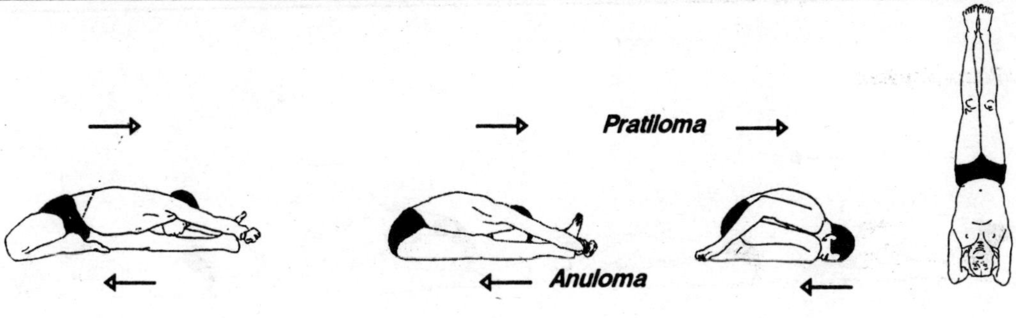
Pratiloma
Anuloma

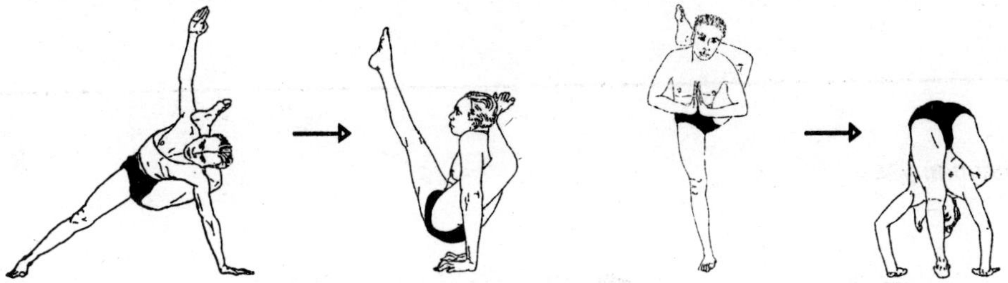

(6) *Viṣamanyāsa krama* - mixed group

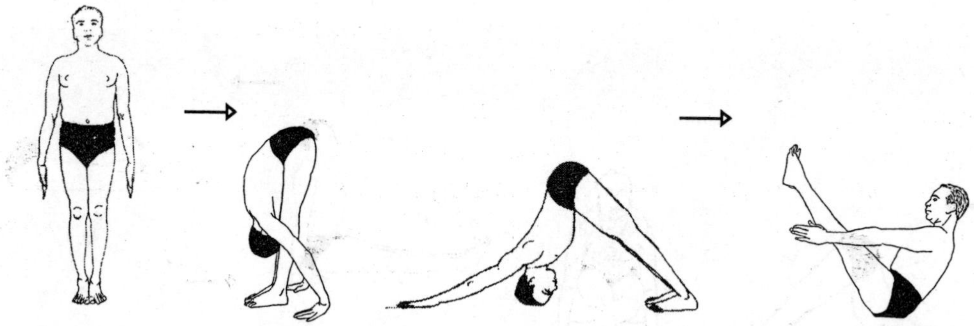

(7) *Viloma vinyāsa*

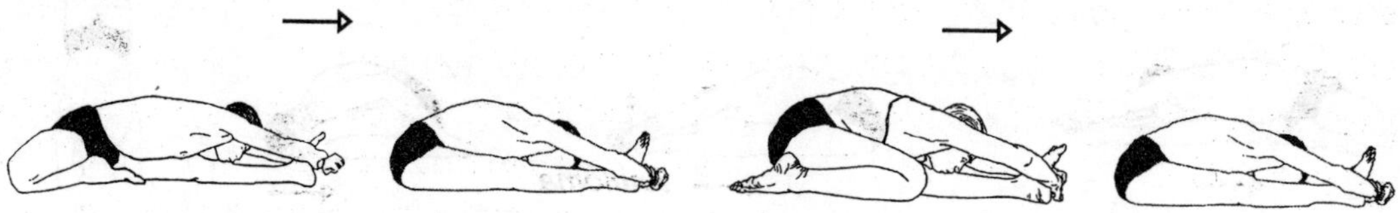

(8) *Viloma viṣam anyāsa*

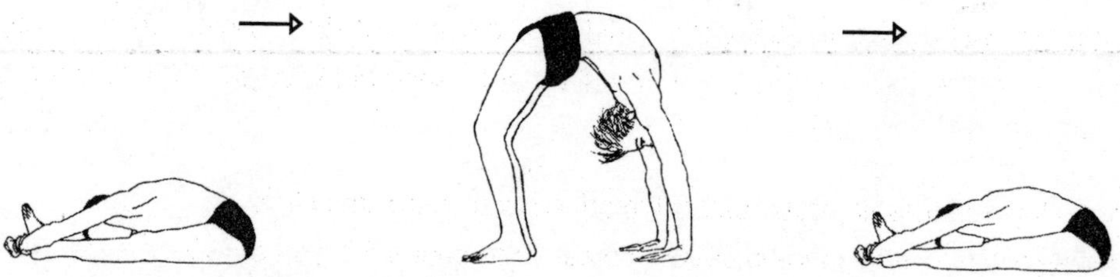

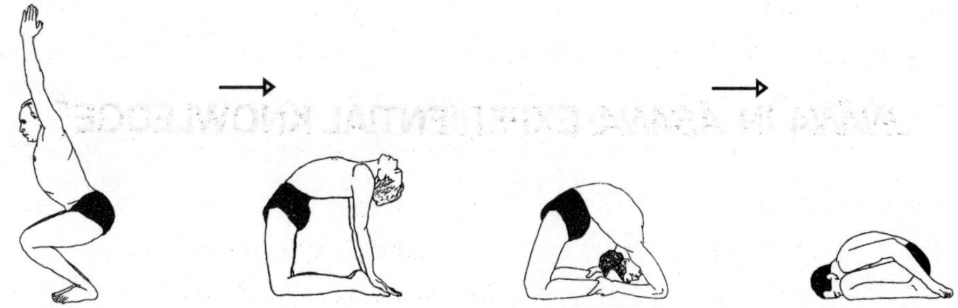

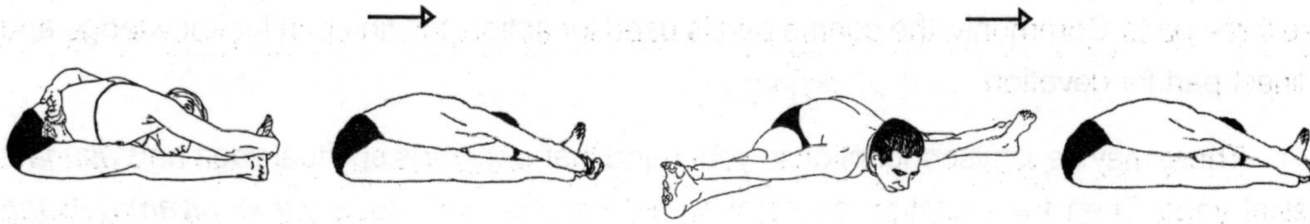

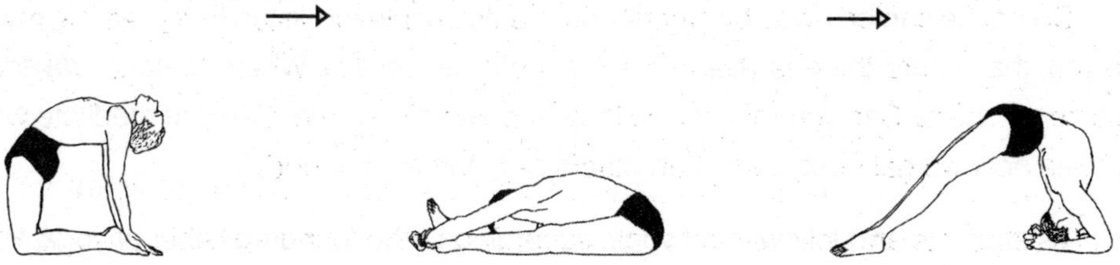

JÑĀNA IN *ĀSANA:* EXPERIENTIAL KNOWLEDGE*

All of you have begun well, and must retain that quality to penetrate from the surface of the physical and the physiological bodies towards the mind – because yogis have divided the body into three parts; the coarse (anatomical) body, the subtle (physiological, mental and intellectual) body and the causal (spiritual) body. In the beginning, at an early stage, we started with the gross body. Now from that gross body let us go to the fine body of the mind, and from the fine body of the mind towards the finest, the core of being. Yoga is the fountainhead for these three parts. Commonly, the coarse part is used for action, the fine part for knowledge and the finest part for devotion.

There may be a misconception in your mind that *dhyāna* is spiritual yoga and *āsana* is physical yoga. Then the question arises, why did Patañjali introduce *yama, niyama, āsaṇa, prāṇāyāma* and *pratyāhāra* before *dhāraṇā* and *dhyāna?* How can we say that we are only taking this part of Patañjali as superior and the other part of Patañjali's words as inferior? Are we better than him? Are we more qualified than him? As *dhyāna* is a part of the tree of yoga (Plate n. 4), so too is *āsana.* So you and I, as practitioners of yoga, should never have that division in ourselves. please know that there is no *sādhanā* by the self for the self, but the *sādhanā* is there for all of us to reach the Self

Do not be carried away by others' comments but please, listen to me, as it is my duty to guide you, that where there is *āsana*, there should be *dhyāna.* Where there is *dhyāna*, there should be an *āsana.* Can you meditate without a posture? Tell me! Can you meditate without a body? See how we get confused when others say, "forget your body".

As students and followers of yoga, according to the founding father of yoga, Patañjali, we should not differentiate these things. Leave these to others who have less knowledge or no knowledge of yoga at all. Let them do whatever they want. Good and bad go together. As we religiously practise, we are true *sādhaka.* But those who say that our practice has nothing to do

---

* Message in American Iyengar Yoga Convention, San Diego, June 1990.

with meditation are hiding their own weaknesses of pride. Let them pride themselves as higher level yogis, let us accept and live in the level we are at and maintain a foundation. Let that foundation be the guide for us, and not the words of bystanders of yoga.

When you do a good and perfect *Paśchimottānāsana,* (Plate n. 5) have you not experienced a state of silence? When you do *Halāsana* with a prop, is your mind silent or not? When you say, "Yes", then is it not meditation? Why do you yourself get confused? Silence is the first goal of yoga. You are experiencing this in *Setu Bandha Sarvāṅgāsana* (Plate n. 5), you are experiencing this in *Halāsana,* as well as in *Paśchimottānāsana* (Plate n. 5).

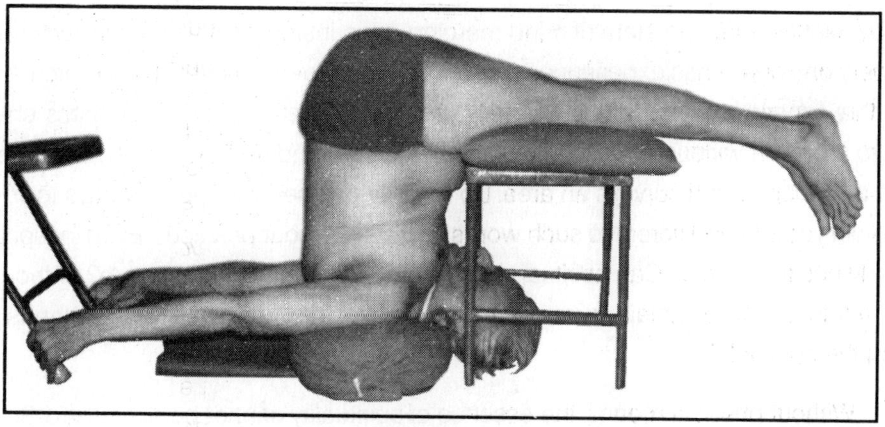

Plate n. 18 - *Halāsana* with a prop

I will tell you the difference between these *āsanas.* They take you to the state of silence, even perfection. But in that silence you find various differences. In *Halāsana,* the silence is passive and makes you pensive. In *Setu Bandha Sarvāṅgāsana,* it is a half-pensive and half-dynamic state of silence. In *Halāsana,* you can go to sleep, but in *Setu Bandha Sarvāṅgāsana* you cannot go to sleep and you cannot oscillate either. In *Sālamba Śīrṣāsana* too (Plate n. 5) you cannot oscillate, you can never be inattentive even for a second, otherwise you lose the balance. Yet you feel cool in the head. In *Paśchimottānāsana* (Plate n. 5) you experience serene silence.

You have to study yourselves, when you do each and every *āsana,* and see what behavioural changes take place in your temperament and mind and where they lead. In *Paśchimottānāsana* (Plate n. 5), the behavioural pattern of the mind is of one type. In *Sālamba Sarvāṅgāsana* (Plate n. 5), the behavioural pattern of the mind is of a different type. In twistings, the behavioural pattern of the mind is different. In backbends, it is different. I say, in backbends

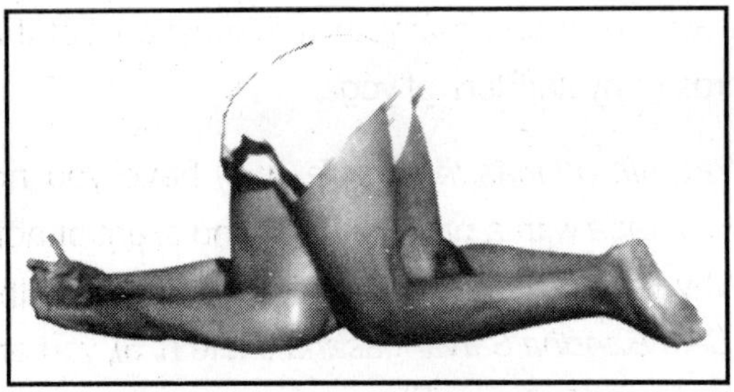

Plate n. 19 – *Karṇapīḍāsana*

your mind is in a full state of awareness and sharp. If your intelligence is not sharp, you collapse. In *Sālamba Sarvāṅgāsana* or in forward bends, you can relax a bit here and a bit there. In *Halāsana* (Plate n. 5) and *Karṇapīḍāsana* you can completely relax.

So you can learn from different *āsana* the three states of consciousness, *jāgrata, svapna* and *suṣupti* (wakeful, dream and sleep). Sometimes, in between these three states you learn by experiencing the state of mind merging deep inside, as if you are in *turīya* state. Each and every one of you has experienced this but your intelligence is not able to catch it. Once you catch this experience, you find in each *āsana* that the states of consciousness change. You begin to survey in various *āsana* the behaviour of your mind and body cells, like a person who flies in a helicopter and surveys an area. Do not be confused if somebody says to you that this is physical yoga, be indifferent to such words and stick to your practices. Even for spiritual yoga, the body has to be used. Can spiritual wisdom be imparted without speech? Without opening one's mouth, can one explain to you what spiritual yoga is? One has to use various means to explain the spiritual life.

Without physical means, the essence of spirituality cannot be expressed. So never get confused. Let this 1990 Yoga Convention open your eyes to see what is a true *sādhanā*, what is a religious *sādhanā* and what is propagandist *sādhanā*. Do not be carried away by propagandist knowledge, but be carried away by your experiential felt knowledge. Develop yourselves from the subjective feeling so that your body, mind and soul feel that each and every individual soul acts as a ray of the Universal Soul. This way you can learn yoga dispassionately.

SAṀYAMA IN *ĀSANA*[*]

Each of the five elements of the human body has its own quality. Earth has odour, water has taste, fire has form, air touch and ether sound. The components of our body, namely, chyle, blood, flesh, fat, bones, bone marrow and semen, are composed of these five elements in varying proportions. Besides these five elements and their five qualities, each human has in his system five organs of action (mouth, legs, arms, excretory and generative organs) and five senses of perception (eyes, ears, nose, tongue and skin). The existence of gross elements is recognisable in our body through their action and traceable through the functions of organs of action, while the qualities of elements are felt by the senses of perception through the network of the nerves. There is a great deal of natural communication between the organs of action and the senses of perception. For instance, the flesh, the bones and the bone marrow exist in the skeleto-muscular body (organs of action); they primarily consist of earth, air and water. To be specific; the flesh is of earth element, bones are earth and air, bone marrow water[1]. The movements of joints, the firmness of arms and legs in the functions such as holding or walking are experienced by all. All these are done or controlled again by the nerves. The nerves are basically made of the element of water and fire. The element of fire carries the message and sensation. Transmission is the quality of the element of fire. So, the conductivity of the nerves is due to the presence of the element of fire on them.

The skin, one of the senses of perception covering the body has the sense of touch (air), carried to the brain and from the brain to the skin (fire). It makes us feel the vibration of the movement (ether and air). Again the sense of touch has its origin in air. After a long *sādhanā (dīrghakāla)* the *sādhaka* feels the sense of touch from within, which otherwise is felt from outside. While performing the *āsana* even if the understanding is limited only to the movements, there is involvement of the gross elements, viz., earth, air and water. There is an involvement of the subtle elements as well. Odour because of the earth element, the feel of touch because of the air element, and sweating because of the water element.

---

* Published in the *Iyengar Yoga Institute Review*, San Francisco, vol. 6, no. 2, October, 1985.

1 Suśruta – *Bhānumati ṭīkā*.

While performing *āsana*, you and I have to carefully observe that if the muscles are extended strongly and heavily with force, then the senses of perception cannot receive the action done by the fibres, the cells and the spindles. The afferent nerves carry the message of pain rather than the actual functional imprint. They do not receive the actual functioning of the inner system which can only imprint on the senses of perception, the skin. Then they are felt later by the eyes and the ears as a pressure or a tension because of over work or wrong work. While performing *āsana,* one has to be careful that the spindles of the motor nerves of our system (the fibres of the muscles) should act without disturbing the fibres of the sensory nerves, which are conceived by the senses of perception (the inner layer of the skin). If the muscle fibres are not overstretched, or jammed against the senses of perception, only then can the perceptory nerves receive the exact action done by the flesh. The efferent and afferent nerves work co-operatively to keep the balance between action and perception, in order to correct the position of *āsana* and bring a healthy sensation. While we are performing *āsana*, we have to adjust in such a way that the fibres of the flesh do not protrude against the skin more than is essential, otherwise the nerves and their elemental chemistry – earth, water and air – get disturbed.

In making contact between the movement and the senses of perception, all the elements have to get involved. The power of intelligence, which you use to make contact, is the element of air flowing in the system (bio-energy or *prāṇa*). The will, the mind, which you use, is the fire; the circulation of blood which takes place is connected to the elements of fire and water, and the mass of flesh within is nothing but the element of earth. While performing *āsana* there is a pause (space) between two actions, similar to the pause or gap between two words or two sounds or between two breaths. Similarly there is an inner space between the organs and the cells of the organs in the human system. In the vibrations of each cell and each organ as well as in the action of each organ and the movements of the body there is a major participation of ether and these vibrations have their origins in sound, which is now recorded as sonography.

When *āsana* is performed, the power of intelligence, (the element of air), should be spaced in such a way that the spindles of the organs of action, the flesh, allow the movement to come in contact with the spindles of the senses of perception, the inner layer of the skin. Then you understand the perfect balance of the presentation of that *āsana*. If there is an overstretch, the spindles turn hard, hit and rub against each other very strongly, jarring the senses of perception making them insensitive. If there is an understretch, there is no feeling; the senses of perception do not receive the action due to distance in space between the *nāḍī* of action and perception. While the senses of perception maintain their sensitivity, the fibres of the flesh, the organs of action, have to be carefully handled using the intelligence, so that the mind (the fire), may not burn or move the fibres too fast or extinguish them. If you do this way, then you know the contacting and balancing of the cells of the senses of perception through the cells of the organs of action: the ligaments and fibres. While performing *āsana*, when they communicate, you have understood the tremendous inner balance that you have, without aggravating the senses of perception or the organs of action. The communication between the senses of perception and the organs of action should convey to the intelligence a certain rhythm and balance while performing. When that is performed, only then have you mastered that *āsana*. Sometimes we overstretch, sometimes we understretch, sometimes we use will, sometimes we use force on our body. These are known as imbalances in our presentations. When these imbalances are worked out to balance rhythmically, the *āsana* is perfect.

We need tremendous reflection because on their own the elements cannot reflect at all, they only act; in acting the flesh and bones send a message to the senses of perception, triggering them to feel the essence of the action. This brings alertness in intelligence and consciousness. All these must be intermingled to create the exact blend. This exact blending of the fibres of the flesh with the fibres of the senses of perception requires attentive repose, rethinking, reflection and sensitivity in intelligence. The flesh acts towards a forward action, the senses of perception should draw back to receive. For this you have to create a pause. A space between the action and the perception is needed for the mind and intelligence to conceive. This spacing is *saṁyama* in *āsana*.

The acting movement requires skilful action. You have to create skilfulness and refine yourself to receive that skilful action with skilful senses of perception. That is why I said you have to communicate with each cell, with the intelligence (air). So, the intelligence (air) acts as a bridge to bring the space (ether), through vibration or sound, so that the senses of perception and the organs of action are brought very near without jarring each other. Each cell of the skin, while performing an *āsana*, should exactly face and be level to the flesh fibre. The cells of the skin have an out-going tendency – a sensitivity to the external world. Here they develop an in-coming tendency – a sensitivity to the internal world. The skin develops the quality or attitude of *pratyāhāra*. If done this way, it is integration *(saṁyama)*. When the cells of perception and the cells of action have become one, the intelligence dissolves in them, making the three vehicles of the consciousness become a single conscious movement in the entire body. This is *saṁyama* in that *āsana*.

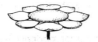

CONFLUENCE OF *ŚARĪRA ŚAKTI, PRĀṆA ŚAKTI* AND *PRAJÑĀ ŚAKTI* (body, energy, awareness)*

The body is like a vessel filled not only with cells, but with energy and consciousness. A body without consciousness and energy is as good as a dead body. For this reason we have three instruments: body *(śarīra)*, energy *(prāṇa)* and awareness *(prajñā)*. *Prajñā* is nothing but awareness of *citta*.

These three *śakti* or powers, namely, *śarīra śakti, prāṇa śakti* and *prajñā śakti*, have to be brought into alignment with *ātma śakti*. The whole practice must be built on this *sūtra* (theme). The practice of *āsana* and *prāṇāyāma* undoubtedly generates a copious *prāṇa śakti* in us. It is primarily this *prāṇa* or bio-energy which combats disease. Therefore, by the practice of *āsana* and *prāṇāyāma*, disease can be prevented.

The tussle begins when this tremendous energy is generated and the consciousness cannot take it. The body is like a small machine, the energy is like electricity. If it receives a voltage which is too high, it will be damaged. If either body or consciousness is insufficiently strong to bear the electrical charge, it can break, and in effect both may suffer damage. Therefore none of us can afford to have even a single extra or unwanted movement in the body or forego the awareness which was created. We must not cheat our consciousness and ourselves or abuse our energy and awareness.

We must differentiate between the expansion of the physical fibre (muscles, bones, nerves and joints) and that of the mental fibre. The body may have the capacity to extend, stretch, flex and increase the physical span of movement as well as its elasticity, firmness, steadiness and so on. But how do we charge it with consciousness? It is through the right utilisation of energy and the awareness of consciousness that we expand it.

When body and consciousness try to go to an *āsana* posture, with all the cellular adjustments, a gap remains between the structural and the organic body. Though one may discipline and coerce them, it has to be done with discriminative intelligence so that we discern

* Notes from classes conducted by Śri B.K.S. Iyengar for students from Bombay at RIMYI, Pune, August 1995.

the under- and over-action in order to get the right action. This gap is like a black hole. One has to fill it by bringing *prāṇic* energy so that the consciousness becomes aware of these gaps in the body. The gap is dark, but through awareness one has to build up.

Mahat (viśva prajña śakti) exists in us as the awareness of consciousness *(prajñā śakti).* It is *vibhu* – all-pervading. But consciousness needs fuel to function. That fuel is the willpower and *prāṇa* is the flame. This *prāṇa* springs out in an individual from cosmic energy *(viśva prāṇa śakti or viśva caitanya śakti).*

Prāṇa (energy) and *prajñā* (awareness) act as friends. Wherever the *prāṇa* goes, the *prajñā* follows and where *prajñā* moves, *prāṇa* follows. Then why does the gap remain? Because the consciousness often is not charged with the willpower of penetration. Only with the power of penetration in the consciousness can intelligence as a messenger reach there and fill the gap with the awareness of consciousness.

Like a couple going together, *prajñā* and *prāṇa* accompany each other. We have to witness this event. Unfortunately we often fail to witness and the gap remains. The function of witnessing is expressed through the will. If one wills, one witnesses. Will is the fuel for consciousness and breath is the fuel for energy. Breath ignites the *prāṇa* and will ignites the awareness in consciousness.

With the practice of *āsana* and *prāṇāyāma* we create space within. Space is freedom. If the space remains dark, it is *avidyā.* As two clouds collide and result in a thunderbolt, the dark space has to be illuminated with the lightning flash of *prāṇa śakti* and *prajñā śakti.* When *prāṇa* and *prajñā* meet, the light of intelligence strikes. If there is more space and less *prāṇa śakti* or *prajñā śakti,* emptiness and dullness set in. In the same way, if there is much *prāṇa śakti* and not enough *prajñā śakti,* the same dullness and emptiness are felt. We have to measure space, *prāṇa śakti* and *prajñā śakti,* and apply them evenly.

The main thing to observe in *āsana* and *prāṇāyāma* is that we have to create space for *prāṇa śakti* and *prajñā śakti* to occupy the frontier of the body from the source body. When practitioners work at the physical level, they do not create this space and do not have the understanding of each cell having its own intelligence with which to establish itself. There they miss the bus. Those who penetrate further feel the space. However, space should not be left empty or it kills the practitioner.

The *prāṇic* energy, when charged with cosmic energy *(viśva prāṇa śakti)* pervades the space, and expresses itself as awareness. The willpower makes this *prāṇic* energy reach the space in the body. Then it is real freedom. Freedom is with fullness and not from emptiness.

In *āsana* and *prāṇāyāma*, whether in stability or mobility, firmness or lightness, expansion or extension, contraction or release, the disparity between cells, energy and consciousness should not be allowed. This is the power of *sādhanā (sādhanā śakti)*. Through right performance of *āsana*, where the mind and self act as a single entity, a union of *prāṇa* and *prajñā* takes place and the gap between *prāṇa śakti* and *prajñā śakti* gets filled in.

Thus, while doing the *sādhanā* of *āsana* and *prāṇāyāma*, the conjunction of *prāṇa* (energy) and *prajñā* (consciousness) has to be like the *tailadhāra*. When oil *(taila)* is poured from one vessel to another, the flow remains uninterrupted. Similarly, the flow of *prāṇa* and *prajñā* has to remain uninterrupted throughout.

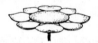

A DIVINE MARRIAGE OF *PRĀṆA* AND *PRAJÑĀ**

Today being *Hanumān Jayanti*, let me say a few words on Hanumān before speaking on *prāṇa* and *prajñā*. Lord Hanumān is a virtuous immortal Soul *(ciranjīvin)*.

He abides in all of us, sitting as a lord on our upper lip below the nostrils, moving in and out in the form of breath, showing us that the nostrils are his gates of *prāṇa*.

In order to understand *prāṇa* and *prajñā*, I have to say something about *prāṇāyāma*. As yoga practitioners, we respect Lord Hanumān because of the deep connection between him and *prāṇa*. Lord Hanumān is recognised by several names. He is known as *Hanumanta* and *Prāṇadeva*. *Hanu* is upper lip and *anta* is its top end. The area between the upper lip and the tip of the nose is the entrance for *prāṇa*, the vital force. Our life is dependent on the flow of breath in our system. In the nose we feel the touch of the breath, hence we explicitly or implicitly, pay our respects to Lord Hanumān. Hanumān, the Lord of *prāṇa,* exists within and moves in us in the form of breath. Therefore, he is our *Prāṇadevatā*, deity of *prāṇa,* who is also known as *Vāyuputra*, or the son of the Wind-God. These qualities of Hanumān are essential for the followers of yoga to emulate. Hanumān was a great devotee of Lord Rāma, so it pleases the Lord if one prays to his *bhaktan,* Hanumān. A servant serves and praises his master in order to get a reward. Similarly, we pray, praise and serve Lord Hanumān, if we want blessings from God. Lord Hanumān is praiseworthy because of his untainted attachment to his Lord – Shri Rāma.

He is an *ārogya kartru* – a giver of health. For *prāṇāyāma* practice one needs health. A pot can only retain the water if it is well baked. Similarly the chest, like the pot, has to be fit enough to hold the *prāṇa* within; therefore we need health. Many yoga practitioners think that *prāṇāyāma* can be done even by weaklings, but that is not true. I have often mentioned that both Patañjali and Svātmārāma have clearly pointed out that unless one practises and masters *āsana*, the body – the container – does not become firm, stable, strong and healthy and therefore cannot take up the practice of *prāṇāyāma*. As Lord Hanumān is the giver of the elixir of health,

---

* Talk given on *Hanumān Jayanti*, Pune, 06.04.1993.

we have to pray to him to grant us the needed health to practise for growth in our understanding of body, breath, mind, consciousness and the self. Lord Hanumān is a *jitendriyan* – one who has conquered the *indriya* (the organs of action, senses of perception and the mind). He is a *brahmacārin* (celibate). His celibacy is natural and not forced like Bhīṣma's. Bhīṣma had to take a vow to remain unmarried and remain truthful to his words. He was a prince and had promised his stepmother that he would neither marry nor claim the throne and remain a lifelong *brahmacārin* (*Mahābhārata*)[1].

Lord Hanumān is also known by these names:

mahābalan	– one who has unequalled strength, and muscular power
dṛḍhan	– of unsurpassable will,
śūran	– a hero with valour,
vīran	– one who has stable will power,
kartan	– a doer, one who does what he decides,
yuktan	– endowed with right thoughts, one who understands the right action at the right time and who is firmly rooted in his undertakings,
prajñāvān	– sensible and judicious,
buddhimān	– intelligent, wise,
kripākaran	– full of compassion,
kṛtārthan	– fulfilled one,
siddhan	– accomplished one,
śuddhan	– personification of virtue and purity,
bhaktan	– a perfect devotee, and
śāntan	– calm, tranquil and free from passion.

He is a great musician filled with the expression of *navarasa*. As food is of six *rasa* (taste), similarly *navarasa* (nine types of taste) are different forms of expression. These are:

Table n. 10 – *Navarasa* – the nine tastes

1.	*śṛngāra*	passion
2.	*hāsya*	amusement, laughter
3.	*karuṇa*	compassion, pity, tenderness
4.	*raudra*	fierceness
5.	*vīra*	valour, heroism
6.	*bhayānaka*	tearfulness, horror, fright
7.	*bibhatsa*	disgust, nausea, hideousness

[1] *Ādi Parva*, chapter 100

8.	*adbhuta*	wonder, marvel
9.	*śānta*	calmness, satisfaction

Śānta rasa is the last one. Peace comes at the end after having tasted all worldly experiences and having renounced them.

Lord Hanumān is always free from passion and therefore his *śānti* is pure. He is a *muktan* - an emancipated one with *brahmatejas* (having the lustre of pure *brahman*). Many of you might have read that Lord Hanumān is considered the next Brahmā, creator of this world, waiting in a queue along with Aśvatthāmā, Bali, Vyāsa, Kṛpācārya, Paruśurāma and Vibhiśaṇa. So we pray to him to grant us emancipation. We, the practitioners of yoga, should bow down to Lord Hanumān since he is a master of *aṣṭāṅga yoga* and can therefore bestow its fruits. As Lord Patañjali is considered a grammarian, so too is Lord Hanumān. He is a *vyākaraṇa paṇḍita* - an adept grammarian, a poet and an embodiment of sound *(nādamūrthi)*. He is skilled in recognising the essence of truth *(tattva vidyā viśārada)*. A perfect master who experienced the effects of *aṣṭāṅga yoga (aṣṭāṅga yoga phalānubhavi)*. All of us as practitioners of yoga should pray to Lord Hanumān since all his qualities are essentially needed by us and at the same time we need his blessings.

Swāmi Vivekananda narrates a story to explain the liberation of the soul. Once, a minister was imprisoned by the King, who had lost confidence in him. The king asked his servants to take the minister to the top of the tower of the city and dump him inside so that he would perish without food and water. This was done. The minister's dutiful wife however called on him every midnight providing him with what he wanted. One night, he asked her to bring a silken thread, a packthread, a long twine, a long rope, a beetle and honey. She brought the demanded items the next night. The minister asked her to tie the silken thread to the beetle, smear honey on its horns and let it climb up the tower. The beetle, once pointed in the right direction, followed the scent of the honey and climbed up. The minister caught hold of the silken thread and asked his wife to tie the pack thread through the other end. Then he pulled the silken thread as well as the pack thread. Then the twine was tied to the pack thread, so that the latter could pull the former. In this way finally the rope was pulled up. The minister tied it at the top, climbed down and escaped. He found freedom. Swāmi Vivekananda narrates the story in the context of liberation of the soul, I connect it to the *prāṇāyāmic* method.

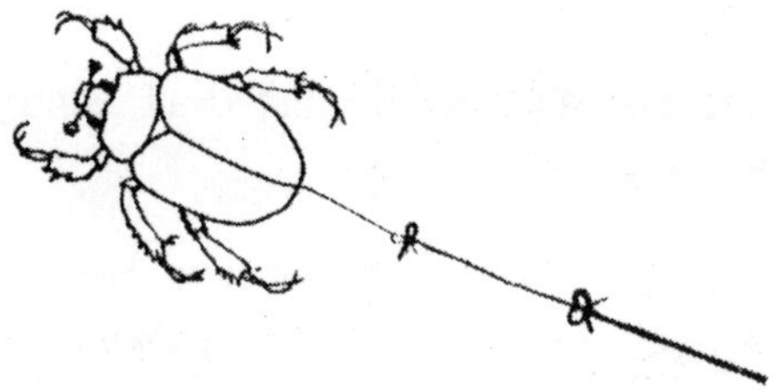

The beetle represents awareness *(prajñā)*, the minister represents *ātman*, the wife of the minister *prakṛti*, which leads either towards *bhoga* (experience) or *apavarga* (emancipation) and the smearing of honey to the horns of the beetle represents the kindling of *śuddha buddhi* – pure intelligence. *Ātman* is imprisoned and therefore it is called *jīvātman* (embodied soul). This *jīvātman* is associated with *prāṇa* and *prajñā*. The various threads up to the rope stand for *prāṇa*. *Prāṇa* can be either subtle (silk thread) or gross (rope). Respiration goes on continuously. This respiration is gross or manifested *(sthūla prāṇa)*. The life force and energy which vibrates within every cell is subtle *(sūkṣma prāṇa)*. Air in the form of *prāṇa* enters into the nose and goes to the trachea (windpipe). The trachea is thick like a rope. It branches into the bronchioles. They are like twine. The bronchioles again spread into a finer network – the packthread and finally the alveoli are represented by the silk thread. The air enters but it is filtered so that only oxygen (life force) is absorbed and unwanted air is evacuated. *Prāṇāyāma* is not merely respiration, but it teaches us how to absorb, retain and utilise energy. In order to do this, a judicious and orderly adjustment of *prajñā* is required. As the beetle climbed up to the minister, *prajñā* reaches *jīvātman*, provided it is charged with pure intelligence *(śuddha buddhi)*. It is pure and illumined *buddhi (śuddha sattva)* and that alone can face *ātman*, and bring freedom from the clutches of sorrow.

First of all, in *prāṇāyāma* the quality of the *prāṇa* is made to vibrate in order to merge the space of the cosmic intelligence (the elemental space or *mahadākāśa)* with space of the Soul (*cidākāśa*).

As the breath is stilled, the mind is stilled. Similarly, if there are no thoughts, then there will be no mind. Even if the mind is quietened, *ahaṁkāra* or the ego poses as a great obstacle for the seeker to go closer to the seer.

Hence the practice of *prāṇāyāma* helps the *sādhaka* to develop *prajñā* in helping to break the speed of the inflow and outflow of breath *(śvāsa* and *praśvāsa)* by deliberate adjustment so that *prāṇa* gains rhythm and smooth flow, and sinks into the system for peace and poise.

By checking *(viccheda)* inhalation and exhalation *(prāṇa* and *apāna)*, a state of soberness in the mind takes place with a vivid state of clarity and a thorough attentive thoughtfulness.

We all hanker for Self realisation. But remember that Self realisation *(ātma-sākṣātkāra)* is not possible unless *prāṇa* and *prajñā* help us to go closer to the Self. For this realisation practice of *prāṇāyāma* is very important.

In order to know the importance of *prāṇāyāma* one has to know the greatness of *prāṇa*. *Prāṇa* and *prajñā* are like twins. They always remain together; but the closeness of *prāṇa* and *prajñā* is realised only through *prāṇāyāma*. *Prāṇa* is the hub of *prajñā*, as the human heart is the hub of life and *prāṇāyāma* is the hub of *aṣṭāṅga yoga*. I refer here to *Praśna Upaniṣad* and *Kauṣītaki Upaniṣad*, which speak of the greatness of *prāṇa*. In the *Praśna Upaniṣad* (II.1-13), Guru Pippalāda is questioned by one of the six pupils called Bhārgava from Vidarbha, now the State of Maharashtra. To him Guru Pippalāda narrates this story: once the arms, legs, eyes, ears, tongue and mind began to fight among themselves to prove their respective greatness. The *prāṇa* within realised that now was the time to prove its greatness. So the *prāṇa* left the body. Obviously the other parts had to leave the body. As the queen bee is followed by other bees, so they had to follow *prāṇa* because they could not exist without it. In the *Kauśītaki Brāhmaṇa Upaniṣad* (II.1-15), *prāṇa* proved its greatness by going a step further. The above story is repeated in this *Upaniṣad* but with the additional remark that one can live deprived of arms and legs or be dumb, deaf or blind, be unintelligent, sleepy or in a state of coma; but one cannot live without *prāṇa*. If *prāṇa* is there, life is there. If *prāṇa* leaves, life is extinguished.

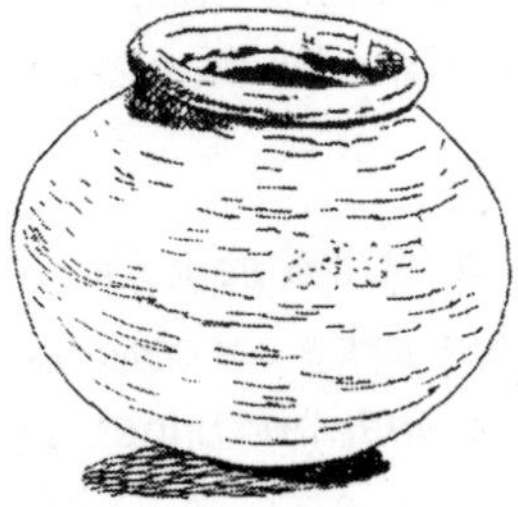

How do we experience this *prāṇa*? *Prāṇa* and *prajñā* (energy and awareness) are in *ākāśa* (space or ether). *Ākāśa* has no beginning and no end. It is infinite. An earthen pot has a space, that can be filled by water. The moment the pot breaks, water vanishes and air occupies the space. The shape of the pot holds the space or gives a shape to the space and when it breaks, the outer and inner space become one. Our body is like a pot. As we have within both *prāṇa* and *prajñā*, similarly these two exist externally as well. *Prāṇa* is *mahadākāśa* and *prajñā* is *cidākāśa*. *Prāṇa* is *mahat-tattva* and *prajñā* is *jñāna-tattva*. *Prāṇāyāma* brings divine unification between *prāṇa* and *prajñā*.

In *pūraka* (inhalation) the breath moves from *mahadākāśa* to *cidākāśa* and in *recaka* (exhalation), the breath moves from *cidākāśa* towards *mahadākāśa*. In *antara kuṁbhaka* (inhalation-retention), the *prajñā* becomes one with *prāṇa* and in *bāhya kuṁbhaka* (exhalation-retention) *prāṇa* merges into *prajñā* and *prajñā* merges into *mahat*. In this way *prāṇāyāmic* action is meant to energise the *prāṇa* and *prajñā*. Though inhalation and exhalation seem to be separate actions, their movement is in fact circular like that of a wheel. Similarly, the *prāṇa* and *prajñā* move together in such a manner that one cannot make out which is the former and which is the latter. *Prajñā* wills and *prāṇa* vibrates. In *prāṇāyāma, prajñā* is awareness in action and *prāṇa* is a flow motion. Bringing *prajñā* (will) and *prāṇa* (energy) into a rhythm is *prāṇāyāma*. *Prāṇāyāma* is a process in which the vibrations of *prāṇa* are lessened and *prajñā* is stabilised.

The space of consciousness and the space between elements are churned and rubbed to produce energy which is carried by the *nāḍī* and cells like electricity. In each cell there is *cidākāśa* as well as *mahadākāśa*. In each cell there is *prajñā* as well as *prāṇa*. The breathing process occurs in the respiratory system, the lungs, the alveoli and so forth, but apart from producing bio-energy it produces *cetana śakti* and that is because *prāṇa* and *prajñā* get unified.

Prāṇa is the supporter of life. It supports *prajñā*, strengthening the willpower. In each breath we carry approximately 500 cc of air. But when we discipline it, we may take in 3000 to 3500 cc. This difference in the amount is measurable. But what about *prajñā?* That cannot be measured. A practitioner of yoga has to take *prajñā* into account while doing *prāṇāyāma*. *Prāṇāyāma* undoubtedly improves respiration, circulation and makes the organic body healthy. But one should not overlook the role of *prajñā*.

Prāṇa and *prajñā* both are precious jewels for us. At the same time they are very delicate and therefore have to be utilised carefully. *Prāṇa* has to be conceived and *prajñā* has to be sharpened and not consumed. We have to see how *prāṇāyāma* brings a divine union of *prāṇa* and *prajñā*.

All of us have experienced the dissipation of energy, but the specific dissipation that occurs in yoga practitioners has been explained by Patañjali in *Samādhi Pāda*. This dissipation of energy can occur in a yogi as it occurs in an average individual. Here one has to refer to *sūtra* 30, 31 and 32 of *Samādhi Pāda*. They explain the causes for dissipation of energy and how one can overcome them. The obstacles in the path of yoga are physical disease, langour, doubt, carelessness, physical laziness, self-indulgence, living in the world of illusion, lack of perseverance and backsliding. Sorrow, despair, unsteadiness of the body and irregular breathing further distract the *citta*. Adherence to single-minded effort of practice in all the eight aspects of yoga alone can prevent these impediments.

The nine impediments *(nava antarāya)* are not merely physical diseases, but mental, sensual, intellectual, emotional and spiritual impediments. These impediments bother the practitioners, shattering their mind and practice through sorrow, despair, dejection, weak-mindedness, inferiority complex, heaviness and shakiness of the body and irregular breathing. They occur at a deep level but their effect can be seen at the outer layers. Disturbance in the innermost consciousness can cause ruffles at the surface.

A yogi, being sensitive, feels deep within and an average individual feels from the outside. In modern terminology one could say that the nine obstacles divert our attention from yoga, causing cardiac problems, Parkinson's disease, mental depression, schizophrenia, asthma, bronchitis or headaches. Sorrow, despair, unsteadiness of the body and irregular breathing accompany all the nine obstacles all the time. Even a single obstacle is enough to cause multiple distractions. If one watches the symptoms of the above mentioned diseases, one realises that they affect *prāṇa* and *prajñā* directly though they vary in degree. Patañjali asks us to treat and correct the defects of *prāṇa* and *prajñā* by *citta prasādanam*, i.e. favourable disposition or graceful diffusion and embellishment of consciousness. In *Samādhi Pāda (sūtra* 33 to 39), Patañjali explains the various methods of *citta prasādanam*, in order to bring a favourable disposition. These methods encompass the eight aspects of yoga in a very subtle form. They embellish the body, the organs of action, the senses of perception, mind, nerves, ego, will, inner tendencies of the mind, intelligence, and so forth. They are:

1. Friendliness towards joy (*Y.S.*, I.33),
2. Compassion towards pain (*Y.S.*, I.33),
3. Joy towards virtue (*Y.S.*, I.33),
4. Indifference towards vice (*Y.S.*, I.33),
5. Maintaining the quiet psychological state of consciousness felt after exhalation (*Y.S.*, I.34),
6. Contemplating an object that helps to maintain the steadiness of consciousness (*Y.S.*, I.35),
7. Contemplating a luminous, sorrowless, effulgent light (*Y.S.*, I.36),
8. Contemplating on enlightened beings who were and are free from attachment (*Y.S.*, I.37),
9. Reflecting on the knowledge obtained while in dream-filled or dreamless sleep during a watchful, waking state (*Y.S.*, I.38),
10. Contemplating on an pleasant object or on an pleasant idea, conducive to yogic practice (*Y.S.*, I.39).

Patañjali asks us to correct the flow of energy by maintaining the passive and pensive state, allowing the outgoing breath to go smoothly and softly and then have a comfortable, passive retention. *Sūtra* 34 indicates its connection with *prāṇāyāma*. If one understands the above mentioned techniques of *sūtra* 33 to 39, he will see that all these techniques correspond not only to *prāṇa*, but also to *prajñā*. To cultivate friendliness, compassion, joy and detachment, one needs *prajñā* (understanding). To contemplate on a sorrowless and luminous state of mind, *prāṇa* and *prajñā* both have to be sharpened. In *sūtra* 39 Patañjali advises us to meditate on any desired object conducive to steadiness of consciousness *(yathābhimata dhyānādvā).* How can one do this unless the *prajñā* has been polished? Finally, to have a total transformation *(samāpatti)* and a matured wisdom *(ṛtambharā prajñā)* accompanied with intense insight, both *prāṇa* and *prajñā* have to be purified.

The practice of *prāṇāyāma* is meant to discipline *prāṇa* and *prajñā* so that at this juncture, when obstacles bother us and the *citta prasādanam* is needed, we can safely overcome them and gracefully embellish the *citta* on the way to Self-realisation.

Knowing the necessity of *prāṇāyāma* while treading the path of Self-realisation, Patañjali devoted five *sūtra* of *Sādhana Pāda* to it. Among them, the first three are on techniques and levels of *prāṇāyāma* and the last two are on effects and fruits of it. The first *sūtra* is: *tasmin sati śvāsa praśvāsayoḥ gativiccedaḥ prāṇāyāmah* (II.49). *Tasmin sati* are very significant words. The literal meaning is: "On being accomplished". It means: "After attaining perfection in *āsana* one has to take up *prāṇāyāma* to regulate the incoming and outgoing flow of breath, interrupted by retention". Here Patañjali indicates very clearly the fact that *prāṇāyāma* should be commenced only after the mastery of *āsana.* But let me tell you something more about this step which he mentions so distinctly.

In the *Samādhi Pāda* Patañjali mentions nine impediments and goes still further by explaining four types of distractions that agitate the mind and consciousness. These impediments not only bother an adept but also a beginner in yoga. One may try to master *āsana,* but still these obstacles may remain. Many times I have told you how in the early days of my practice I faced and fought with these problems. Physical disease limits and stops us from the practice of *āsana.* Languor, laziness and lethargy are a common experience for every one of us. Doubt exists and we think that all we do is perhaps futile and may not give us anything. We practise but we are casual and callous. We practise *āsana* but the mind may roam. Our body may bend nicely and people may appreciate our performance but as long as we do not get the essence, it is like living under an illusion. We do *Utthita Trikoṇāsana* (Plate n. 8), but the performance may not be of the same quality on both sides. What we do on the right, we may not do on the left and what we do on the left, we may not do on the right. We miss the point on many occasions. We may touch the peak of the best performance in *āsana,* but we prove unable to hold on. How many people practise for a few days and give up? Even after achieving something, having made progress, the mind oscillates. Whether one fails or succeeds, the unsettled mind stops one from practising the *āsanas.* Whether in progress or regression, if one is lacking in firm decision, one cannot keep up the practice. Wrong and mechanical practice of *āsana* can lead to pain. The failure to master what one wants to achieve may bring sorrow, dejection and despair. While doing *āsana* you all have experienced that if you overstretch in one place you may understretch at another place. Does it not lead towards shakiness of the body? While doing *āsana,* when you stretch unused muscles for the first time, they tremble. Is it not *angamejayatva?* Do you not become breathless when you make an effort? The breath settles in *āsana* when the body is properly adjusted. In a wrong pose the breath never moves rhythmically. Are these not the obstacles that Patañjali mentions? Can we neglect them? Why do we demand precision? We demand precision so that we overcome these obstacles. In fact it is the way to safeguard oneself from future problems, which are inevitable if one does not pay attention for the right way of practice.

Therefore the words *tasmin sati* are very meaningful. They convey the necessity of *āsana* in order to overcome the obstacles at the preliminary stage. Patañjali devotes three *sūtra* to *āsana,* which are full of potency. *Sthiratā* is stability, which is not only of the body but also of the nerves and the mind. *Sukhatā* is the spread of consciousness *(prajñā).* One has to see whether the intelligence has touched all the frontiers. *Prayatna śaithilya* is not laxity or effortlessness, but seeing whether the efforts are properly directed to overcome the above mentioned obstacles. When there is no impediment, *prayatna śaithilya* follows. *Ananta samāpatti* is to reach the infinite within. Compare this to *ekatattvābhyāsa.* When the single-minded effort and the cessation of fluctuations take place, the opposing pairs of dualities disappear. Then there is no room for doubt.

One will find the same obstacles *(antarāya)* in the practice of *prāṇāyāma.* But those who practise *āsana* in a proper way can practise *prāṇāyāma* safely. They develop an inner capacity, courage and discrimination to eradicate the obstacles in *prāṇāyāma.*

Prāṇāyāma is a fascinating subject, but at the same time quite a lot of practitioners get bored quickly. The few enthusiasts who practise may invite problems because of wrongdoing, want of knowledge and lack of understanding. People attempt and give up. The *Haṭhayoga Pradīpikā* mentions that those who do improperly will invite severe respiratory problems, pain, fever and so on, as the three humors of the body are vitiated.

The practice of *āsana* clears the channel for *prāṇa* to move freely and uninterruptedly. In this sense, practice of *āsana* brings perfection. It breaks the rigidity and hardness of the inner body. The unrhythmic breath becomes rhythmic. The outbreaths and inbreaths become deep, slow and soothing.

In *sūtra* II.50, Patañjali explains the technique of *prāṇāyāma: Bāhya ābhyantara stamba vṛttiḥ deśa kāla saṁkhyābhiḥ paridṛṣṭaḥ dīrgha sūkṣmaḥ. Prāṇāyāma* has three movements:

prolonged and fine inhalation, exhalation and retention; all regulated with precision according to duration and place. He states *deṣa,* which means place. It is a very significant word as it places the elements of *prāṇāyāma,* namely: inhalation, inhalation-retention, exhalation and exhalation-retention.

The varieties of *prāṇāyāma* are meant to introduce us to different parts of the body. The *prāṇa* is absorbed through different avenues to different areas of the body. *Prāṇa* cannot reach anywhere in the body unless *prajñā* reaches there. Duration *(kāla)* is a factor to be thought of as well. The *prāṇa* may penetrate for a moment, but that is not enough for *prajñā* to get awakened. Here, *kuṁbhaka* plays a great role. If *prāṇa* has to energise one, then one has to hold on to *prajñā* for some time, so that the distribution of energy takes place and one can reflect on what has been done in order to have precision *(saṁkhya). Dīrgha* and *sūkṣma* relate to the quality of the breath. The breath cannot be extended, expanded or made finer unless one develops a special awareness and intelligence to penetrate.

To know the unknown, one has to know the known properly. In *sūtra* II.49-50, Patañjali asks us to learn first the known before trying to understand the unknown. *Sūtra* II.51 conveys how to know the unknown. When the inhalation, exhalation and retention *(bāhya* and *antara)* transcend the limitations of *deṣa, kāla* and *saṁkhyā* and go beyond, volition ends, efforts end. *Prāṇa* and *prajñā* both reach maturity. Patañjali explains *prāṇāyāma* at the physical level in II.49, at the mental and intellectual levels in II.50 and at the spiritual level in II.51. *Sūtra* II.52 and 53 convey the effects of *prāṇāyāma* saying that it uncovers the light of intelligence and so the mind becomes fit for concentration. In terms of *prāṇa* and *prajñā,* I would say that it is the consummation of *prāṇāyāma.* The *prāṇa* is trained like a winning racehorse so that it is consumed to reach the goal, i.e. the soul. At this stage the *prāṇa* and *prajñā* both get united and this divine couple becomes one, losing their separate identities, and leads the *sādhaka* towards the Self.

We can trace this explanation of Patañjali's in the fourth chapter of Svātmārāma's *Haṭhayoga Pradīpikā.* Brahmānanda calls it *Samādhi nirūpaṇa.* He explains the relationship, dependence and co-operation of *prāṇa* and *prajñā.* When a practitioner suspends the breath or checks the movements of the breath, then the movement of the mind is also checked. If *prāṇa* is restrained, *prajñā* too is restrained.

When *prajñā* remains in a state of absorption, *prāṇa* remains quiet. It does not disturb the *prajñā. Prāṇa* helps *prajñā* by itself remaining motionless. If the husband is engrossed in work, then a faithful wife does not disturb him. Similarly, *prāṇa* being faithful to *prajñā,* does not disturb the latter since it is in a state of absorption.

The inner space and outer space become one, like an empty pot in an empty space. The elemental *ākāśa,* i.e. *prāṇa,* is empty. If the pot is kept in a space, the emptiness within and the emptiness without become one. Similarly, if the space of consciousness is full, then the space of the elements is also full. If the pot is kept in a sea, the water enters in the pot. The water in the sea and the water in the pot are the same. Since the sea is full and the pot is full, the water in the pot remains in the pot and the water in the sea remains in the sea. Similarly, when *prāṇa* and *prajñā* are both full, they remain in their places. Svātmārāma too says that when both *prāṇa* and *prajñā* are full and steady, external thoughts do not enter and internal thoughts do not creep out. If *prāṇa* is steady, internal thoughts cannot creep out. *Prajñā* guards so that external thoughts do not enter in. If one remains without thought and does not allow internal thoughts to extrude and then excludes all thoughts whether external or internal (objective or subjective) and puts an end to all, one remains a witness without allowing any thinking force to disturb one. Then both *prāṇa* and *prajñā* remain checked.

Yoga is the union between *prāṇa* and *prajñā*, equilibrium between *prāṇa* and *prajñā*, fullness and completeness in *prāṇa* and *prajñā*. *Prāṇa* is vital energy. It can be developed and multiplied, but when *prajñā* also develops along with *prāṇa*, it is virtuous *(śīla)*. With the practice of yoga we have to develop *śuddha buddhi*. That is why Patañjali advises us to practise *prāṇāyāma* in order to unveil the light of *sattva*. This is very significant. If *prāṇāyāma* was meant for developing *prāṇa śakti*, he would have said so. Duryodhana had tremendous power and valour. Even King Dhṛtarāṣṭra had tremendous *prāṇa śakti*. He embraced the iron statue of Bhīma and crushed it into pieces, as his anger flared up. But they both lacked *prajñā*. Whereas the Pāṇdava had *prāṇa* and *prajñā* both. *Prajñā* is the faculty of insight. As *prajñā* gets matured, the intelligence gets seasoned. *Ṛtambharā* is a seasoned intelligence. *Ṛtambharā* is knowledge full of truth. The truth-bearing *prajñā* is always full of virtue. Therefore, *prāṇāyāma* illumines one to get the vision of the Self. *Prāṇāyāma* certainly gives physical as well as vital strength *(prāṇa śakti)*, in order to develop *prajñā*, so that it leads towards the ultimate freedom.

Lord Hanumān had tremendous valour, strength and power, and at the same time he was wise His intelligence was incomparable. He is described as *buddhi matam variṣṭham*, the wisest among the wise. He is the best example of one in whom *prāṇa* and *prajñā* were both balanced and united divinely to serve his master Rāma, the Lord within.

I conclude this talk by praying Lord Hanumān to bestow the same virtue on us so that we may serve the hidden *antarātman* with *prāṇa* and *prajñā*.

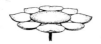

PRACTICE OF *PRĀṆĀYĀMA**

Besides mind, intelligence, ego, consciousness and soul, the human body is made of five elements; earth, water, fire, air and ether. The five elements have a grip on the five organs of action. Similarly, the subtle qualities *(tanmātra)* of these five elements viz., odour, taste, form, touch and sound are felt by the five senses of perception. In *Chāndogya Upaniṣad,* it is said that the eyes belong to *prāṇa vāyu,* ears to *vyāna vāyu,* tongue to *apāna vāyu,* nose to *samāna vāyu* and skin to *udāna vāyu.*

Table n. 11 – *Mānava śarira* (the human being)

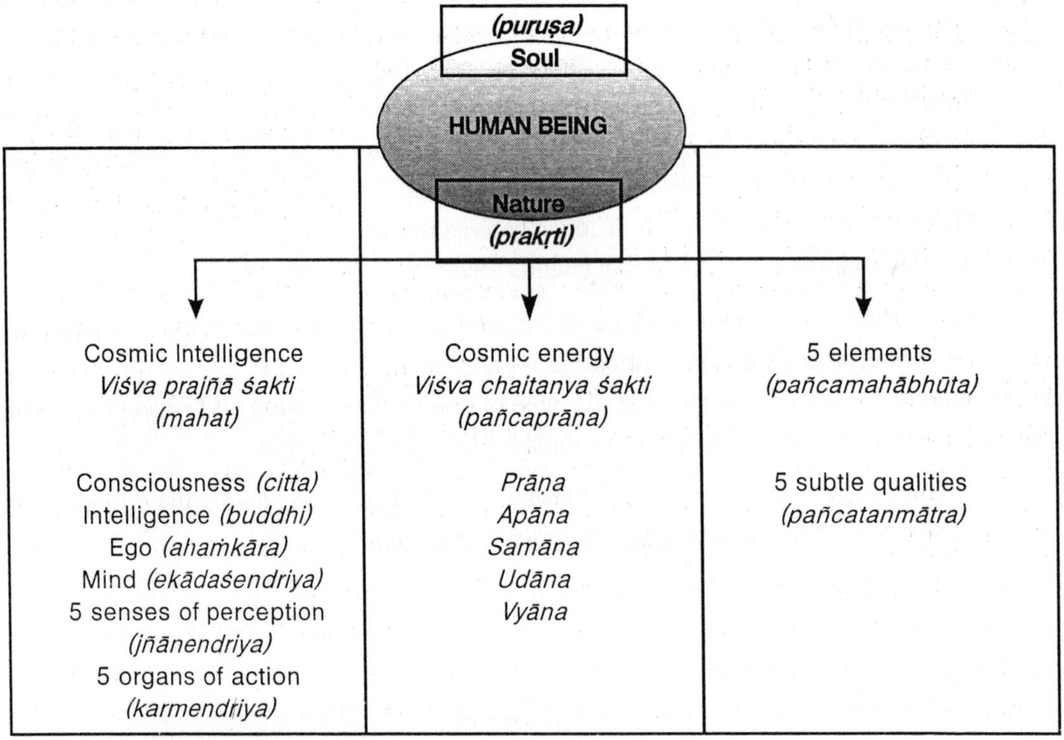

* Also published as: *"Introduction to prāṇāyāma",* in *Yoga Rahasya*, vol. I, no. 2, July 1994

The *mahat* or the cosmic intelligence *(viśva prajña śakti)* is transformed in an individual as *citta* (consciousness). The cosmic energy *(viśva caitanya śakti)* divides itself as *prāṇa, apāna, samāna, udāna* and *vyāna* in the body. The five gross elements *(pañcamahābhūta)* correspond to the five sheaths *(pañcakośa)* of the human being. Wherever the five elements exist, the subtle qualities *(pañcatanmātra)* accompany them. Thus, the anatomical sheath *(annamaya kośa)* corresponds to earth and odour; the physiological sheath *(prāṇamaya kośa)* corresponds to water and taste; the mental sheath *(manomaya kośa)* to fire and form; the intellectual sheath *(vijñānamaya kośa)* to air and touch, and the sheath of bliss *(ānandamaya kośa)* to ether and sound.

Table n. 12 –*Pañcaprāṇa* and *bhūta*

***PAÑCAPRĀṆA (PAÑCAVĀYU)*, THEIR PROVINCE AND THE ELEMENTS THEY REPRESENT**			
Pañcaprāṇa	**Province as per *āyurveda* and yoga**	**Functions of *prāṇa* in our body**	***Bhūta* they represent**
Prāṇa	Brain, chest	Respiratory	*Āp* (water)
Apāna	Waist, thighs, uterus, testicles, rectum	Excretory, reproduction	*Pṛthvī* (earth)
Samāna	Intestines, stomach	Digestion, integration of other systems	*Tej* (fire)
Udāna	Throat, nose, bronchioles, diaphragm	Spiritual Enlightenment	*Vāyu* (air)
Vyāna	Heart, entire body	Nervous and circulatory systems	*Ākāśa* (ether)

PAÑCA PRĀṆA (FIVE VITAL ENERGIES)

The brain and the thoracic region are the centre or the main province of *prāṇa.* They control the breathing process and cause the vital energy of atmospheric air to be absorbed through the respiratory system. *Apāna* has its abode at the lower abdominal region and controls and eliminates urine, semen and faeces. *Samāna,* with its seat at the navel, stokes the gastric fire, aiding digestion and harmonising the functioning of the other vital airs. This energy integrates all physiological systems in man. *Udāna,* at the seat of the throat, controls the vocal cords, the intake and output of air, and acts as the gate to the fourth state, *turīya. Vyāna* exists everywhere pervading the entire body and distributes energy to the necessary parts of the body.

Chāndogya Upaniṣad (VII.1) explains the greatness of *prāṇa* through the dialogue between Nārada and his preceptor Sanatkumāra. Sanatkumāra, before accepting and initiating him as a pupil, wanted to know what he knew. Nārada said that he knew all the *veda, itihāsa* (history), *purāṇa,* grammar, rules of worship, mathematics, science of logic, ethics, etymology, science of war, stars, fine arts and so on but he was not the knower of the *puruṣa.* With all this knowledge, he said, "I am in grief and it does not leave me. Guide me, so that I am free from grief and know the *puruṣa".* Sanatkumāra explained that *veda* are names, and names through speech help the aspirant towards higher knowledge. He went further and said that speech is greater than name, mind is greater than speech, will greater than mind, consciousness greater than will, contemplation greater than consciousness, discriminative power greater than contemplation, strength greater than discriminative power (as truth gets revealed), food greater than strength, water greater than food, fire greater than water, ether or space greater than fire, memory greater than space, aspiration greater than memory and *prāṇa (vāyu)* greater than aspiration. Because when *prāṇa* departs, all these things depart. Therefore, *prāṇa* is all these.

Life force or energy and absolute consciousness *(prāṇa + prajñā)* together are known as *jīvātman* or individual self. To know the mortal self or *jīvātman* you have to understand energy or *prāṇa.* Even in various *Upaniṣads* we find how sages and yogis came out with the greatness of *prāṇa* and how the techniques were built around *prāṇa* as *prāṇāyāma.*

PRIME FORCE

We are born with the three components, viz., 1) nature *(prakṛti)* and matter or elements of nature *(bhūta* and *tanmātra),* 2) energy *(viśva caitanya śakti)* commonly called *prāṇa,* and 3) absolute consciousness or absolute awareness *(viśva prajña śakti).* The prime force for activation is energy. This energy exists in every thing as universal or cosmic energy *(viśva caitanya śakti).*

Hence, matter, energy and absolute consciousness create action and stability, motion and mobility, as well as understanding and creativity respectively. Without this cosmic energy, nothing moves. It acts as a hidden force within us, as well as embracing the world outside us. Yogis of yore, after study, understood the value and the essence of *prāṇa* and gave importance to it. They framed methods to master *prāṇa* and named them *prāṇāyāma*.

Unless the inner latent energy is understood and tapped, it is a very difficult process to practise *prāṇāyāma*. This latent energy manifests itself as breath and becomes the promoter to receive the cosmic energy in the form of inhalation and at the same time, it is the power that helps to release the drawn in breath in the form of exhalation. When the cosmic energy is fully drawn in, the inner latent energy expresses itself as individual energy or *vaiyaktika śakti*.

In inhalation the cosmic energy *(viśva caitanya śakti)* unites with the individual energy *(vaiyaktika śakti)* and in exhalation the individual energy *(vaiyaktika śakti)* unites with the cosmic energy *(viśva caitanya śakti)*. One learns to control through matter, energy and absolute awareness, the rhythmic intake of cosmic energy, its utilisation and its release, in the form of outbreath.

Prāṇa, the self-energising force[1], makes the body function, creating potency and power in the *prajñā*. It is *prāṇa* that acts as a bridge connecting matter *(bhūta)* and total awareness in the consciousness *(prajñā* of *citta)*. *Prāṇa* helps *prajñā* to discover matter *(bhūta)* and consciousness *(citta)*. Thus matter *(bhūta)*, energy *(prāṇa)* and absolute awareness or consciousness *(prajñā)* become one. *Prāṇāyāma* practices make one see how all these three get united, as a single united force.

PRĀṆĀYĀMA

For *prāṇāyāma* practice one has to sit in an *āsana*, so let me explain what an *āsana* means. *Āsana* means a posture. It means positioning the body in various ways. After posing, the doer has to reflect carefully on the position with its reactions and again repose to experience the harmony, the balance and the sense of touch of the intelligence *(buddhi sparśa)*. If posing is the element of earth, reflection is the element of water. Reaction and reposing belong to the element of fire. If the feeling of uniform touch of intelligence is felt at once in the entire body, then it belongs to the element of air; whereas, extension, expansion, contraction and diffusion of the body as well as the consciousness are the works of the element of ether. When concord of these five elements is traced, then the *āsana*, according to Sage Patañjali, brings stability in the body *(sthiratā)* and poise in the self *(sukhatā)*. In this state begins *prāṇāyāma*.

---

1 See the Author's *The Tree of Yoga*, Harper Collins, London, pp. 125-128.

Table n. 13 – *Āsana, bhūta, tanmātra, jñānendriya* and *karmendriya saṁbhanḍha*

THE RELATIONSHIP BETWEEN THE *BHŪTA, TANMĀTRA, JÑĀNENDRIYA* AND *KARMENDRIYA* IN THE PRACTICE OF *ĀSANA*				
***Pañca-mahābhūta* (5 elements)**	***Tanmātra* (5 qualities)**	***Jñānendriya* (5 senses of perception)**	***Karmendriya* (5 organs of action)**	**Function and expression in *āsana***
Pṛthvī (earth)	*Gandha* solidity, odour	Nose	Excretory organs	Posing or structuring
Āp (water)	*Rasa* fluidity, taste	Tongue	Generative organs	Reflection
Tej (fire)	*Rūpa* heat, shape, form	Eyes	Mouth	Attention of Intelligence
Vāyu (air)	*Sparśa* mobility, touch	Skin	Legs	Touch and trace of intelligence
Ākāśa (ether)	*Śabdha* volume, sound	Ears	Arms	Extension, expansion, contraction, diffusion of intelligence

The *sādhaka* has to learn to observe, mould and adjust the five elements and their subtle qualities, so that they balance evenly for the five *vāyu* (Plate n. 6) to move without any hindrance in the practice of *prāṇāyāma*. The subtle qualities *(tanmātra)*, viz., sound, touch, form, taste and odour *(śabda, sparśa, rūpa, rasa, gandha)* are felt by the senses of perception. These are ears, skin, eyes, tongue and nose.

Prāṇāyāma is a compound word made up of *prāṇa* and *āyāma*. *Prāṇa* means self energising energy and *āyāma* means stretch, regulation, restraint, control, check, exercise, prolongation, extension, expansion, length, breadth and circumference. It also means maintenance of self-energising energy in a healthy state at all ages and in all circumstances. This exercising of *prāṇa* helps physiologically in toning the cells, sinews, tendons, ligaments, muscles and nerves, and stimulates the heart muscles to function rhythmically with proper circulation and ventilation. Psychologically it builds the intelligence and consciousness to remain in an optimum level of efficiency in awareness without signs of fatigue in the body or the feeling of boredom in life.

Before the practice of *prāṇāyāma*, the *puruṣa* guides the senses of perception to build up passivity and receptivity. Then it teaches them to receive *śakti* in *pūraka* and release *śakti* in *recaka*. From this the *sādhaka* learns the ways of using the senses of perception in *prāṇāyāma*. He uses ears to check and control the vibration or sound in *pūraka – recaka*; feels from the skin the resonent and exhilarating sensation of touch and controls the flow; adjusts the energy to a conditioned form within the body. The roof of the palate notices the coolness or the hotness and guides the other three subtle *tanmātra* to go slowly; while the nose receives and smells the fragrance of both the *viśva caitanya śakti* and *vaiyaktika śakti*.

This is how the five *bhūta*, the five *tanmātra*, the five organs of action, the five senses of perception and the five *vāyu* (Plate n. 6) interact and intermingle in unison with energy *(śakti)* and awareness *(prajñā)*, to make the body the abode of the nectar of life.

While walking on a straight avenue, we do not like to zigzag or deviate from one end to the other. Though walking like this may be fun, later on one loses the balance of mind and gets dizzy. Similarly, we should know that we have different roads or paths in our respiratory organs for inhalation and exhalation. Firstly, we have to learn to observe and trace these paths that are there but go unnoticed. As we walk on the roads carefully by using the intelligence of our eyes to guard ourselves from accidents, we have to make use of the intelligence of the consciousness to make the breath flow in and out on the allotted avenues formed by nature.

The entry for the inbreath is the passage underneath the cheekbones, whereas for the outbreath, it is the lower eyelids and above the rings of the cheekbones. We have to know these different passages of inhalation and exhalation before we begin to practise *prāṇāyāma* with open nostrils.

In digital *prāṇāyāma*, or nostril breathing, the breath or *prāṇa* moves in inhalation, touching the surfaces of the septum areas, whereas in exhalation, it touches the inner membranes of the outer walls of the nostrils[1].

While doing *prāṇāyāma*, the *sādhaka* has to create mental dykes so that the breath does not gush in or gush out, but is allowed to seep and soak in gradually through the windpipe,

[1] For details, see the Author's *Light on Prāṇāyāma*, Harper Collins, London

trachea, bronchial tubes and aerial cells. At the same time, he has to feel the rhythmic and smooth pattern of the incoming energy and outgoing energy throughout the practice of *prāṇāyāma*.

JĀLANDHARA BANDHA OR CHINLOCK

In open-nostril or non-digital *prāṇāyāma* like *ujjāyī* and *viloma*, the practitioner has to construct the dykes on the body with the help of *prajñā* at the entry gates for inhalation. They are at the bottom cheekbones, upper palate and the top of the windpipe. In order to build natural dykes for *prāṇāyāma* practices, *Jālandhara Bandha* or the chinlock was introduced by the yogis. This judiciously helps the *prajñā* of the inner *prāṇa* to receive the incoming *prāṇa* as well as check the incoming *prāṇa* to flow in rhythmically and later on be distributed. Dykes are to be built at the diaphragm, external intercostal muscles, the windpipe and the top rings of the cheekbones for smooth release of the outgoing breath or energy.

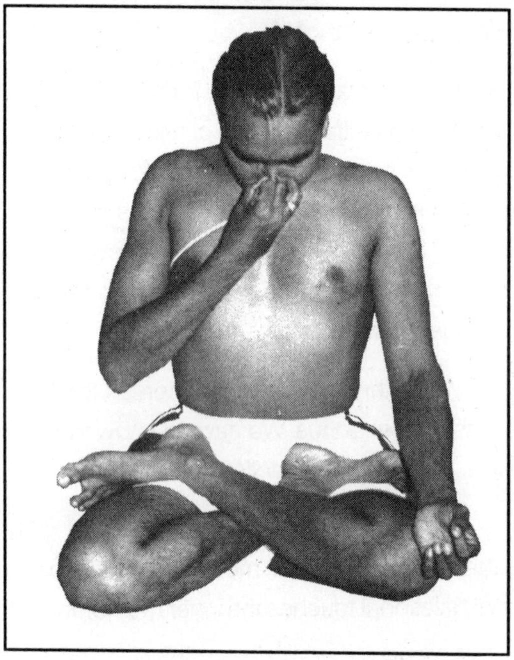

Plate n. 20 – Digital *Prāṇāyāma* showing *Jālandhara Bandha*

In controlled nostril or digital *prāṇāyāma* such as or like *Anuloma, Pratiloma, Sūrya Bhedana, Chandra Bedhana* and *Nāḍī Śodhana*, the practitioner has to construct the dykes at the inner edge of the roof of the nostrils for inhalation and the outer edge of the roof for exhalation. He has to know these above mentioned places in order to form the dykes before beginning digital *prāṇāyāma*.

If the breath deviates from its conditioned paths, it enters forcibly and goes out forcibly. This type of deep breath cannot be termed *prāṇāyāma*. In *prāṇāyāma*, the job of the *sādhaka* is to see that in inhalation the energy gets filled in deeply and soaked into the body and in exhalation, the energy is released through the sluice gates of the nostril formed by the fingers and the thumb so that time is given for it to be absorbed and stored in the system.

In inhalation *(pūraka)*, the outer skin of the back moves down first and then towards the body while the inner frontal skin expands and opens up without disturbing the outer frontal skin of the chest box. The back inner skin and front inner skin act as a mirror and a reflected mirror.

In exhalation *(recaka)*, the skin at the inner back and inner front of the trunk is lifted up and alerted to keep it steady. Then the breath is released in the form of *recaka* through the outer skin of the front chest. When passivity is felt evenly in the inner and outer skin of the front and back trunk without shrinking and caving in the chest or stooping the spine, *recaka* is complete.

ART OF SITTING

Before sitting for *prāṇāyāma*, you should know how to sit, so that turbulence in the body does not take place. Know exactly the end middle portion of the tailbone and sit in such a way that it runs perpendicular to the floor. Treat this point as the South Pole, and the centre portion of the head of the spine as the North Pole. *Jālandhara Bandha* (Plate n. 20) helps to spot this area to adjust clearly for the rest of the spine to float in line, as if you had placed one vertebra of the spine over the other, like a mason planting one brick over the other. This adjustment helps the *sādhaka* to understand the movement of the five elements in the process of *prāṇāyāma*. Any forward movement or backward stretch of the body means disturbance or imbalance in the elements.

In order to learn *Tāḍāsana* (Plate n. 8), we place and spread the bottom mounds of the feet evenly. Similarly, we have to learn to use the buttock-bones as if they are the mounds of the seat in the sitting position. Do not strain but relax the groins. Position the centre of the buttock-bones and the crown or the middle portion of the ankles that touch the ground, so that the water element of the body finds its level on the seat, groins and feet. In the same way, keep the back and front of the floating ribs running parallel to each other.

BHŪTA, *VĀYU* AND THEIR MOVEMENTS

The five elements of the body, viz., earth, water, fire, air and ether *(pṛthvī, āp, tejas, vāyu,* and *ākāśa)*, relate to the anatomical, physiological, psychological or mental, intellectual and blissful sheaths. While performing *āsana*, these five elements and five sheaths are interwoven, observed and tended (Plate n. 6). Similarly, the five *vāyu (prāṇa, apāna, vyāna, udāna* and *samāna)* are interlinked with the five elements. *Apāna vāyu* relates to the element of earth *(pṛthvī)*, *prāṇa vāyu* to water *(āp)*, *samāna vāyu* to fire *(tejas)*, *udāna vāyu* to air *(vāyu)* and *vyāna vāyu* to ether *(ākāśa)* (Table n. 12). While doing *prāṇāyāma*, observe carefully and adjust the five elements with *vāyu*.

Table n. 14 - Interaction of the *anyonya bhūta, kośa, prāṇa, krama anyonya kriyā* (Interaction of the five elements with the *kośa* and *prāṇa*)

pañcamahābhūta **(5 elements)**	***pañcakośa*** **(5 sheaths)**	***pañcavāyu*** **(5 vital airs)**
Pṛthvī (earth)	*Annamaya kośa* (anatomical body)	*Apāna*
Āp (water)	*Prāṇamaya kośa* (physiological body)	*Prāṇa*
Tej (fire)	*Manomaya kośa* (psychological body)	*Samāna*
Vāyu (air)	*Vijñānamaya kośa* (intellectual body)	*Udāna*
Ākāśa (ether)	*Ānandamaya kośa* (causal body)	*Vyāna*

In *pūraka* (inhalation), *apāna (pṛthvī-tattva),* with the help of *samāna (tejas-tattva),* acts as a base for *viśva caitanya śakti* to move in and up so that *prāṇa (āp-tattva)* can be accepted and received, while *udāna (vāyu-tattva)* fans the energy that is received by the body and *vyāna (ākāśa-tattva)* spreads it. This means that *pūraka* is complete. In *pūraka, puruṣa* evolves through *vāyu* towards the *prakṛti* covering the five *bhūta* and merges with the *prakṛti.*

In *recaka* (exhalation), *samāna vāyu (tejas-tattva)* is quietened, *udāna (vāyu-tattva),* with the help of the *apāna vāyu (pṛthvī),* upholds and converts the *viśva caitanya śakti* into *vaiyaktika śakti,* and *vyāna vāyu* controls and releases *prāṇa (āp-tattva)* till it reaches the inner space *(ākāśa-tattva).* Thus the passivity and quietness are felt in all the five *kośa.* The five *vāyu* get stabilised. In *recaka, prakṛti* moves through *vāyu* towards the *puruṣa* and merges in the *puruṣa.*

ESSENCE OF *PRĀṆĀYĀMA*

Thus, *prāṇāyāma* is to regulate through intelligence *(prajñā)* the flow of life giving energy *(prāṇa).* Through *pūraka, viśva caitanya śakti* is absorbed, along with *viśva prajñā śakti.* This nourishes and enriches both *prāṇa* and *prajñā* within. These two are already existing in a very subtle and radical state. The *prāṇa* is charged with *viśva caitanya śakti* and *prajñā* of *citta* is charged with *viśva prajñā śakti.* The *viśva caitanya śakti* is converted to *vaiyaktika śakti* and *viśva prajñā śakti* is converted to individual *prajñā.* Through the technique of *prāṇāyāma,* the dykes are created within the body for *viśva caitanya śakti* to have its harmonious flow and distribution as *prāṇa* and for *viśva prajñā śakti* to have its harmonious pervasion as *prajñā.*

In *prāṇāyāmic* inhalation it is not only the length or the breadth of the breath and chest that are important, but the communication and communion of *viśva caitanya śakti* with the causal body, subtle body and gross body *(kāraṇa, sūkṣma* and *kārya śarīra* respectively*).* When *viśva caitanya śakti* enters the inner body, a latent *śakti* of the same nature, which is lying in the body, arises and awakens to receive the incoming *śakti,* making the *viśva caitanya śakti* spread in order to touch all the frontiers of the trunk up to the skin. When the skin feels the touch, that means the *viśva caitanya śakti* has reached its zenith in inhalation. In *prāṇayamic* exhalation, the *viśva caitanya śakti* manifests into *vaiyaktika śakti* (individual energy) and releases the breath as exhalation from the gross body towards the subtle body and from the subtle body towards the causal body. From here, it proceeds further and loses its manifested form into unmanifested form (the *prajñā puruṣa).* This state conveys the end of *recaka* (exhalation).

TRACING THE ORIGIN OF BREATHING PROCESS

In *prāṇāyāma,* before we begin *pūraka* (inhalation) we make our lungs and brain passive by releasing residual breath through *recaka* (exhalation). The reason for passive release of inner residual breath is to make the awareness in *prajñā* to reach the element of ether. This feeling brings a state of passive silence and emptiness *(śūnya)* in the lungs as well as in the intelligence of the brain. At the same time passive alertness *(aśūnya)* is experienced in the seat of the *puruṣa* (the intelligence of the heart). At this moment *śūnya* and *aśūnya* mingle together where all five *bhūta* and five *vāyu* come closer to each other like the petals of the lotus, which close when the sun sets, and open at sunrise. This state of poise creates dykes at the gates of *pūraka* to allow the energy of atmospheric air to come into the system without hardening the body or creating harshness in the sound *(nāda)* of the breath.

ART OF INHALATION

After the exhalation of residual breath, in *pūraka* we observe sensitively how this *viśva caitanya śakti* comes in contact with *vaiyaktika puruṣa* (individual self) through the element of ether (space, *citta),* air (touch, intelligence), fire (form, mind), water (balance of fluidity) and earth (fullness and firmness). Here, *pūraka* first communicates with the individual self and then follows *citta, ahaṁkāra, buddhi, manas, jñānendriya* and *karmendriya.* With the touch of the inner space *(ākāśa)*, *pūraka* comes in contact with the *sūkṣma śarīra* consisting of *citta, ahaṁkāra, buddhi* and *manas (vāyu* and *tejas)* through extension. Then it begins to expand *(āp-tattva)* and extend to encase the *kārya-śarīra* or the *annamaya kośa*, the anatomical body *(pṛthvī-tattva)* (Table n. 4). When the latent inner *śakti* and *viśva caitanya śakti* unite and lose their identities, *pūraka* is complete. All the elements in the body become dynamically active.

ART OF EXHALATION

Before exhalation *(recaka)* begins, the drawn-in energy changes into individual energy *(vaiyaktika śakti)*. The dykes are built up at the top of the cheekbones in the reverse order to that of inhalation *(pūraka)*.

In the process of *recaka*, the *vaiyaktika śakti* which is in contact with the *prajñā puruṣa* is allowed to recede from the element of earth (gross body) towards the element of ether (causal body) via the elements of water, fire and air (subtle body). Then the energy which may be still remaining inside unknowingly is further made to move, so that the *sādhaka* feels the spark of the *puruṣa*.

In *pūraka*, the *śakti*, first as an abstract, touches the subtlest element ether and ends with the gross element – the earth – and becomes concrete. In *recaka*, the same "concrete" *śakti* releases from the gross element *(pṛthvī-tattva)* and moves towards the subtle element *(ākāśa-tattva)* and transforms into the abstract.

Vyāna vāyu maintains the hold on the other elements to receive and release the *śakti*, both in *pūraka* and *recaka*, with smoothness. In *pūraka*, all elements expand on the path of evolution along with the *puruṣa*, and in *recaka* they recede to reach a state of passivity on the path of involution and merge with the *puruṣa* within.

In *pūraka*, *vaiyaktika puruṣa* (individual self) is exposed and expanded to unite with *mahadākāśa* which is outside the body. In *recaka*, *prajñā puruṣa* (individual *prajñā*) recedes to unite with *hṛdayākāśa* or *cidākāśa*, which is within the body.

At the end of *pūraka* but before *recaka* and at the end of *recaka* but before *pūraka*, one feels wholeness *(pūrṇatā)*. This *pūrṇatā* is nothing but the spark of divinity. These sparks of divinity evolve in *pūraka* and involve in *recaka*, yet never diminish.

Table n. 15 – Evolution *(pravṛtti)* and involution *(nivṛtti)* of energy in inhalation and exhalation

PŪRAKA* – INHALATION** ***Pravṛtti mārga	***RECAKA* – EXHALATION** ***Nivṛtti mārga***
Viśva caitanya śakti becomes *vaiyaktika śakti*	*Vaiyaktika śakti* becomes *viśva caitanya śakti*
Abstract becomes concrete	Concrete becomes abstract
Cosmic energy unites with the individual energy	Individual energy unites with the cosmic energy
Puruṣa towards *prakṛti*	*Prakṛti* towards *puruṣa*
Ether to earth	Earth to ether
Takes towards *mahadākāśa*	Takes towards *hṛdayākāśa* or *cidākāśa*

ART OF *KUṀBHAKA*

Caution

Before going into the art of *kuṁbhaka* let me give you a hint not to do *kuṁbhaka* before getting well established in *pūraka* and *recaka*. See that no jerks or disturbances are created in the inner elements of the body while doing *prāṇāyāma*. Measure and maintain an even balance between activity and passivity and mobility and rigidity. The moment disturbances are felt, turbulence takes place in the *viśva caitanya śakti* shaking the poise not only in the five *vāyu* but also in the five sheaths of the body bringing exhaustion, shakiness and fear.

Kuṁbhaka is commonly known as retention of breath or maintaining a pause between *pūraka* and *recaka* as well as *recaka* and *pūraka*. The void or space between these two is *kuṁbhaka*. But the real meaning of the practice of *kuṁbhaka* is the process of holding and prolonging the sparks of divinity that flash after *pūraka* and *recaka* with steadiness and calmness. Thus, the performance of *kuṁbhaka* is an art.

TYPES OF *KUṀBHAKA*

Kuṁbhaka is of two types, *antara kuṁbhaka* (retention after *pūraka*) and *bāhya kuṁbhaka* (retention after *recaka*). Again, they have deliberate and non-deliberate qualities[1].

[1] For details, see the Author's *Light on Prāṇāyāma*, Harper Collins, London.

Antara kuṁbhaka is inhalation-retention, where *udāna* and *samāna* support the drawn-in *śakti* with the help of *apāna* to uphold with *prajñā*, while *vyāna* lifts and sustains it. In this *kuṁbhaka*, *prakṛti* and *puruṣa* are kept dynamically tranquil as a single unit being actors and witnesses at the same time.

Bāhya kuṁbhaka is exhalation-retention, where *prāṇa* releases, *udāna* upholds, *vyāna* sustains, *samāna* appeases and *apāna* supports so that all the five elements and the five sheaths of the body *(prakṛti)* come close to each other to involute quietly towards the *puruṣa*, experiencing a passive state of tranquillity.

Table n. 16 – *Kṛti krama* in *prāṇāyāma*

FUNCTIONS OF *PRĀṆA* AND *BHŪTA* IN *PRĀṆĀYĀMA*					
Pañca-Mahābhūta (5 elements)	*Pañca vāyu*	*Pūraka* (Inhalation)	*Antara Kuṁbhaka* (Inhalation Retention)	*Recaka* (Exhalation)	*Bāhya Kuṁbhaka* (Exhalation retention)
Pṛthvī (earth)	*Apāna*	base	helps *vyāna/samāna*	helps *vyāna*	upholds/ supports
Āp (water)	*Prāṇa*	receptacle	upholds	passive	comes close to *apāna*
Tej (fire)	*Samāna*	movement to help *apāna*	supports the drawn energy	quietens/ pacifies	appeases
Vāyu (air)	*Udāna*	spreads/ extends	grips/sustains	controls/ releases	sustains
Ākāśa (ether)	*Vyāna*	ends	extends and distributes the drawn energy	upholds/ converts	contracts space and upholds nature to be close to *puruṣa*

While doing *prāṇāyāma*, if the element of earth gets disturbed, then tremors in the nerves are felt and *prāṇa vāyu* is drawn fast; if the brain and eyes are strained, it means the fire element is aggressively used or *samāna vāyu* is over activated. In that case, you have to learn to use the *udāna vāyu* that tries to maintain the other elements in order to remain steady.

In *prāṇāyāma*, the contact or touch of energy *(prāṇa sparśa)* is felt by the touch of intelligence *(buddhi sparśa)*, through the element of air. Vibrations in *prāṇāyāma* (*śabda sparśa* or sound of breath) are felt through the element of ether. These two elements play major roles in learning *prāṇāyāma* with accuracy. The shaping of the breath in the body is looked after by the element of fire and the levelling of energy is adjusted by the element of water. The element of earth throughout remains stable. In this way, the *bhūta* and the *vāyu* act in unison in *prāṇāyāma*.

KARMA, JÑĀNA AND *BHAKTI* IN *PRĀṆĀYĀMA*

As we use matter *(bhūta)* for action *(karma)*, energy for knowledge *(jñāna)* and live in the sparks of divinity to use the *saṁprajñā* (auspicious awareness) for *bhakti*, *prāṇāyāma* becomes the source for *karma*, *jñāna* and *bhakti*.

The art of sitting, the cultivation of dykes, the usage of body and the adjustment of *pañca bhūta*, *pañca tanmātra* and *pañca vāyu* make us understand *karma*. *Pūraka* and *antara kuṁbhaka* develop *jñāna*. *Recaka* and *bāhya kuṁbhaka* lead us towards *bhakti*.

See that the *viśva caitanya śakti* moves in and out like the smooth flow of oil from one vessel to another. Body is the vessel. *Pūraka* – *recaka* is the oil. The holder (or owner) of the vessel is the *puruṣa*. The oil, the vessel and the holder of the vessel should move in unison according to the needed adjustments. This is the secret of mastering *prāṇāyāma*.

The practice of *prāṇāyāma* is a *homa kuṇḍa* (sacrificial altar). The *prāṇa* kindles awareness in *buddhi* and *citta* to experience the *puruṣa* as *prajñā puruṣa*, not as an object to be known but to live in it as a subject. Finally the *prajñā puruṣa* is surrendered to the Supreme God. This is a journey from matter to consciousness and from consciousness towards God, and the vehicle that takes us from the nadir of life to the zenith of uniting with God is *prāṇa*. Hence the importance of *prāṇāyāma*.

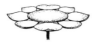

ŚAVĀSANA: THE GLIMPSES OF THE STATE BETWEEN *JAGRATĀVASTHĀ* AND *TURYĀVASTHĀ* *

Our society seems to rest upon sedatives and tranquillisers. We adopt a "reach-for-that-pill" attitude towards almost every problem of life. The tempo of modern life is such that its maintenance makes the taking of sedatives imperative for most people. As the giddy pace increases, tensions build up in our systems, our nerves get frayed, and haggard remnants of humanity are left to seek solace in some form of drugged sleep.

This is strange, for modern men have all the leisure at their disposal. Machines have taken the drudgery out of life and the forty-hour week gives men enough time to relax. The art of relaxation, however, eludes modern man; it seems to be something past and beyond recall.

Relaxation is necessary, for it is recuperation. The draining of energy has to be counteracted in some way. The yogic art of relaxation known as *Śavāsana* puts down in precise steps how relaxation and recuperation take place. *Śava* means a corpse, a dead body. *Āsana* means a posture. *Śavāsana* is thus the posture of emulating the dead and out of apparent death comes life. (Plate n. 3)

Śavāsana is not simply lying on one's back with a vacant gaze or flopping on a foam rubber mattress. Nor should it end in snoring. It is by far the most difficult of yogic postures, but it is also by far the most rewarding and refreshing one. It is a very precise method of disciplining both the body and the mind.

TECHNIQUE

Śavāsana begins with placing the body accurately on the floor. An even place has to be chosen for this, that is clean, free of insects, loud noises and noxious smells. Spread a blanket or rug on the floor so that the body can lie full length on it. These precautions are necessary because a cold or an unclean floor can disturb the depth of relaxation.

---

* *The art of relaxation*, first printed in *Bhavan's Journal*. October 20th, 1968.

Sit on the blanket with the knees drawn up and the feet together, so that a straight line can be drawn from the place where the heels, the big toes and the knees meet, along the anal mouth, the navel, the sternum (breast-bone), the throat, the chin, the bridge of the nose to the centre of the forehead. Then gradually stretch one leg forward after the other so that both legs lie on the straight line in the median plane. Rest the buttocks evenly on the floor to either side of the anal mouth. If one buttock feels broader, place the hands on the floor to either side of the hips and lift the buttocks off the floor and adjust them. With palms on either side of the hips, slowly slide them downwards and sideways to rest on the floor so that they lie evenly on either side of the coccyx and the anal mouth. Then turn the palms towards the ceiling and take the arms sideways to rest well on the elbows.

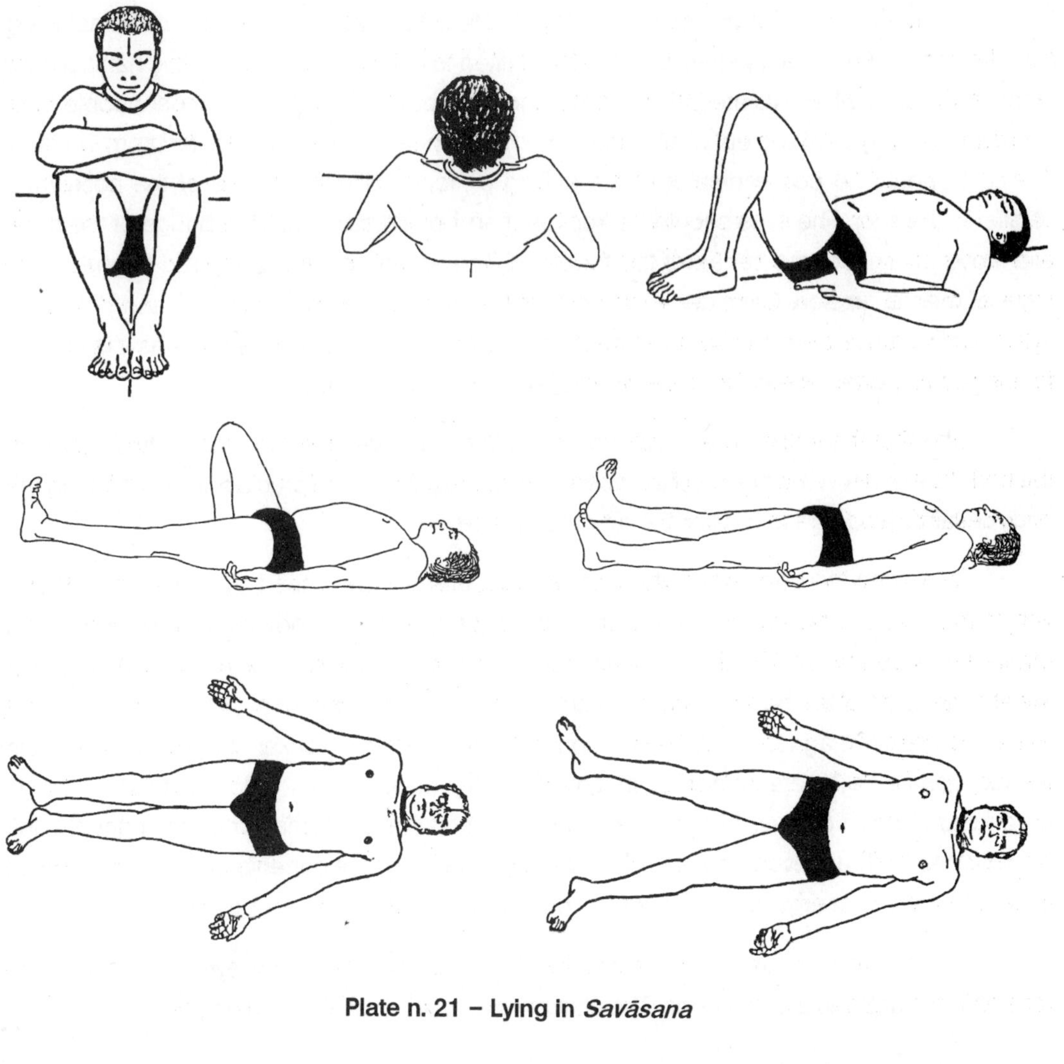

Plate n. 21 – Lying in *Savāsana*

Make the spine convex and lower the body, vertebra by vertebra, to the floor so that the entire spine rests on the floor equally and does not tilt to one side or the other. The bottom points of the shoulder blades, like the buttocks and the hips, should rest evenly on the floor to either side of the spine.

Once the spine is placed on the floor, bend the arms and touch the shoulders with the fingers. From this position, gently extend the back of the upper arms towards the elbows on the floor so that the back of the arm rests and elongates evenly. Afterwards lower the hands to the floor to rest the palms, but facing upwards. Keep the median plane of the wrists resting on the floor. The arms and hands should form angles of not more than fifteen degrees from the sides of the body.

Unlike the rest of the body, which is adjusted from the back, the head should be adjusted from the front. Babies usually sleep with the head tilted to one side. Because of this habit, a dent forms in the skull when we are babies, and hence, the back of the head in most people gets misshapen and its centre is out of alignment. Hence the head should be adjusted from the face. The chin should be perpendicular to the ceiling or floor, while the bridge of the nose runs parallel to the floor. The eyes should be kept shut and equidistant from the bridge of the nose and move away from the centre of the forehead. The squint and the puckered forehead are signs of mental tension. Consider each pore of the skin as a "conscious eye" and delicately adjust and balance the body from within with the help of these conscious eyes, as it is difficult for the normal, external eyes to observe and rectify the body position.

See that the entire body is placed on the floor with precision so that the two halves of the body lie evenly on either side of the spine. Attention to detail and precision in positioning the body certainly lead one to master the art of relaxation.

Very often the body tilts to its stronger side; this is experienced by many. This tilt may vary from person to person; in some people the right side of the body may tilt while in some others it may be the left. The tilt is experienced as a sort of magnetic pull of the earth towards the stronger side of the body. Once the practitioner knows the dominant side of the body, that exerts the greater magnetic pull, he can consciously adjust the weaker side of his body from the very start by deliberately placing it in a more intelligent way on to the floor. In this way the tilt is obviated. If the tilt occurs, there is a drain of energy on the tilted side. When the right and left halves of the body are evenly balanced, the positive and negative currents of the body are held in equilibrium, the energy is kept within the body resulting in quick recuperation.

A load on any corner, in the middle side or anywhere on the eyebrow may cause tension in the brain as a concussion. The chin on one side brings the load on the eyebrow. If the magnetism is at the centre of the eyebrow, the intelligence is very strong, so extend it to the side. Keep the crown of the head parallel to the wall. With the spinal column touching the ground, move the skin sideways from the centre of the spine, so that the spinal column remains in the centre. The extreme ends of the heels remain above the ground and the flesh between the ankles and the heels remains well extended. Here the feet relax better.

The bottom of the sternum goes down in *Śavāsana*. Alert the sternum from empty space so that both edges of the sternum are level. By this adjustment you will not go to sleep but remain alert and attentive. If the top and the bottom of the sternum are lifted properly the intellect descends; otherwise the intellect ascends and the self descends; the intellect bumps and the frontal brain becomes active. Alert the sternum bone without disturbing the back spine from the ground. Extend the back of the skull towards the crown of the head, and the frontal brain relaxes. Mentally measure the distance from the corner of the left eye and from the corner of the right eye to the ground. If one is above and the other below, there is no *samasthiti* of intelligence. The intelligence reamins active on the side of the corner that is above. Drop the skin there. The intelligence settles by itself.

CONTROL OF THE SENSES

The next step in *Śavāsana* is the control of the senses and stilling their outward movement towards objects of desire. *Śavāsana* is a descending psychosomatic movement. It is a descent of the body and the mind deep inwards tracing the source of energy. *Śavāsana* is not a rigid state of stillness. No doubt it blocks out the external world, but know that the doer should not remain egotistical but humble. *Śavāsana*, properly performed, brings not a simple stillness but a divine silent state of stillness. It helps to surrender one's ego with the receptive awareness of divinity. For achieving this state, the brain cells have to "descend" passively. The brain cells will not experience this descending movement if the senses are not controlled and have not learnt to withdraw within themselves. Most of our senses of perception are located on the face and the entire struggle for control takes place on the face from the throat upwards, where the impressions gathered by the senses are experienced. *Śavāsana* is said to be complete if the breath, the eyes, the eardrums and the root of the tongue at the palate are all in a relaxed state yet under control. (Plate n. 22)

The beginner slowly begins to observe that not only do the senses of perception not stay quiet, but the eyelids flicker and the eyeballs move upwards. These are sure signs that the eyes are tense and that the brain is being disturbed by thought waves. The appearance of saliva in the mouth and the constant desire to swallow it are an indication of tension in the tongue. Hardness in the ears can also be experienced as tension around the temples. The beginner should consciously search out these tensions and, by knowing where they exist, learn to relax them.

DESIGN T HE CIRCUIT OF ENERGY

To descend and relax the senses delicately, elongate the back of the neck towards the crown of the head so that there is an upward movement of energy. This flow of energy is then to be directed downwards from the top of the head by descending the bridge of the nose so that the bridge is parallel to the ceiling and the floor. In elongating the back of the neck and descending the bridge of the nose care should be taken that a tense chin-lock does not result; so as to offset a tense chin-lock (where the chin would dig into the top of the breast bone), the beginner must learn to lift the chin gently upwards, so that the chin is at a right angle to the floor or ceiling. This ascending movement of the chin must balance the descending movement of the bridge of the nose. Then a sense of tensionlessness is felt in the throat *(viśuddhi cakra)* and lightness on the forehead *(lalāṭa cakra)*. When the bridge of the nose and the chin are held in equilibrium, the head and the brain feel light and the throat relaxed.

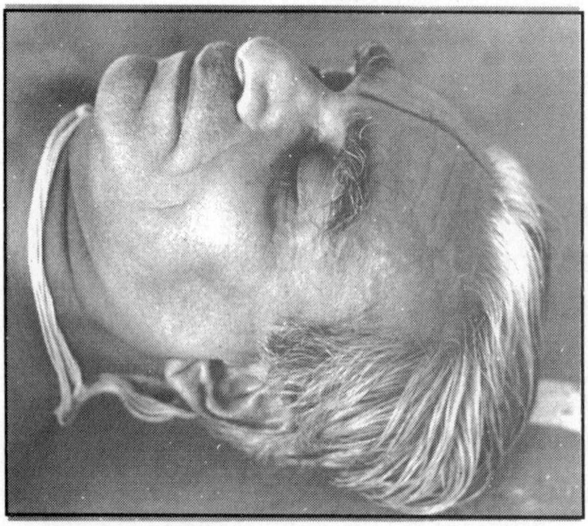

Plate n. 22 – The face in *Śavāsana*

In *Śavāsana* the energy flows in a circular motion over the back of the head, down the nose, towards the toes and then back to the crown of the head. In this way the circuit of energy is well designed and the flow of energy is kept within the body and the dissipation of energy and consequent exhaustion are avoided. This leads to faster recuperation and refreshment of body and consciousness.

Once the flow of energy is correctly directed, the pupils of the eyes must be made to passively descend towards the bottom of the breast bone or the seat of the mind, which is the centre of emotions *(manas cakra)* and above the solar plexus *(sūrya cakra)*. The eyeballs should shrink pleasantly inside the sockets. A shrunken eyeball is a relaxed eyeball. Bulging eyes reveal tension. The optical nerve must be drawn towards the centre of emotions, so that in the single "eye of awareness" of the soul, the physical eyes lose their identity. This "eye of awareness" of the soul is found in the *manas cakra*.

Descend the body energy from the throat in such a way as though the energy is being filtered through the *viśuddhi cakra,* the purifying wheel, at the base of the throat. The current should not move above the neck to the head. If it moves, you become active. You get lost in the ocean of thoughts wherein you are neither aware of the movements of the mind, nor aware of silence. The mental current flows without direction. In this situation descend the lower eyelids by bringing the upper eyelids down. Then the mental current along with the body energy is kept down and no vibration occurs in the intellectual centre. Stay in this state. This is true *brahmacarya. Brahma* means Self, *carya* means movement. To move towards *Brahma* is *brahmacarya.* Do not run away from the *ātman.* If intellect runs away from *ātman,* bring it back to the Self. Spread the skin on the forehead horizontally and descend it. First the self should move deep into the body, so that the appearance of the body becomes as subtle *(sūkṣma)* as the self. The 'eye of awareness' should move with the movement of the self; and at the same time do not waver the physical eyes. Otherwise, the wavering takes place in the intellectual eye, and you will be far away from the self.

EARS

The ears should be kept relaxed and the throb of nerves at the temples must also cease. The auricular, the auditory nerve and the skin of the temples must be drawn towards the centre of emotions. This joint movement of the eyes and ears is felt as a quiet and cool movement downwards, which is infinitely relaxing.

SKIN

The facial skin is a sensitive gauge of relaxation. It should be made to descend towards the centre of emotions. At the same time the facial skin should be adjusted as if it is separate from the flesh that is below the skin. The two sides of the palate at the uvula should passively come together. Then there is shrinkage and dryness in the mouth, especially at the uvula and the tongue, and relaxation is experienced.

Each pore of the skin of the chest should send the message to the brain as to whether it has opened or not. Keep the back of the head completely quiet and able to receive. When the attention drifts away from observation, come back. The brain should be thoroughly mingled in breath with one pointed attention. The top portion of the collarbone should be up but the eyes should not move up. The eyes have to penetrate the lungs. Do not allow the eyes to go up or to go outside the brain. To live totally with the body is to live totally with the Self. Often we do not live totally with the body, our sensitivity to existence does not penetrate even skin-deep. When one feels total presence and total existence one is with the self.

Do not inflate the root of the tongue. Then only you can peep in. All *jñānendriya* should be alert to peep in with an extraordinary alertness. With what curiosity we see a thing which we have never seen before, so see within with that same curiosity. Penetrate with that curiosity and not with a mechanical approach. Watch the new awakening coming in the body. The body, the senses and the mind should be supersensitive to feel this new awakening.

RECAKA TO SURRENDER THE EGO

The control of breath is necessary and rhythmic breathing at the beginning helps towards good relaxation. Inhalation *(pūraka)* should not be deep, but should be of normal duration. Exhalation *(recaka)*, however, should be with a soft smooth flow and of longer duration than inhalation. During *pūraka* as well as *recaka*, the brain cells are made to descend towards the centre of emotions. This downward movement is more difficult in *pūraka* than in *recaka*. For about three-fourths of the duration of inhalation, one can experience the descent of the brain cells, but at the last quarter the brain cells start slightly moving upwards on their own. Watch and avoid this upward movement. *Pūraka* reflects the dominance of the ego, while *recaka* denotes surrender of one's ego to the divinity within us. *Recaka* empties the brain and the ego. Surrender of the ego is accelerated in *recaka*.

"ECHO EXHALATION"

After a period of time there occurs, by slow and smooth exhalation, what might be described as "echo exhalation". This is a fine and subtle exhalation and may be likened to the exquisitely pure and delicate top notes of a string instrument in the hands of a master musician that seems to echo back gently from nowhere. This "echo exhalation" empties the brain completely and results in withdrawal of the nerves and senses within oneself. Conscious and deliberate surrender of the ego is hard to achieve. That is why the texts of yoga recommend thinking upon the name of the Lord whilst practising *prāṇāyāma*. The practitioner then feels that the source of all energy is entering within himself with each inbreath, and while he is exhaling, surrenders to the Lord through his very life-breath, the self within. Then one experiences purity in thoughts, feelings and desires.

MOVEMENT OF EYES, BRAIN AND INTELLIGENCE

However, as soon as the intellect moves towards the brain, bring that intellectual energy towards the heart without disturbing the attentive passive state of the body. The thinker should move to the centre of the mind. Intelligence and self should both involute towards the Self. Movement of consciousness is movement of life. *Manomaya kośa* and *vijñānamaya kośa* should not waver. They should be silent. Nothing should disturb your breath. Doing normal breathing, remain in a state of passivity in body, mind, intelligence, ego and consciousness.

When the eyes move up, the current of intelligence also moves up. You are living in your brain if the lids of the eyes feel heavy. Watch your brain without opening your eyes. Bring the intelligence back to its original position for a tranquil state. Motion and motionlessness go hand in hand and the senses follow that which is stronger. The act of drawing the intelligence towards the Self and of consciousness holding on to the Self is *dharma*. The life in the eye should not move to one side. If the eyes are away from each other, the flow of intelligence stagnates. The eyes therefore have to be withdrawn from the centre of the nose, the ears and tongue, so they spread horizontally. This creates the feeling of non-existence of the eyes as space will be created behind them. Without tracing this space at the back of the eyes, one cannot release the other senses.

Thoughtless bumping of the intellect is a movement. So discipline it so that it does not bump. Stop it consciously. Touch the seat of the Self in each *pūraka* and *recaka* without allowing the mind to waver. Whether in *pūraka* or *recaka*, always keep your attention on the core.

Learn to remain intellectually silent, without allowing any fluctuation to take place in the brain. Then it is real relaxation and recuperation. As soon as the fluctuations come, let loose and relax the nerves immediately. This is neuro-psychology.

Be a watch dog to your own self. Do not think that the intellect should be supreme. Deliberately train the ears, facial muscles, membranes and the tongue to be without fluctuations. Drop the eyebrows to the eyes, then there will be no intellectual fluctuations. As soon as the distance between the eyebrows and the eyes increases, there is a fluctuation. The 'I'-ness and the intelligence move from position to position. The mind being the eleventh sense, let us stop its movements, moment to moment and enter into the twelfth sense, the intelligence, and then the thirteenth sense, 'I'-ness. Do not create any vibrations. Even the thinking of the self itself creates movement. Just the word "think" creates movement. Thought being negative, and thinking being positive, both should be made not to act at all. Not only does the negative become completely negative, but the positive too becomes negative. This is the beginning of spiritual discipline.

SAHAJĀVASTHĀ AND MENTAL *PRĀṆĀYĀMA*

Dullness and leaning on the side of the brain indicates that you cannot find that *sahajāvasthā* – the natural state of equanimity. Empty the brain along with the exhalation and see that it merges into passivity. This stops the brain from leaning on one side. When the brain is passive and centred, there is a suspension of breath, which leads towards *sahajāvasthā*. This state may not prolong itself chronologically, so do not try to grip it psychologically. Turn your mind to the breath. Do the *pūraka* and *recaka* mentally, and not physically. The nostrils should not feel the warmth of *recaka* from a forceful breath. When the air is released from the brain softly, the brain becomes empty. That is mental *prāṇāyāma*.

DEEP BREATH AND *SAHAJA KUṀBHAKA*

In a good *Śavāsana* the body rejects deep breathing. However, when you are disturbed mentally and emotionally, when you are weak and morose you need to have the support of deep, soft and gentle breathing. If you do deep and sharp breathing in *Śavāsana* then it makes you feel at times as though you are frozen. Start slowly, thoroughly, completely, doing *recaka* and *pūraka*. After complete *pūraka*, you need not do *kuṁbhaka* purposely or intentionally, but observe the small pause following *pūraka*. This is called *sahaja antara kuṁbhaka*, in which the body gets adjusted, and a certain type of biochemical change takes place. The longer the *pūraka*, the firmer will be the mind. You shed your laziness, no more do you feel weak or morose. You are free from fear, you become courageous and gain self-confidence. You develop a positive attitude. But when you are mentally and emotionally disturbed and find yourself unsteady do not do longer *recaka*. Otherwise the diaphragm becomes hard and you lose the firmness of mind.

Do slow *recaka*. In *recaka*, there is no support for the mind to imprint on the self. The slow, thorough *recaka* is the way of purging the brain and the mind. Purging the mind is a supreme movement by which to live in the Self. In *recaka*, as you are mentally quiet, you experience a state of non-being. This is the *sākṣātkāra* of *jivātma*. After the end of *recaka* and in the beginning of *pūraka*, there is a small pause. This pause is a passive *sahaja bāhya kuṁbhaka*. It appears as a physical meditation, but when you progress mentally and intellectually to peep inside the body, it transforms into spiritual meditation. With quiet normal *recaka* and passive *sahaja bāhya kuṁbhaka*, find out how the brain and mind get quietened. Observe the purity of yourself after *recaka*. Extend that pause. Elongate it; spread it; not with the intelligence, but with the self. Build that purity at the end of *recaka*, so that *jivātmā* is free from contact and touches the feet of *paramātmā*.

A WELL-PERFORMED *ŚAVĀSANA*

The Self is pure consciousness, free from thoughts, feelings and desires. The mind is the vehicle of consciousness. When the intellectual centre is active, the mind reveals itself as intelligence. When the brain is perfectly quiet and the intellectual centre is stilled, the mind appears as the self in the centre of emotions. Here one is gathered up and yet suspended, empty yet perfectly satisfied, serenely balanced, neither free nor bound. This is stillness in pure awareness. The awareness of 'I' is transmuted into the awareness of the Creator. There is emotional stability and mental humility.

There are several signs of a well-performed *Śavāsana*. A few indications may help the beginner to test the depth of his relaxation. Yoga is not an intellectual game. It is a sharing of real experience. In a good *Śavāsana* there is a feeling of shrinkage of skin and muscles, for *Śavāsana* is after all a movement of inward withdrawal. At the same time there is a feeling of elongation of the limbs and the body. Sometimes, this elongation is experienced as a twitch of the nerves. A pleasant feeling of heaviness and constriction is experienced through the whole body, especially in the upper arms just above the elbows and in the calves below the knees. At these four places one can experience the beating of the pulse. The balance of the body can be tested by watching the evenness of the pulse at these places. Dryness is felt in the bones and the joints. A feeling of being suspended on a thin line of awareness is also present.

The best sign of a good *Śavāsana* is a feeling of deep mental peace and pure bliss. *Śavāsana* is alert surrender of the ego. In forgetting oneself, one discovers oneself.

DISTURBANCES OR OBSTACLES IN *ŚAVĀSANA*

Any movement of thought creates a kind of hardness on the face. Movements come deliberately creating vibrations that make the brain expand. Activity and a load on the brain bring emotional fluctuations. This leads to hypertension and cardiac attacks. Deliberately see that no vibrations go beyond your throat to *sahasrāra*. This tautens the face and brain and hardens the nerves. Psychologically the body commences from the throat and moves towards the crown of the head *(sahasrāra cakra)* and you get disturbed.

SATKARMA

Treat thought movement as a movement of the consciousness. Unless it is quietened, the gate of the *Brahman* will not open. Release the skin at the centre of the *lalāṭa cakra*. Bring the *ajñā* to *anāhata*. *Anāhata* is a seat for *bhakti*, the abode of the Lord. He is in the centre of the chest. Like a *bhaktan,* devote yourself on that centre, allowing the senses of perception *(jñānendriya)*, mind, intelligence and 'I' to descend to the centre of the chest. Remain silent and feel the Lord resting in your Self.

Body, mind and intelligence should be silent without the wavering eyes. The life force of the eyes should not go away from the mind and senses. Learn to remain without movement. As intelligence is still, there is no *karma*, so you are free from *kleśa*. If intelligence is quiet, no *karma* is generated. The *karma* going towards the Self is pure *karma (satkarma)*. Keeping the intellect away from residual action brings *akleśa*. If you react to action, it brings *kleśa*.

MIND, CONSCIOUSNESS

Check the mind through the mind. But the mind, due to lack of discriminative power, has no power to know the mistakes of itself. Therefore check the mind through the intelligence and consciousness.

The mind is a sheath to the self. As long as the brain is not silent, the mind remains insignificant. The sheath cannot be opened – so the Self cannot be visualised.

As the snake charmer tames the snake by tapping its hood as soon as it is raised, similarly, when the mind and consciousness raises its hood, tap it with your superconsciousness that is hidden within you, so that it does not raise the hood but goes towards steadiness and silence.

Whenever the hardness in the body or mind is felt, learn to let go the hardness immediately. This empties the consciousness, so the self remains as a witness. Feel each inhalation consciously but do not feed the mind or consciousness to raise its hood.

Continue the intensity of descending the consciousness in *recaka*. Consciously bring the mind to the state of silence. If the breath is strong, it touches the extreme ends of the nostrils, and consciousness becomes rigid. If the breath touches the empty space of the nostrils, the consciousness gets pacified. So work deliberately to see that the air moves only from the empty space of the nose which is known as *ākāśa-tattva*. Leave off *pṛthvī, āp, tej, vāyu*, which have frontiers. *Ākāśa* has no frontier. The middle portion of the nostril is *ākāśa*. In inhalation, if the air does not touch the frontier, you lose your identity and you are in *ākāśa-tattva*. You are one with the Lord. Chronologically living in that state, psychologically bring the consciousness to that state of stability. When this state of stability is prolonged without feeling the bondage of time, the state of *dhyāna* and *samādhi* is sensed, felt and experienced. When the sense of time is lost in that pure state of *Śavāsana* (Plate n. 3) your existence without taints becomes pure. Such *Śavāsana* brings a glimpse of *samādhi.*

According to *Yoga Upaniṣad,* twelve seconds of *dhāraṇā* is one second of *dhyāna* and twelve seconds of *dhyāna* is one second of *samādhi*[1]. That is how it is explained. The moment there is fluctuation *dhyāna* is interrupted. A single thought wave *(ekāgra)* is necessary, otherwise *dhyāna* is broken. This indicates to what extent past yogis stressed the conquest of chronological time.

PURṆATĀ IN *ŚAVĀSANA*

Experience of *pūrṇatā* in *Śavāsana* is essential. *Pūrṇatā* means fullness and wholeness and at the same time quietness. Bring down the senses to the seat of the heart and remain without the sense of existence, I or me. There should be no movement in the brain or nerves. When the intellectual current moves up, immediately bring that down by submissive will towards the heart. When one is silent in head and heart, the current flows in a subterranean level and thought does not arise nor are the organs disturbed. Remain silent and quiet without ruffles.

SĀTTVIC ASMITĀ

In *Śavāsana* one experiences freedom in imprisonment. The body and its movements as well as the mind and its movements are arrested. As the prisoner has freedom to move in a limited place within the prison bars, one has the freedom to penetrate the unlimited and unknown area within, which is fathomless. If your thoughts go out, you have broken the prison bars. In freedom, all the senses are cut off completely from currents of thought. It is a thoughtless state. In that state what is left is the grip of the internal self *(sāttvic asmitā).*

THE FOUR STAGES AND FOUR STATES IN *ŚAVĀSANA*

In *Śavāsana* one undergoes four stages and also experiences four states. In *ārambhāvasthā* of *Śavāsana,* as the body and the mind begin to relax, sleep is inevitable. As relaxation commences in *Śavāsana,* many go to sleep. This is the state of *suṣupti.*

In *ghaṭāvasthā,* one relaxes the physiological or organic body. The consciousness *(citta)* remains closer to the organic body. It is a state where one is neither sleepy nor wakeful. This is *svapnāvasthā.*

---

[1] This kind of explanation on conquering chronological time is found in *Skanda-Purāṇa* and *Yogacintāmaṇi Upaniṣad.*

Gradually, one comes to the wakeful state from the sleepy or dreamy state. One learns to recede the energy from the periphery towards the deep interior body. In this *paricayāvasthā* the intelligence observes the receding flow of energy. This is *jagratāvasthā*.

Finally one transcends even this wakeful state. *Citta* dissolves into the source and experiences quietitude. In this *niṣpattyāvasthā* one gets the glimpse of *turiyāvasthā*. One experiences freedom from bondage.

COMING OUT OF *ŚAVĀSANA*

Think of the Lord, feel his presence and surrender yourself to Him. While coming back to the wakeful state from *Śavāsana*, watch how the consciousness comes from passivity to activity. Open the eyes gently: watch everything from inside. Listen to what the body says to the brain, whether it is in a state of restlessness or restfulness. Observe how the brain reacts. These observations are nothing but *svādhyāya*. Find out what brain says to brain and body to body.

After *Śavāsana*, to come back to the conscious state, do not create movement to bring the mind to the surface but allow it to go towards the depthless place within. Remain in this *pūrṇa* (fullness) state. The external light should not disturb your eyes and brain. Watch the space between two thoughts. The mind does not want to accept any thought.

You have to watch those changes taking place within you. Be as though you are blind and pray for the Lord's grace. Feel the grace falling on you. Then turn the whole body to the side and remain there while the brain is cool. When the brain becomes warm, move to the other side and allow the other part of the brain to experience that coolness. Do not get up suddenly, but after a while.

This is *Śavāsana*.

ŚUDDHI SĀMYATĀ[*]

ILLUMINED *BUDDHI* AND LUMINOUS *ĀTMAN*

YOGA – THE *GURU*

First let me salute my *guru*, on this *gurupūrṇimā* day. Yoga is my *guru*. The *guru* I adore is yoga. As yoga is guiding my life, it is my *guru* and I salute that *guru*. It is yoga alone that has enticed me and I have stuck to it since 1934, the year I was introduced to its practice, and I would like to continue its practice as long as my consciousness *(citta)* maintains its awareness. Yoga has bound me to my present life and I am yoked to yoga by yoga.

I am grateful to all of you, who have an equal share in yoking me to yoga. It is your demand that made me penetrate yoga in its depth further and further.

All pupils who come to me are not in the same physical and mental category. All do not partake of the same frame of mind. Some are arrogant, some very intellectual, some dull, some stupid and some lazy. I have come across students who are of various or multiple states of mind. Some do not adhere to the same state always, but show different expressions and different moods. As a teacher, it is very hard for me quickly to uplift students from lower categories to higher ones, from a low state of mind to a high state of mind, from an uncultured state to a cultured state.

Just now you heard the prayer:

Gururbrahmā gururviṣṇu gururdevo maheśvaraḥ /

Guru sākṣāt para brahma tasmai śri gurave namaḥ //

Guru is Brahmā, the creator. *Guru* is Vishnu, the protector. *Guru* is Maheśvara, the destroyer. Let us salute the *guru* who represents all the three Gods. Why is a *guru* compared to this trinity? It is because he plays three roles while teaching and treating the *śiṣya*.

---

[*] Gurujī's message on *Gurupūrṇimā,* July 14, 1992.

The *guru* generates power and intelligence – so he is a creator (Brahmā). The *guru* keeps the pupil alert to maintain and sustain interest in the subject – so he is a protector (Vishnu). The *guru* destroys the quality of intoxicated intelligence, inflated ego and arrogance in his pupils – so he is a destroyer (Maheśvara).

The *guru* continuously guides the pupils without break. He tries to transform the *tāmasic* pupil to become *rājasic* and a *rājasic* pupil to become *sāttvic*. Like the Creator (Brahmā), the *guru* uplifts the *tāmasic*, dull and uninterested pupils to attain a *rājasic* nature. As a maintainer, he protects the good and auspicious qualities that have been achieved by the pupils, so that their interest may grow further. As a destroyer, he destroys the unwanted, harmful qualities of the pupils and makes them pave the path of practice from a *rājasic* to a *sāttvic* pure nature. *Guru,* as a destroyer, destroys the ego and transforms the *ahaṁkāra* into *asmitā,* the auspicious state of *ahaṁkāra*. This auspiciousness of 'I' leads towards enlightenment. This way the *guru* plays the role of the Trinity as he sets the lamp of enlightenment in his pupils.

This day is also known as *Vyāsa pūrṇimā*. Without paying my respects to *Maharṣi* Vyāsa, I cannot proceed. Vyāsa is a *ciranjīvi* (an immortal person). He is ever-present, everywhere. As far as knowledge is concerned, he occupies the highest seat. He is the first and foremost teacher for all of us. Even this dais on which I am sitting is called *Vyāsapīṭha*. I do not think I can sit on this high dais without his grace and guidance.

Pūrṇimā means full moon. This signifies that the intelligence, which is covered by want of knowledge or misunderstandings and misconceptions, has to be unveiled so that the intelligence glows clearly like the full moon that you see today.

Can this veil covering the intelligence be eradicated? Can the discriminative intelligence be made to surface everywhere? Here a *guru* is needed to enlighten the intelligence.

Take the example of a pot and a light. The light inside the pot cannot spread unless the pot is broken. Similarly, the *guru* breaks the cover that enshrouds the pupils' intelligence and makes it shine and spread. The moment ignorance *(ajñāna)* is eradicated, awareness *(prajñāna)* takes its place. Removing ignorance through the practice of yoga is rapid. The teaching of the philosophy of yoga – *yoga darśana* – is the only straightforward method that can lift off this veil over the intelligence, and yoke the intelligence of the mind to the soul. Everything which is not visible to the physical eye, but is felt, can be united with the intelligence. What we need is the matured eye of intelligence *(jñāna cakṣu)*.

GURU IS WITHIN

This morning, in the intensive class, I was telling pupils that today being *Vyāsa pūrṇimā*, let me give you something as a gift. Let me give you some enlightenment. While stretching the body on one side, say in *Utthita Trikoṇāsana* (Plate n. 8), do you observe the other side? While stretching on one side, you expose the awareness as on a full moon day, whereas you keep the other side in the dark like a waning moon. It is true that it requires great attention to spread awareness everywhere and to diffuse the intelligence evenly all over the body. Hence, practice of yoga is not as easy as many think, though it is a straight path. As you continue your practice with tremendous attention, yoga brings in you the quality of tolerance and forbearance to accept and take the load with ease. This load is taken by the *sva* and not by the *svāmi*. *Sva* is *prakṛti*, the *svāmi* is *puruṣa*. That means the principles of nature take the load and not the master. *Sva* separates, disintegrates and creates division in man, because his body, organs of action, senses of perception, mind, intelligence, ego and consciousness are all parts of *sva*. Each part thinks that it is the lord without an overlord, and hence does not integrate with the others to become good companions to *svāmi*, the inner lord. So first the *sva* has to integrate and unite to serve the *svāmi*[1]. For this purpose the matchstick of intelligence has to be struck and to ignite[2].

While we practise *āsana*, the intelligence "evolves" on one side and it "involves" on the other side. As this process flourishes, we learn to look within. If the practice of *āsana* is a torture, who wants to do it? If you practise to learn and understand yourself, it is a joy and an eye-opener. It not only generates life-giving force, but acts as an inspiration to earn the nectar of knowledge. The cycle of evolution and involution continues and the intelligence does not stagnate. That is why you always find a newness in my practice and in my teachings. I want in you this type of *śodhaka* mind. *Śodhaka* means the searcher – the one who searches and cleanses his whole being.

---

1 *Sva svāmi śaktyoḥ svarūpopalabdhi hetuḥ saṁyogaḥ* (*Y.S.*, II.23). The conjunction of the seer with the seen is for the seer to discover his own true nature.

2 *Vivekakhyātiḥ aviplavā hānopāyaḥ* (*Y.S.*, II.26). All pains are avoided through uninterrupted awareness of discriminative knowledge.

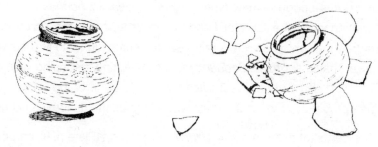

The *Upaniṣads* recognise three types of *guru* - *codhaka, bodhaka* and *mokṣaka* - the prompter, the awakener and the liberator. I add one more type to it: the *śodhaka guru*. It is not enough to do merely that which is known, you have to search further to find out what is still left beyond the known. That is *śodhana*. *Śodhana* means searching, cleansing, refining, sifting and investigating. The *śodhaka guru* reinvestigates the subtle parts of the known, cleanses and refines them, then proceeds towards the unknown and finds the fathomless knowledge.

When we say, stretch the arms in *Utthita Trikoṇāsana* (Plate n. 8), can they stretch on their own? Or does your mind go with the action? You have to yoke your mind to the action and in this way the arms are stretched. Can you do this without yoking your mind to it? Can you do it without volition? Can you do it without an initial impetus? When the mind goes there, it stretches. But what alerts the mind? You stretch the arms and when you are questioned as to where they stretch, the intelligence has to wake up and become involved in the search for where they are extended from. Mind stretches the known parts, the intelligence stretches the unknown parts. Mind indulges in acquired knowledge, i.e. the stretches, extensions or actions that are known to it. But the intelligence goes beyond, to experience by searching the unknown and hidden parts of the body. Normally the mind repeats the experience of acquired knowledge whereas the intelligence searches for unexperienced knowledge and that is the attitude of the *śodhaka guru*. The *śodhaka guru* makes the mind and the intelligence get involved in the work and makes them realise that they too work under the light of the Self.

EVOLUTION AND INVOLUTION

While performing *āsana*, the Self has to guide the individual self, the individual self the intelligence, the intelligence the mind and the mind the body. The body then expresses the *āsana* accordingly. This is evolution. This is *śodhaka vṛtti*, which investigates and searches. On the other hand, when experienced knowledge is reflected back from body to mind, mind to intelligence and intelligence to individual self and then to the Self, it becomes involution. This *śodhana vṛtti* cleanses and purifies. When the intelligence faces the body, it is evolution, and when the intelligence faces the Self, it is involution. While doing the *āsana*, the journey from the self to the skin is evolution and when it moves from the skin towards the Self, it becomes involution. Both evolutionary and involutionary observations are, in truth, evolutionary methods.

While doing *Utthita Trikoṇāsana* (Plate n. 8) on the right side, the evolution is on the right side and involution is on the left side. On the right side, which is perceivable by the senses, you penetrate outwards to watch with the eyes to see what you do and how you do it. On the left side, which is not perceivable by the senses, you need to penetrate with the mind to that side and watch mentally what you do, and how you adjust. In order to watch on the left side, you need to take your mind along with your intelligence in order to penetrate that area. Mind and intelligence have the capacity to know either outside through the senses of perception or inside through mental penetration. When they know through the senses of perception, it is evolution; when they know through mental penetration, it is involution.

Similarly, let us consider the *āsana* from its anterior and posterior sides. Adjustment of the anterior body is evolution, since the mind and intelligence use the senses of perception to reach the surface, which is visible. Whereas adjustment of the posterior body is involution, since the intelligence can use only mental penetration to reach that part which is invisible. Though it seems to be a body-related action, the intelligence is thus trained in both ways, in the path of evolution and of involution.

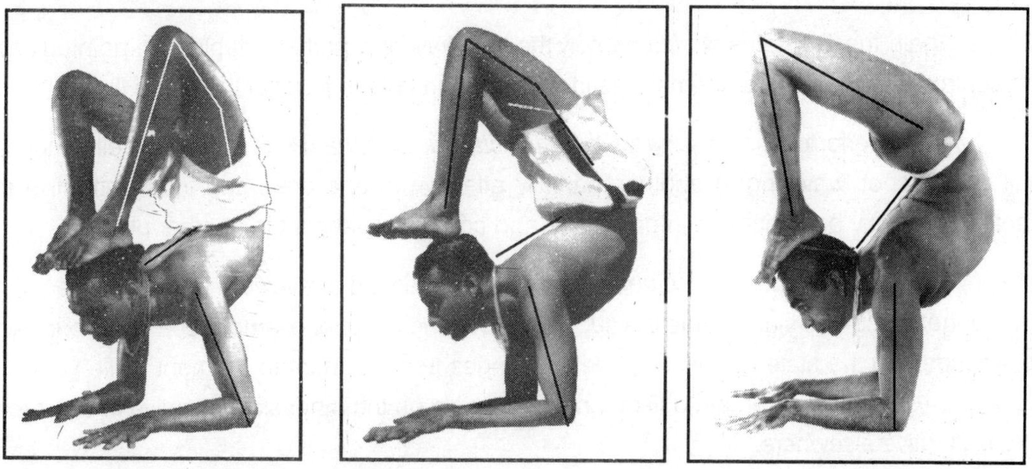

Plate n. 23 - Evolution in *āsana* (*Vṛśchikāsana*) – The evolution in this *āsana* can be observed in the space of the triangle formed with the spine, backs of the thighs and lower leg, in the final *āsana* (on the right) this space as well as a vertical ascension of the spine is achieved.

When the intelligence expands to reach its optimum level, it is evolution. Involution is at optimum level when the intelligence recedes and touches the Self. This oneness of space hidden in the stretch of the body in *āsana* is *dhyāna*. Until one reaches this state, the teacher holds the pupil in the first stage like a kitten carried in the mouth of the mother cat. Evolution is like the mother cat carrying the kitten so that is does not fall. The four aspects; *yama, niyama, āsana* and *prāṇāyāma,* together belong to the path of evolution, as they connect the Self to the periphery (nature). With the practice of these four disciplines, the intelligence surfaces to its highest level from the self to the skin.

When this state is reached, it becomes *pratyāhāra*, since there is the experience of the withdrawal of the senses. Here *guru* and *śiṣya* become like a mother monkey and a baby monkey. The baby monkey holds on to the mother monkey in the second stage.

Dhāraṇā, *dhyāna* and *samādhi* belong to the path of involution. Here the intelligence makes a return journey and moves from the skin towards the Self. In this involutionary process, the intelligence remains alert and illuminative at all times like the eye of a fish. This is the third and final stage of *sādhanā*, where the *guru* and *śiṣya* relationship comes to an end as the *śiṣya* has reached the level of the *guru* in his *sādhanā*.

When I said that evolution and involution constitute a simultaneous process, it means that one has to keep one's eyes, mind and intelligence like the eye of a fish while practising, to experience the process that is going on.

Again, the five states of *citta*, namely the dull, wavering, partially stable, one-pointed and the controlled state express themselves in different parts of the body at the same time.

While performing an *āsana* such as *Utthita Trikoṇāsana*, (Plate n. 8) the intelligence is dull in one spot, wavering in another, partially attentive in one area, and totally attentive in another; or it may be controlled in one place and completely absent in another place.

The states of one's consciousness change as fast as a revolving wheel and as such one cannot grasp one state before it is superseded by the next. For example, see from your own experience that the state of consciousness changes from moment to moment while you are doing the *āsana*, as you remain dull on one side, active on the other side, attentive to one area and inattentive elsewhere.

The question is, how to change this quality of mind, so that it may lead us towards tranquillity. I do not mean just a dull or *tāmasic* quietness. It is tranquillity of mind with sharp attention that is needed; that is the state to be achieved.

EXTERNAL AND INTERNAL PROPS

Here I should like to mention something about "props". You all use the props to do *āsana*; but are you using them intelligently? For example, when you use a belt for tying your legs in *Sālamba Śīrṣāsana*, do you use it as a guide for better action or use it as a supporter to stretch the legs? Do you see whether the legs hit the belt, or the belt hits the legs? You all rest on *Setubandha Sarvāṅgāsana* benches (Plate n. 11). Do you use the bench for resting or use it to act with discrimination? Is yoga meant for resting always? Remember that yoga is *agni* (fire). Props are meant to ignite that fire: unless that fire of intelligence is ignited, what is the use of these props for yoga? Can you not even think how to work constructively on the support given by the props so that energy may be generated and invoked in the body?

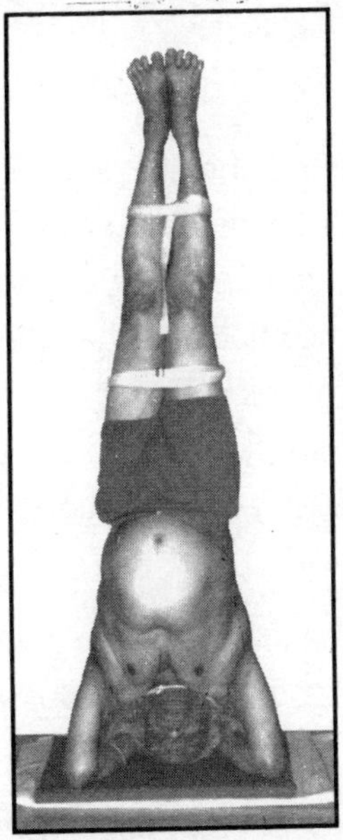

Plate n. 24 – *Sālamba Śīrṣāsana* – with belts

I invented these props to help those who are aged, disabled and invalids. But now my pupils who are healthy and fit have started using them as though they themselves are invalid. The use of props should not become a habit. Why do you not think the other way, "Let me do the *āsana* today without using props". Use your own body, mind and intelligence as if they are props. This nature *(prakṛti)* is also intended to help you as a prop for Self-realisation. Use props to reach the optimum level in the poses. Then practice independently and see whether you can do as well as you practised with the help of props. This way of study takes you to your optimum level of intelligence, which can carry on growing for ever.

Let all the qualities that Patañjali mentions such as faith, valour, memory, keen intellect and power of absorption, be your props (*Y.S.,* I.20). These are the real props to build a natural bed in your system to rest the intelligence. When you do not know your *sva* (all layers or sheaths of being), how will you know that you are the *svāmi* (Lord)? You should know that you are the *svāmi* of *sva*, i.e. you are the master of these. The body is your assistant which helps you through its service to know your own Self.

In fact, when I place emphasis on *āsana*, I mean this. *Āsana* makes you realise exactly the difference between *sva* and *svāmi*. The soul is the *guru* here. The duty of the Self is to build the body up to the level of exalted intelligence – i.e. *vivekaja jñāna*.

If you rest, letting yourself loose in the *āsana*, how can exalted intelligence develop? While doing *āsana*, either by depending on external props, or by letting loose your own natural props and lacking any firmness, you do not conquer nature but you become dependent on it. You are neither supposed to depend upon the external props forever nor are you supposed to depend upon the internal props such as body and mind by making yourself a slave of them. The body, mind, intelligence, ego and consciousness have to depend upon the *puruṣa*. They are slaves of *puruṣa.* They are supposed to serve the *puruṣa.* When nature depends upon your Self, you are actually free; you are not bound. And that is the *mokṣa* state. *Mokṣa* means liberation from dependence.

ŚUDDHI SĀMYATĀ – A BALANCED PURITY

The light of intelligence flows uninterruptedly only on attaining this liberated state, engulfing the five sheaths of the body and of the self. At this stage, the mind, intelligence, ego and consciousness listen to you, obey your orders, and behave as you want them to behave. Duality vanishes and from then on no longer does the body fight with the mind or the mind with the body. No longer does the mind fight with the ego or intelligence and they with the mind. The ego vanishes as the intelligence matures. No longer does the intelligence fight with the self and the self with the intelligence. Your *sādhanā* should be of that type, leading you towards liberation. I do not want you to transform this Institute into a resting place or a health club.

I stayed with my *guru* for a very short period of two years. But the little knowledge that he gave me was enough to ignite my inner fire of *jñāna (jñānāgni).* My inner *svāmi* guided me to reach this level.

You have all seen my *āsana* practice and so you know. But if you see the way I do the practice of *prāṇāyāma*, you will be surprised. You may be able to see my *sādhanā* externally, but how can you see my internal practice of *prāṇāyāma* or my internal adjustments of my *āsana sādhanā?* The internal practice cannot be externalised. External practice is evolution whereas internal practice is involution. Evolution can be perceived but involution cannot be perceived. However involution is not possible without evolution, so also without externalised practice it is impossible to have an internalised practice. Those who can see the evolution can sense the involution.

But these days yoga is popularised the other way. They teach *dhyāna* – meditation – first, and say that the rest of the practices are absolutely unnecessary. Remember, the ultimate freedom is impossible unless one frees oneself from the bindings *(bandha)* of nature.

The river flows from the mountain to the sea as one single unit. Similarly, *āsana* too can take you to that level of flow when intelligence qualitatively improves. To improve yourself qualitatively, you must touch every aspect of your existence qualitatively as well as quantitatively. If the evolution is optimal, the involution too will be optimal.

The practice of yoga makes the intelligence penetrate deeper and deeper into the body. As the intelligence penetrates, dualities are diminished. This is the real meaning of *tatodvandvānabhighātaḥ* (*Y.S.,* II.48). From then on, the practitioner is undisturbed by dualities.

But you attend partially to your practice and hence the intelligence unfortunately does not penetrate and does not flow uninterruptedly. When the mind has no intention or volition, then the intelligence has no incitement and will; even the first step of learning becomes impossible.

A goldsmith weighs gold very carefully, a diamond seller weighs a diamond carefully. You also, as practitioners of yoga, have to weigh each cell as if it were a diamond, and the intelligence as if it were gold. The mind gets carried away with action since it is always moving forward, while the brain, as a thinking power, reverses this onward process and makes you wait and look back. The alert consciousness tutors the intelligence to become sharp and very sensitive. At that time, it does not take you backward or forward, but towards purity. Then the intelligence remains the same inside, outside and in the middle. Weigh yourself with this intuitive intelligence, so that there is no difference or variation in practice.

You take any *āsana* of mine, or see *Light on Yoga*[1]. Some people say that each *āsana* appears clear-cut, like a diamond. In case you think that it is an exhibitive expression, let me inform you that the inhibitive expression of the posture is that I weigh each and every cell evenly with that intuitive intelligence. I do not spend, waste or invest unnecessarily the vital energy. The energy too finds equilibrium. Remember, without the inner experience there cannot be an outer expression. That is why my approach to yogic *āsana* is not merely one of performance, but a performance in which the body and the intelligence remain in an exalted state, equal to that of the Self. In this way, the cells of the body, the intelligence of *prakṛti* and the Self remain in a state of equilibrium. There comes *śuddhi sāmyatā*. All the evolutes of *prakṛti* remain pure and therefore equal.

Sattva puruṣayoḥ śuddhi sāmye kaivalyam iti (*Y.S.,* III.56). When the exalted intelligence is as pure as the seer, there comes the indivisible state of existence.

So, my dear friends do not imprison your body and mind in the shackles of the props. Use the props when your body is tired, when the mind is dull, when you are sick or when you lack will power.

Yoga teaches you independence. Dependence is *bhoga*, independence is yoga. Do not pollute the subject by over-simplifying it. If you want a real transformation, then use the body, mind and intelligence as props, so that they may become transformed to the state of purity.

People do question, why one should do difficult and advanced *āsana*. Can one not stick to some simple *āsana*, which to their minds are uncomplicated and non-harming? But they do not know that by this way of thinking, they are caught in the net of body and mind

[1] Harper Collins, London.

limitations. Yoga cannot be done by cajoling. It teaches endurance and strength of the nervous system. The practice of backward bending makes you realise how much stress the nerves can take. The backward bendings build up a strong will power. The difficult *āsana* are a challenge to help you to progress.

Use the props, if this is giving you "feed-back". Props give you understanding in measuring an action and how to correct a mistake. There too, you need a searching eye – the *śodhaka vṛtti.* When my own pupils use the props as an indulgence, I feel like blaming my own improvisation in developing them as it acts as a thorn in intellectual growth. Yoga is meant to make you an illuminated person and not a dull one. Do not use the props to rest but to awaken your intelligence like a *bodhaka guru.* When I taught standing *āsana* against a wall, I called this practice "the wall – my *guru".* I used the wall to guide me, but I do not mean to rest on the wall. You have to learn how to activate yourself when taking a support. The props should be used as *pravṛtti* for *nivṛtti;* evolution for involution. So when using them, learn to minimise the support and maximise the independence; learn to minimise the mistakes to go towards correctness.

In olden days, children were sent after the thread ceremony to a *gurukula* in order to study. The pupils were controlled by the *guru.* The *guru* was like a father, and the *gurupatni* (the wife of the *guru)* was like a mother. Since the pupils were away from their parents, they were not corrupted, spoiled or pampered. In these days, you cannot withstand and face a *guru* like me because you want to be pampered and cajoled. For me, the art of yoga is important. I see whether the very purpose of yoga is served or not. I do not change the principles of yoga for your sake. I shall not corrupt the subject, nor shall I myself become corrupted. This is a message for today from me, that you should not pamper yourselves but strengthen your nerves to withstand hardships. That in itself will be a great service to me.

When education was given in the *gurukula, gurupūrṇimā* was considered a very significant day. This was the only day on which pupils could show or express gratitude towards their *guru.* There are three ways to serve the *guru,* i.e. serving him financially, serving him physically and propagating the knowledge given by him. From my heart of hearts I feel satisfied, since I myself have served my *guru* in all three ways. I do not expect the first two types of service from you. I want only the third one. Propagate yoga in its real spirit, and carry on the Light of Yoga. Teach others with the same zeal and zest, ignite them with your knowledge, take them from dependence to independence, from the finite to infinite and from impurity to purity.

Let the flame of yoga burn in you constantly so that you may give that Light to others.

God bless you.

FROM *MOHA* TO *MOKṢA* *

(Enamouration to emancipation)

This subject, the upliftment from enamouration to emancipation, is really a very serious 'soul-searching' one. Therefore tune your ears attentively, passively and pensively, so that the words you hear penetrate deep into your heart. At the same time keep your eyes quiet with enthusiasm but no tense, so that you absorb the fragrance *(rasa)* of what you hear on the matter and it reaches you with clarity. If the eyes are taut, the ears get blocked and you tend to lose the faculty of listening and miss the track as you follow and grasp the flowing wisdom of the garland of *aṣṭadaḷa yoga*.

I have churned my body, mind and intelligence for more than sixty-five years, filtering and re-filtering repeatedly my experiences each time. These experiences enable me to verbalise and share them now with you all. The experience of today has to become a focal point to work for the future. The present acts as a guiding star though it moves to the past. As knowledge is infinite, the wheel of experiential knowledge should continue along with *sādhanā* for further exploration. Try to internalise the senses and the mind through *sādhanā* so that your understanding saturates and settles in the seat of the wisdom of the heart, so that you move from *moha* towards *mokṣa* or emancipation and liberation.

In olden days, *guru* used to test the calibre of students to find out whether they were fit or unfit *(pātran* or *apātran)* to receive spiritual knowledge. But the disciplines of yoga were an exception. It was taught to one and all in the form of *āsana* and *prāṇāyāma,* hoping that one day the raw body and the unripe intelligence might develop ripeness, through the integration of body, mind and self in order to understand the ultimate aim of life and to proceed towards the subtle aspects of yoga.

Moha means infatuation or enamouration; while *mokṣa* means emancipation and freedom from the turbulence of nature *(prakṛti)* or change from its natural state *(vikṛti)* with its first evolute, – cosmic intelligence *(mahat)* –, ego, elements and their qualities.

---

* Talk given on the 14.12.1999

Practice of yoga develops the art of knowing *(veda)* and aims to reach the ultimate in knowledge, that is *vedānta*. Hence, *veda* means knowledge, to know, and *anta* means the end. *Vedānta* means pursuit of spiritual knowledge and its culmination. To put objective knowledge into a subjective experience and transmit the subjective experience into objective knowledge is *vedānta*. For this, one has to filter and re-filter the experiences in order to develop discerning intelligence *(prajñāna)*. This needs a lot of vigorous and rigorous disciplined practice.

One should not take the first experience as "fool-proof truth." One should go on churning the same experience until profound, unshakeable knowledge *(prajñāna)*, surfaces. Until then the subjective word *prajñāna* remains an unknowable entity in our vocabulary *(vikalpa)*.

Jñāna is knowledge. *Vijñāna* is experimental knowledge while *prajñāna* is experiential knowledge that has been re-filtered through *vijñāna*. *Prajñāna* is an intense, total knowledge. It is something like the nectar *(amṛta)*, that came by the churning *(maṅthana)* of the ocean. The *ṛṣis* and yogis found the churning rod in *aṣṭadaḷa yoga* to bring out the nectar of wisdom.

We are endowed with the five elements *(pañcabhūta)* and seven ingredients *(saptadhātu)*, as material to bring out the elixir of life *(sañjīvanī)*. To stir this elixir one has to rub one's body, senses, mind, intelligence and self with the *puruṣa śakti*, the *ātman*.

Pātañjala yoga is a necklace containing 196 gems of wisdom, woven together in the form of aphorisms. As a necklace has two hooks to link together, so too this wisdom of yoga has two ends to hook together. One is *anuśāsanam* (means) and the other is *cīti śakti* (power of *ātman*). *Anuśāsanam* is intended to make *jīvātman* recognise its own power – *cīti śakti* – in order for one to become a *jīvanmuktan*.

Patañjali says that when *sādhanā* has reached perfection, the matured, truth-bearing knowledge and wisdom *(rasātmaka prajñā)* sprouts from it. Patañjali calls this *rasātmaka jñāna* as *ṛtambharā prajñā*. When this sprouted wisdom percolates evenly and harmoniously, there is *ātma-prasādana*.

Before going into the disciplines of *āsana* and *prāṇāyāma*, one has to know *prakṛti* and its five elements. Those are: earth, water, fire, air, and ether *(pṛthvī, āp, tej, vāyu* and *ākāśa)*. If *pṛthvī*, *āp* and *tej* are nature's gross elements, *vāyu* and *ākāśa* are its subtle parts. These five elements have their infrastructures *(tanmātra)*, odour, taste, form, touch and sound *(gandha, rasa, rūpa, sparśa* and *śabda)*. The human body contains all these five elements and their infrastructures. The organs of action *(karmendriya)* are connected to the *pañcabhūta*, and the five senses of perception *(jñānendriya)* are connected to the *pañca tanmātra*. If the *pañcabhūta* are felt by the organs of action, the *tanmātra* are tangible to the senses of perception. *Karmendriya* and *jñānendriya* are *sthūlendriya*. Then comes *sūkṣmendriya* – the subtle senses, namely *buddhi, ahaṁkāra, citta* and *antaḥkaraṇa*. *Buddhi* is intelligence, *ahaṁkāra* is the one that impersonates or dramatises as Self, *citta* is consciousness and *antaḥkaraṇa* is conscience. The mind *(manas)* is the medium between the *sthūlendriya* (gross) and the *sūkṣmendriya* (subtle). All of these are controlled by *mahat* or cosmic intelligence *(viśva prajñā śakti)* and cosmic energy *(viśva caitanya śakti)*. These two stir and comb nature either for silence or turbulence. If turbulence ensues, the evolution is slow or nil. If silence is built up in *mahat*, *prāṇa* then becomes rhythmic, and *buddhi, ahaṁkāra, citta* and *antaḥkaraṇa* develop quietude (*Y.S.*, II.18 & 19).

The body has five *kośa*. The anatomical body *(annamaya kośa)*, is the solid sheath or *pṛthvī-tattva*, the physiological vital body *(prāṇamaya kośa)*, is *āp-tattva*, that keeps up the fluidity in the body. The mental body *(manomaya kośa)* is ruled by the *tejas-tattva*, which is vibrant like fire. The body of intelligence *(vijñānamaya kośa)* belongs to the element *vāyu-tattva* or air, which fans and keeps the body cool. The ethereal body *(ānandamaya kośa)* creates space for the air to move in and out. In modern terms it is called contraction, expansion, abduction, adduction, circumduction and so on. The practice of *āsana* and *prāṇāyāma* fans the body as muscles move circularly.

COSMOLOGY

Cosmology is well explained in the systems of *śāṁkhya* and *āyurveda*. They sing the same tune as yoga. In *āyurveda*, more ideas are added, such as the seven ingredients *(saptadhātu)*. They are: chyle *(rasa)*, blood *(rakta)*, flesh *(māṁsa)*, fat *(meda)*, bone *(asthi)*, marrow *(majjā)*, semen *(śukra)* in men and ovum *(śoṇita)* in women. Chyle *(rasa)* is formed with the intake of food, from which blood is formed. The blood produces flesh. Flesh protects the bones by generating fat. Fat acts as a lubricant while the bones produce marrow. Marrow not only gives strength, but also produces semen and ovum. These *dhātu* are again the chemical combinations of the *pañcabhūta* and *tanmātra*. For instance, chyle is mainly the juicy water *(āp* and *rasa)*, formed with the intake of food; blood, the combination of fire and water *(tejas* and *āp, rūpa* and *rasa)*; flesh is earth *(pṛthvī* and *gandha)*, fat is earth and water *(pṛthvī and āp, gandha* and *rasa)*, bones are earth, air and ether *(pṛthvī, vāyu and ākāśa*, and *gandha, sparśa* and *śabda)* bone marrow, semen and ovum are water and fire *(āp* and *tejas, rasa* and *rūpa)*. That is why *āyurveda* recognises the importance of the seven *dhātu*. In addition to these *dhātu*, there is one extra *dhātu* in us. This is *puruṣa śakti*. Without this *dhātu*, nature *(prakṛti)* cannot function. This is known as *tejas śakti* or *ojas śakti*, the eighth *dhātu* in our system. If the seven *dhātu* are from nature, the eighth *dhātu* is from the inner core of being. From the union of these eight *dhātu* sprouts the conscious force and the life force.

I call the *puruṣa śakti* as *dhātu* for the simple reason that it alone upholds, maintains and supports the body and life force. The meaning of *dhātu* is to hold, *dhāraṇāt dhātavaḥ,* meaning the one that holds the body. Though the *puruṣa* is above all the elements, it is the source, which holds and energises the elemental body.

As you use a mixer to blend vegetables, all these seven *dhātu* are mixed with gross and subtle senses *(sthūlendriya* and *sūkṣmendriya),* blended with the five *tanmātra,* along with *ojas śakti.* This new blend in the body is known as life force *(jīva śakti).* Hence, our survival is dependent upon this *jīva śakti.* As long as *jīva śakti* stays, we will be in a position to strive to reach the higher and deeper state of consciousness. Unfortunately, due to our ignorance, taking for granted the non-permanent as eternal, pain as pleasure, the impure as pure and non-self as Self, we block our intelligence. With this perverted intelligence *(viparyaya)* and delusive knowledge *(bhrānti darśana)* we mistake the 'I' for the Soul[1]. The practice of *āsana* and *prāṇāyāma* develops the sense of differentiation in the seeker so that he distinguishes the real from the unreal, the unbiased joy from pleasure, and minimises the ignorant character of *viparyaya, vikalpa, bhrānti darśana* and attachment with lust and cultivates indifference towards hatred and malice.

We all know that the body has nine outgoing gates *(navadvāra).* They are the two eyes, two ears, two nostrils, mouth, generative and the excretory organs. However, yogic science explains four incoming gates, namely, *buddhi, ahaṁkāra, citta* and *antaḥkaraṇa.* Unless and until one closes the outgoing gates, one cannot open the incoming gates. The closure of the outgoing gates is possible only by cleansing them. Rather the cleansing or purification itself is the closing of the gates. The incoming gates are opened one by one through the practices of *aṣṭadaḷa yoga.*

These gates are inter-linked, inter-related and inter-woven, but finally lead one towards the indweller – *puruṣa* (Soul). Until one cleanses the gross (structural) body or the distinguishable and the undistinguishable or non-specific parts of nature *(viśeṣa* and *aviśeṣa),* they do not allow the *sādhaka* to see the incoming gates of *liṅga* (phenomenal) and *aliṅga* (noumenal)[2]. It is not easy to enter the intellectual and the spacial bodies. These gates cannot be opened by listening to a talk. They have to be opened and cleansed only by internalising the practice of *āsana* and *prāṇāyāma,* combined with *yama, niyama* and *pratyāhāra.* The actual scope of *āsana* and *prāṇāyāma* is that they enable us to reach the holder of the body, the *ātman* (Soul).

---

1 See the Author's *Light on the Yoga Sūtras of Patañjali,* I.8; II.5,30,32 and 34, published by Harper Collins, London.

2 *Ibid.,* I.4, 18, 19; II.19 and 33.

PURUṢA

The body is the container and the content is the *ātman,* or the holder of the body. In order to reach the content, all the inner gates of the body have to be opened one after the other, to reach the dweller, the content *(ātman).* Then one experiences the state of eternal, unalloyed, untainted, absolute, independent, bliss *(sānanda),* that springs out from a regular and reverential *sādhanā*[1].

HEALTH: PHYSICAL, MENTAL AND SPIRITUAL

Health is soundness of body, a condition in which its functions are duly discharged. It is qualified as bad, good or delicate. Maintenance of health is an art against a background of body and mind knowledge. It is a re-planning of one's way of living.

Health is classified as moral health, physical health, environmental health, emotional health, intellectual health and spiritual health.

Mind is the seat of thoughts, feelings, desires, sentiments, love, devotion and courage. Health is a combination of heart, head and hand. If head is the seat of sensation, thinking, memory and imagination (*jñāna*), heart is the seat of love, devotion and courage (*bhakti*), while hands are for action (*karma*). It is like a river, flowing with fresh energy moment to moment. We are told that health is dependent on the three humours *(tridoṣa),* namely, *vāta, pitta* and *śleṣma,* which are element oriented. *Vāta* contains air *(vāyu* and *sparśa)* and ether *(ākāśa* and *śabda).* *Pitta* contains fire *(tej* and *rūpa)* and *śleṣma* contains earth *(pṛthvī* and *gandha)* and water *(āp* and *rasa).* The physiological body of modern medical science corresponds to the element of water *(āp),* the psychological body to the element of fire *(tej)* and the neurological body to the element of air *(vāyu).*

The specialists of *āyurveda* test *tridoṣa* by placing their fingers on the side of the right thumb below the wrist for men and on the left side for women. It is said that *vāta nāḍī* on the top edge represents Brahmā, *pitta nāḍī* in the middle represents Shiva and the *kapha* or *śleṣma nāḍī* at the end is Vishnu. The movement of *vāta nāḍī* is like a snake, that of *pitta nāḍī* like a frog and *śleṣma nāḍī* like a swan.

The *tridoṣa* of *āyurveda* have a bearing on the *triguṇa* of the yoga *śāstra;* these are luminosity *(sattva),* vibrancy *(rajas)* and inertia *(tamas)*[2]. If the *tridoṣa* or *triguṇa* are imbalanced,

---

1 *Ibid.,* I.3; II.21, 22 and 25.

2 *Ibid.,* II.18, 12 and 31.

they cause ill health, restlessness and spiritual disturbances. If they balance perfectly, they bring perfect physical health, mental poise and spiritual bliss. The mingling of the *tridoṣa* and *triguṇa* generates *tāpa* or torments. In order to be rid of this process one has to use *abhyāsa* and *vairāgya*, the two wings of *sādhanā*[1].

These *tāpa* are of three types – *ādhidaivika*, *ādhibhautika* and *adhyātmika*. Today's AIDS can be termed as self-inflicted or *adhyātmika* disease, which later turns into *ādhidaivika*. The *ādhidaivika tāpa* includes hereditary, congenital, viral or allergic diseases. The *ādhibhautika tāpa* causes imbalance in the *pañcabhūta* and in the *pañcatanmātra*, due to snake bites, mosquito bites, dog bites, bee stings and so on. Yoga, as *tapas*, plays a major role in fighting these three afflictions and torments. If practice *(abhyāsa)* is study or understanding of one's own body, from the skin to the self and from the self to the skin, then detachment *(vairāgya)* is the knowledge of developing restraints from the attachments *(rāga)* and aversions *(dveṣa)*. It is a way to cultivate non-attachment towards the sensual joy of pleasure and pain, longing and desires. Hence, the yogic *abhyāsa* and *vairāgya* combined together are called *tapas*.

Tapas is a determined effort with a calm head and heart to build up intellectual fervour and body tolerance to face environmental calamities as well as mental disturbances such as lust *(kāma)*, anger *(krodha)*, greed *(lobha)*, infatuation *(moha)*, pride *(mada)* and jealousy *(mātsarya)*.

The *tridoṣa* and *triguṇa* are closely linked with and correspond to the three elements, water *(āp)*, fire *(tej)* and air *(vāyu)*. *Āp-tattva* corresponds to *sleśma doṣa* and *sattvaguṇa*. *Tej-tattva* corresponds to *pitta doṣa* and *rajōguṇa*. *Vāyu-tattva* corresponds to *vāta doṣa* and *tamōguṇa*. *Pṛthvī-tattva* acts as the foundation for these three elements to function. *Ākāśa-tattva* acts as a distributing agent. In modern terminology it is 'survey and marketing' or 'demand and supply'.

The three elements water, fire and air either contribute harmony in the maintenance of perfect health in body, mind and intelligence or disharmony between the physical, physiological, neuropsychological or psychoneurological and psychospiritual fields. These three elements are the three spokes of the wheel of life which are activised, balanced and made to function properly in the body by the practice of *yogāsana*. While doing *āsana*, if one uses the *sūkṣmendriya (buddhi, ahaṁkāra, citta* and *antaḥkaraṇa)* to focus on the core of the being, then one experiences unalloyed bliss, emancipation and freedom from suffering[2].

Patañjali says that when the three spokes of life, *tribhūta*, *triguṇa* and *tridoṣa*, move in the wheel of lust, anger and greed, they bring sorrow *(duḥkha* or drying of *āp-tattva)*, fickleness

---

1 *Ibid.*, I.30, 31 and 32.

2 *Ibid.*, I. 48; II.15, 18, 19, 20, 21, 25, 26, 28, 46, 47 and 48.

or weakness in mind *(daurmanasya* or diminution of *tej-tattva),* shakiness or trembling in the body *(aṅgamejayatva* or diminution of *vāta-tattva),* and fearful breathing *(śvāsapraśvāsa* or diminution of all three *tattva),* expressing the symptoms of various psychosomatic problems springing out from the above three. They are bodily ailments *(vyādhi),* body inertia *(styāna),* doubt *(saṁṣaya),* heedlessness *(pramāda),* mental laziness *(ālasya),* indiscipline of the senses *(avirati),* erroneous views *(bhrāntidarśana),* lack of perseverance *(alabdhabhūmikatva)* and backsliding *(anavasthitatva)* (*Y.S.,* I.30 and 31). The two processes of yoga – *abhyāsa* and *vairāgya* (*Y.S.,* I.12) act like wings for the seeker of a valued life with sound health in body, mind and self. They bring *ṛtambharā prajñā, dharmamegha prajñā* and *puruṣa prajñā.*

In our body, the *sūkṣmendriya* are like *jñānapuṣkariṇi* (lakes of knowledge), generating sensitivity, feeling and awareness of the life force. Our bodies have lakes filled with intelligence, but do we swim or dive in these lakes is the question. Before going into these lakes of *buddhi, ahaṁkāra* and *antaḥkaraṇa,* we need to swim in and cross the lake of *manas* or mind.

Mind *(manas)* can be either the unifier or the breaker of the *sthūlendriya (karmendriya* and *jñānendriya),* with the *sūkṣmendriya* (intelligence, 'I'-ness and *antaḥkaraṇa).* The mind is in between the *sthūlendriya* and *sūkṣmendriya.* It acts like a mirror between them. It is an agent that carries the messages between the observer and the observant, or the seeker and the seer (*Y.S.,* I.3 and 4). It carries the imprints of *jñānendriya* and *karmendriya* to the *sūkṣmendriya.* Thus it does a two-way job – the thinking process and the thought process. The thought process is from the past experiences of the motor nerves, and the thinking process is on the sensory nerves. This interaction between sensory nerves and the motor nerves is the cause for the generation of *vṛtti* (fluctuations or modifications). That is the reason why Patañjali begins yoga with *citta vṛtti nirodhaḥ* (restraint of the generation of *vṛtti* in the consciousness) (*Y.S.,* I.2).

The *vṛtti* are like the rays of the sun. As one cannot count the rays of the sun, similarly, countless *vṛtti* sprout from the consciousness either bringing pain and pleasure or taking one beyond pain and pleasure.

The *vṛtti* are five-fold. The consciousness *(citta)* fluctuates and emits the rays of modifications as *vṛtti,* which could be either afflicting and painful or non-afflicting and non-painful. The five modifications *(citta vṛtti)* are: correct knowledge *(pramāṇa),* illusion *(viparyaya),* delusion *(vikalpa),* sleep *(nidrā),* and memory *(smṛti).*

Citta vṛtti can modify in sleep, memory, imagination, doubt, inference, indifference, opposition, restraint, dream, perverse thinking, tranquillity and single pointed attention. It can also have fissures and holes. It may be charged with right-conception. It could be free from passion and filled with divine thoughts. As the range of modifications are from knowledge to sleep, the range of transformation is from out-going thoughts *(vyutthāna citta)* to incoming divine thoughts *(divya citta).*

The painful and non-painful *vṛtti* go hand in hand. Even with all the impediments that come in *sādhanā*, the *sādhaka* continues to pursue his *sādhanā*, because he realises that there are also the non-painful modifications. The painful ones create obstacles and non-painful ones clear the path for moving ahead. In other words, if the painful *vṛtti* create obstacles, the non-painful *vṛtti* lead us on the path of yoga. For instance knowledge *(pramāṇa)* or memory *(smṛti)* can both make or break us. They help us to build ourselves up in the yogic path or they distract us[1]. The two faceted, five-fold *vṛtti* accompany the consciousness from the fluctuating state towards a divine, attentive and conscious state, keeping one healthy, positive, dynamic, constructive and contented.

I just gave the example of various rays of *vṛtti* carrying innumerable thought waves from the disc of the *citta*. If you can work out and count how many would diminish and how many would remain, you would be wonderstruck. However, you can do so when you swim into the lake of consciousness *(citta)* and conscience *(antaḥkaraṇa)*.

Patañjali explains the method to stop the *vṛtti* through the eight aspects of *aṣṭāṅga or aṣṭadaḷa yoga*, namely, *yama, niyama, āsana, prāṇāyāma, pratyāhāra, dhāraṇā, dhyāna* and *samādhi*. He shows how they work as antidotes to painful *vṛtti*. Not only do they keep the various afflictions and torments of psychosomatic *vṛtti* at a standstill, but at the same time help us to develop a composed state of consciousness *(samādhāna citta)*. Without *samādhāna citta*, we cannot go to the higher subtle aspects of consciousness.

Now, let me explain *aṣṭadaḷa yoga* in brief.

AṢṬADAḶA YOGA

YAMA

Yama being the Lord of death, Patañjali might have deliberately used this name for the moral disciplines of life so that a *sādhaka* might realise that unethical practices destroy one's character and honour which is as good as death *(amaratva)*. Then he explains the ten facets of wrong and right behaviour, placing them in counterpoint as *yama* and *niyama* for the conquest of deadly mental and intellectual perversions.

Patañjali explains the ten principles of *yama* and *niyama* as *ahiṁsā, satya, asteya, brahmacarya, aparigraha and śaucha, santoṣa, tapas, svādhyāya, Īśvara praṇidhāna*. Due to our own motives and desires, we are often prone to go against these ten healthy mental and

[1] *Ibid.*, II.12, 13 and 14 in order to understand the making and breaking of the turbulence of life.

spiritual currents through violence, untruth, stealing, libertinism, greed, uncleanliness, unhappiness, indiscipline, enamourment by mental joy and disbelief in God. These being very common in man, they mar our growth. These tendencies are a very destructive force in man's life. Patañjali guides us not to fall prey to unhealthy thoughts, which are opposite to the principles of *yama* and *niyama;* he wants us to keep away from these unwanted practices through *yama* by not allowing the *karmendriya* to participate, even though thoughts ignite them.

Niyama

Through *niyama* Patañjali speaks of *śauca, santoṣa, tapas, svādhyāya* and *Īśvara praṇidhāna* which are filled with constructive ideas for a better, auspicious state of life. They train and guide man to be free from *aśauca, asantoṣa, atapas, anadhyayana* (non-study) and *nirīśvaravāda*[1].

Niyama helps one to develop healthy thoughts by disciplining the senses of perception and makes one more inward, by keeping the mercurial mind passive and quiet through the right usage of *karmendriya* and *jñānendriya.*

Āsana

The growth and understanding of intelligence are not the same in all practitioners. Vyāsa divides mind into five categories. They are: dull *(mūḍha),* distracted *(kṣipta),* agitated *(vikṣipta),* one-pointed *(ekāgra)* and restrained *(nirūddha).* These five types of practitioners are again subdivided into dull *(mūḍha),* mild *(mṛdu),* moderate *(madhyama),* keen *(adhimātra)* and intensely intense *(tīvra).*

Today's practice of yoga is in a *mūḍha* state. This can be further divided as *mṛdu mūḍha* or *ati mūḍha yogābhyāsa* (mild, dull or excessively dull practice of yoga). Beyond this we have not opened our eyes.

The *mūḍha* or dull *sādhaka* is satisfied with triggering the motor nerves, which becomes a conative action. He thinks that is yoga. The *mṛdu sādhaka* is happy when the sensory nerves are triggered by action and the *madhyama sādhaka* is one who is satisfied when the motor and sensory nerves get fused causing sensual pleasure in the mind. This type of practice of *āsana* may be called *bhogābhyāsa.* This again becomes a destructive practice. Here the *sādhaka* thinks that the aim of yoga is a play of giving and taking pleasure. That is why Patañjali introduces *śauca* and *santoṣa* in *niyama* first and then takes one towards *tapas, svādhyāya* and *Īśvara praṇidhāna* which are constructive when one undertakes the practice of *āsana.*

[1] *Nirīśvaravāda* – The doctrine which denies the existence of *Īśvara.*

Being a psychologist and parapsychologist, Patañjali knew that people would be satisfied with health and happiness *(śauca* and *santoṣa).* Beyond that they seek nothing. So he advises the *sādhaka* to become an *adhimātra sādhaka.* This is the category of students who study prudently, bringing the intelligence *(buddhi)* to mingle and act by observing the fusion between the *karmendriya,* the *jñānendriya* and the *manas* and the reaction of the motor nerves with the sensory nerves and their reaction upon the central nervous system by involving the *sūkṣmendriya.*

The central nervous system functions with the *sūkṣmendriya.* By using *sūkṣmendriya* one refines the practice by re-evaluation of the right re-adjustments, right realignments, right feelings and right movements of inflow and outflow of breath. Here begins the pureness in *āsana sādhanā* as the intelligence *(buddhi)* is refined. This comes when you are in an *adhimātra* state. *Tīvrasaṁvega* is the anchoring of the noblest path of all practitioners, who are cheerful, sharp, vigorous and connect the *indriya* for the inward journey. This is possible only when one practises, not only as a doer *(kartan),* but as a devotee *(bhaktan).*

Practice of *āsana* not only keeps one healthy, but it also puts a halt to the mind's perennial wandering. That is the reason why Patañjali says that firm ground is established only when one practises uninterruptedly with proper application, devotion, attention and awareness. Today, yoga has become just like fast food. Which fast food gives nourishment? Practice of yoga for a week, or a month or two does not give one even a taste to feel the essence or flavour of yogic knowledge.

You have all experienced the incoming and outgoing thoughts having several breaks or pauses in between. Similarly, while doing *āsana* and *prāṇāyāma* you might have experienced, but not cognised that the dormant imprints *(saṁskāra)* surface and diminish. As I am saying this, you recognise that at times the *vṛtti,* which flow like a turbulent river, drop on their own or you deliberately put a halt now and then, while practising *āsana.* This natural and automatic, sporadic restraint is nothing but mind control, which has to be watched and prolonged in chronological time. In fact, prolonged psychological silence is the effect of *āsana.*

What is an *āsana?*

Patañjali defines *āsana* as *sthira sukhamāsanam* (*Y.S.,* II.46). An *āsana* is assuming a certain position in the body, bearing in mind the physical rhythmic form and discriminative mental attitude. To feel the *āsana,* one has to be in the *āsana* by placing the different parts of the body in a right position with perfect carriage and use the body accurately and evenly with the pressures and counter pressures. It is from this state of performing the *āsana* that one dips into the *jñānapuṣkariṇi* (the lakes of knowledge) to move towards *dhyāna.*

Here the *sthirāsana* stands for silencing the turbulence of *prakṛti* (*Y.S.*, II.19) and *sukhāsana* for *ātma-prasādanam* (Y.S., II.20, 21 and 25). When the turbulence *(vikṛti)* of nature *(prakṛti)* is silenced and transformed into a noumenal state it is considered as the end of effort *(prayatna śaithilyatā)*. From this serene quiet state, if we intensify the *yogāsana* (I.20) we experience the self without its echo *(manas, buddhi, ahaṁkāra)* and Patañjali defines this state as *ananta samāpatti* (II.47).

Each *yogāsana*, has to be done from the seat of conscience and should express the state of meditation *(dhyāna)* and action *(karma)* going together. The grip of each *āsana* must be like a *yoga paṭṭa*, binding the container with the content, or the body with the seer.

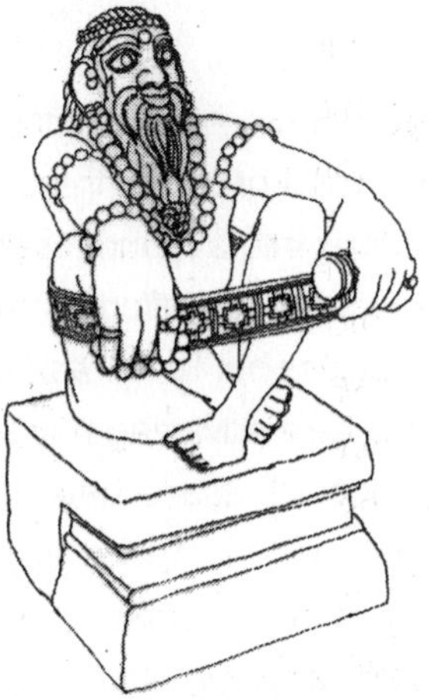

yoga-paṭṭa

As one feels the existence of the invisible God in anything, everything, anywhere as well as everywhere, the *yogābhyāsi* treats all creations of God as God's children. He visualises these creations. He tries to imitate them by assuming those shapes and forms in his body using the *sthūlendriya* as well as the *sūkṣmendriya* to feel the sense of them and to cultivate universality in himself.

The feeling in the spiritual heart must be, "I am not separate from *āsana*, *āsana* is not separate from me, I am *āsana* and *āsana* is me." I hope you understand how the practitioner visualises these various shapes while in *āsana*. I am giving a few names of *āsana* that resemble creation; they represent animals, birds, mountains, flowers and trees such as, *Vṛkṣāsana, Parvatāsana, Dhanurāsana, Padmāsana, Nakrāsana, Śalabhāsana, Vṛśchikāsana, Bhujangāsana, Matsyāsana, Kūrmāsana, Bhekāsana, Kukkuṭāsana, Gomukhāsana, Tiṭṭibhāsana, Mayūrāsana, Haṁsāsana, Śvānāsana, Vātāyanāsana, Uṣṭrāsana, Kapotāsana, Rājakapotāsana, Ganḍabherūṇḍāsana*. The practitioner does not forget *Garbhapīṇḍāsana*, the human embryonic state. Heroes, like *Vīrabhadra, Hanumān* and *Ṛṣis* and divine beings, like *Matsyendra, Gorakṣa, Bharadvāja, Marīci, Kapila, Vaśiṣṭa, Viśvāmitra, Buddha, Kapiñjala, Dūrvāsa, Kāśyapa, Kauṇḍinya, Gheranḍa, Aṣṭāvakra, Vāmadeva*, are revered and remembered through *āsana* as a salvation. Even the incarnations of God are not forgotten. The yogis perform *āsana* like *Anañta, Anañtaśayana, Matsya, Kūrma, Siṁha, Trivikrama* and *Naṭarāja*. This is just to give you a glimpse of how the yogi sees oneness in the creation of God. A yogi sees God in everything and everywhere. *Āsanāni ca tāvanti yāvantyo jīvarāśayaḥ*. It is said that *āsana* are innumerable.

Now I hope you understand why so many *āsana* are there. As there were many species of created beings, the yogis visualised, practised and presented them for us to feel the divinity of God and divinity in His creation throughout practice.

Practice of *āsana* builds one to make the body fit to take the load of spiritual *sādhanā*. When the *sādhaka* gets the precise positioning in the *āsana* and silences the turbulence of *prakṛti*, spiritual maturing comes to him and he feels the unity in diversity and universality in individuality, expressing strength, shape, power, inner beauty, nobility, majesty, excellent dignity and joy. This conveys another facet of *ananta samāpatti*.

In *Darśana Upaniṣad* and *Triśikhi Brāhmaṇōpaniṣad* it is said, *āsanam vijitam ena jitam tena jagatrayam*.

It means that when all *āsana* are perfected, as they should be perfected, then the *sādhaka* has conquered the three worlds: earth, space and heaven. For us, the three worlds are our body, mind and soul. Here forceful effort *(prayatna)*, transforms into a natural *(sahaja)* state, where the feeling of effort automatically dissolves and we no longer feel effort as effort. Know that the above *upaniṣadic* statements are not meant for one *āsana* but for all *āsana*, whether they are easy, difficult, complex or seemingly unnatural. Do not take advantage by saying that seemingly unnatural *āsana* are not possible. The yogis say that all *āsana* have to become natural. When effort *(prayatna)* transforms into a non-enduring, non-struggling and effortless condition, a state of serene tranquillity from nature's turbulence is felt in each and every *āsana*. Patañjali puts the effects of *āsana* in a capsule, *tataḥ dvandvāḥ anabhighātaḥ* – gain or loss, victory or defeat, fame or shame, body or mind, mind or soul, disappear. Actually the space and pause is created between *prakṛti* and *puruṣa* when the presentation of the *āsana* reaches the ultimate state of precision and divinity.

This state and this experience is possible only when you can distinguish *samānāsana* from *viṣamāsana*. *Viṣamāsana* is like a brook with no direction and control, whereas *samānāsana* is like a river flowing within its banks steadily and smoothly. In *prāṇāyāma*, people speak of *samavṛtti prāṇāyāma* and *viṣamavṛtti prāṇāyāma*. But nobody speaks on *āsana*. *Śthira sukham āsanam* of Patañjali, is totally misunderstood and misinterpreted saying that *āsana* means a comfortable sitting position in accord with the limitations of the body and *karmendriyas*. It is like "things move as the wind blows." This way of doing *āsana* becomes *viṣamāsana*. Here, there is no proper adjustment, or alignment of nature's elements or the *tanmātra*. The energy is not balanced properly. The functions of the *sūkṣmendriya* are not properly incorporated. Thus, the actions in *viṣamāsana* are limited to the structural body only.

The practice of *samānāsana* requires a tremendous disciplined, discriminative study. The effects of *āsana* are deeply penetrative of the five sheaths of the body. One has to use intelligence *(buddhi)* and consciousness *(citta)*, with an optimum level of attention and awareness.

An *āsana* is well defined when the *pañcabhūta* and *pañcatanmātra* are used with intelligent attention and awareness to place millions and trillions of cells along with precise distribution of their electro-magnetic power.

The practitioners of *samānāsana (samānāsanābhyasin)* have to intensify their attention *(dhāraṇā)*. Attention and awareness *(dhāraṇā* and *dhyāna)*, with the synthesis of yogic *prajñā* – *vitarka*, *vicāra*, *ānanda* and *āsmitā*, are made to function in every motion, action and feeling on the level of the structural, organic, biological, neurological, mental and intellectual sheaths. When this state is achieved, it becomes *samānāsana*.

Vitarka prajñā functions on the frontal part of the brain and body, *vicāra prajñā* functions on the back of the brain and body. When *vicāra prajñā* is active, *vitarka prajñā* is in shadow. And when *vitarka prajñā* functions, the *vicāra prajñā* fades. When both are attentively internalised and interpenetrated towards the conscience *(antaḥkaraṇa)*, *ānanda* sets in. This *ānanda* does not sprout from the senses but from the inner core. You can call it *sāttvic asmitā*, which in turn flashes the subtlest particle of *prakṛti jñāna*. While practising various *āsana* in sequence, glimpses flash now and then resulting into *sāsmitā jñāna*. This flashing is the feel of the merging of the individual intelligence in the cosmic intelligence, known as *mahat*. Thus, the *jñānapuṣkariṇi* (lakes of knowledge) are full of *sāsmitā jñāna*.

I hope by now you have understood how to practise *āsana*. The body, which is a finite vehicle, acts as a mirror to feel the infinite *ātman*, as it loses the sense of division. All elements and ingredients or evolutes of *prakṛti* lose their individuality or self-identity for the indivisible *puruṣa* to glow in glory. This is the meaning of Patañjali's *prayatna śaithilyatā* that takes one to feel *anañta samāpatti*. If one reads and refers carefully the *sūtra* of Patañjali in IV. 2, one realises that the conjunction of *prakṛti* with *puruṣa* is not a painful process (II.17) since nature's energy flows abundantly and uninterruptedly in one who has reached *sthiratā*, *sukhatā* and *prayatna śaithilyatā* in *āsana*.

Āsana takes you to *anantānanda samāpatti*. Therefore, I feel that *āsana* and *prāṇāyāma* act as two wings of *aṣṭadala yoga* to make the *abhyāsin* move towards the inner, deeper or higher consciousness. The combined practice of *āsana* and *prāṇāyāma* brings the *tribhūta (āp*, *tejas* and *vāyu)*, with their counterparts, *tritanmātra (rasa*, *rūpa* and *sparśa)*, to blend with the *sūkṣmendriya (buddhi)*, so that the pure crystal *(abhijātamaṇi)*, the *ātman*, is traced. This is the end feeling when *āsana* and *prāṇāyāma* are practised with a religious heart in *sādhanā*.

PRĀṆĀYĀMA AND PRATYĀHĀRA

Prāṇa (energy) and *prajñā* (awareness) are interconnected. Where there is *prāṇa*, *prajñā* will be there; and where *prajñā* is, there *prāṇa* rests. In the practice of *prāṇāyāma*, *prāṇa* draws the energy from *viśva caitanya śakti* and *prajñā* draws the awareness from *viśva prajñā śakti*. The drawn in *viśva caitanya śakti* (cosmic energy) and *viśva prajñā śakti* (cosmic intelligence) stir each other. *Prāṇāyāma* charges and energises both *prāṇa* and *prajñā*[1]. *Prāṇa* is energy and *āyāma* is a combination of *dairghya* (extension), *āroha* (expansion) and *viśālatā* (spreading).

Prāṇa śakti can be increased or decreased according to prolongation or curtailment of the inbreath *(pūraka)*, outbreath *(recaka)* or stillness of the breath *(kumbhaka)*. By increasing or decreasing or silencing the *prāṇa vṛtti*, the *citta vṛtti* too can be increased, decreased or silenced[2]. Actually, in *pūraka*, the inner core *(sāsmitā)* expands, extends and spreads while in *recaka* the *bhūta*, *tanmātra*, *sthūlendriya* and *sūkṣmendriya* retrace their path towards the core. In *kumbhaka*, the *ātman* is held in a state of stillness and silence. Thus, *prāṇāyāma* helps the *sādhaka* to hold *prāṇa* and *prajñā* by internalising *buddhi*. *Pratyāhāra* is the steady maintainance of this acquired state of inner quietude and attention. The cloud *(ajñāna)* that darkens the *buddhi* (intelligence) gets removed; the mesh of sensual pleasure that covers *buddhi* disappears and makes it a fit instrument for *dhyāna*.

If *āsana* helps for a firm foundation and stabilises the element of earth *(pṛthvī-tattva)*, *prāṇāyāma* helps us to understand cosmic intelligence *(mahat)* through *buddhi* and to stabilise the elements of air and ether *(vāyu-tattva* and *ākāśa-tattva)*. *Āsana* and *prāṇāyāma* together fuse water, fire and air with their counterparts, taste, form and touch, to sharpen the *sūkṣmendriya* and comprehend *sāsmitā*. Each *āsana* or each stance of *prāṇa śakti* takes shape so that *asmitā* becomes *sāsmitā*. This is what Patañjali explains by the term *anugamāt* – to become that *(sāsmitā)*, and to be that *(sāsmitā)* in the *āsana*. This means the quality of *sattva* totally pervades the *buddhi*. Thus, the effects of *āsana* and *prāṇāyāma* are far, far deeper than our intellectual capacity and capability can grasp.

Prāṇa śakti and *citta śakti* are totally linked in *prāṇāyāma*, destroying the veil of *ajñāna* and making one gain *prajñāna* in order to experience the state of purity *(śuddhatā)*, sanctity *(pavitratā)*, auspicious delight *(sānanda)* and the luminous 'I'-consciousness *(sāsmitā)*. This is just the feel of *pratyāhāra*.

---

[1] *Ibid.*, II.51 and 52.
[2] *Ibid.*, I.34; II.49, 50 and 51.

As students of yoga, we have to observe the five sheaths of the body and at the same time feel the movements of the *tanmātra*, namely, the right touch *(sparśa)*, correct vibration *(śabda)*, the fragrance *(gandha)*, right posturing *(rūpa)* and taste or the flavour *(rasa)*, and feel in *prāṇāyāma* how *ānanda* oozes from the inner core that is bereft of sensory mind.

Dhāraṇā and *dhyāna*

Dhāraṇā means focus of attention and *dhyāna* total absorption. In this state, the intelligence of the head and the intelligence of the heart are blended together to become a single intelligence and a single consciousness. This singleness occurs when *jñāna* is thorough and ripe.

In *dhyāna*, both intelligence and consciousness spread from the source to the periphery, without centripetal or centrifugal force.

The beauty of *dhyāna* is the dissolution of *ahaṁkāra* (impersonator of the Self), and the conscious intelligence changing from a complex state to a single virtuous state.

Hence, *dhyāna* is a means to plough the inner body with intelligence and consciousness so that the weeds in the form of lust, anger, greed and jealousy, do not grow and these two get purified and sanctified with virtuous illumination[1].

In *dhyāna*, the windows of knowledge, namely, the senses of perception, which hanker for objective knowledge, are made to reverse their currents inwards towards the core of being, to gain a subjective state of knowledge through experience. Hence, *dhyāna* is not an expressive theme but a wordless experiencing state. *Dhyāna* traces silence in silence[2].

Samādhi

When awareness of chronological time is lost and the attention of *buddhi* flows uninterruptedly like *tailadhāra* (oil poured steadily from one vessel to another), *dhyāna* automatically becomes *samādhi*. Here, the *guṇa* of nature return to their source leaving the seer to live in his emancipation *(mokṣa)*[3].

---

1 *Ibid.*, I.23, 27, 33, 35, 36, 37, 38, 39, 40, 41, 42; II. 44, 45, 47, 48 and III.1, 2and 55.

2 Please note that *dhyāna* is of three types, namely, *prakāśa* (*sāttvic*), *krīya* (*rājasic*) and *sthiti* (*tāmasic*). Kumbhakarṇa's meditation was *tāmasic*, Rāvaṇa's *rājasic* and Vibhiṣaṇa's *sāttivc*. They were all well versed in the *vedas*. Rāvaṇa and Kumbhakarṇa did penance and won boons from Brahmā. Rāvaṇa carried Kailasa in his hands and Kumbhakarṇa was in deep inertia, while Vibhiṣaṇa was always in the thought of Lord Rāma. Therefore, be careful that though one can reach great spiritual heights, ego and pride may create confusion, and one may lose the path of emancipation.

3 See the Author's *Light on the Yoga Sūtras of Patañjali*, I.3, 17, 18, 19, 48, 51; II.2, 45; IV.34. Published by Harper Collins, London.

Yoga begins with the development of equilibrium, both within and without. It subdues *ahaṁkāra* and sanctifies *buddhi* and *citta,* and then makes the *ātman* spread gracefully in its empire, the body, with splendour. Here, body, mind, intelligence and consciousness become one, pure and divine. This is the *vedānta* of yoga *sādhanā* that makes one transform oneself from *moha* (enamouration) towards *mokṣa* (emancipation).

ENIGMA

Dhāraṇā and *dhyāna* are the *parama sūkṣma* parts of *aṣṭadaḷa yoga.* Here, there is the stage where one may go blank and empty, creating a state of void. One may remain as *videhin* or *prakṛtilayin.* In this state one may feel the loss of body, like angels, or remain an inanimate thing. Stunned in this state with astonishment, one is stupefied. Fear, confusion, perplexity may set in leaving the *sādhaka* in frustration and doubt. This level is the real acid test, known as the touchstone *"kasoṭi"* of the yoga *sādhaka.*

Here the enigma for the *sādhaka* is that he has to test the state of *videhin* or *prakṛtilayin* by rubbing *jñāna* and *prajñā* by appropriate methods or efforts *(abhyāsa)* to come out of this enigma. Those are zeal *(śraddhā bhāva),* vigour *(vīra bhāva),* friendly approach to come back into the body *(maitrī bhāva),* showing compassion *(karuṇā bhāva)* and linking the body *(śarīra)* to the soul *(śarīrī)* and *(muditā bhāva)* to work once again with gladness, break the enigma and go ahead to reach the unalloyed state of *kaivalya.* The *sādhaka* has to conceive the qualities such as zeal, vigour, friendliness, compassion and infuse or instil them in mind. This is known as *bhāva.*

As far as my experience goes, *āsana* and *prāṇāyāma* act as a touchstone to help the *sādhaka* in re-educating and re-building confidence and power, to reach and experience the seasoned and matured intelligence *(ṛtaṁbharā prajñā).* Sage Patanjali also explains in clear terms that as the farmer builds banks in the fields for water to soak in, he wants the energy of *prakṛti* to be controlled and stored so that it is utilised at the time of essential needs (*Y.S.,* IV.3)[1]. Hence, the *sādhaka* has to realise the importance of *āsana* and *prāṇāyāma* even after spiritual achievements.

From here one can move towards *nirbīja prajñā.* When *ṛtaṁbharā prajñā* dawns, non-painful *vṛtti (akliṣṭa vṛtti)* begin. Hence, no painful afflictions *(kliṣṭa kleśa)* will be there at all. With this *ṛtaṁbharā prajñā* he further practises to use the ingredients of *prakṛti* to sharpen his *jñāna* and *prajñā* towards *vivekaja jñāna.* This undoubtedly takes the *sādhaka* to experience the *kaivalyāvasthā,* or *mokṣāvasthā.*

---

[1] *Nimittaṁ aprayojakaṁ prakṛtīnāṁ varaṇabhedaḥ tu tataḥ kṣetrikavat*

Before concluding, let me remind you all that our kingdom *(śarīra* and *citta)* is like the kingdom of Rāvaṇa. He had ten heads which represent in us the five organs of action and the five senses of perception. Though Rāvaṇa had powerful boons from Brahmā, he was caught in lust, and his pride had no bounds which caused his downfall. God has blessed us, turning us towards Him through yoga. But our own nature may take us away from Him.

Probably, all of us have qualities such as vanity, pride and ego in the form of *ahaṁkāra,* which represent the demonic nature hidden in us. Hence, we have to know about another king demon, Hiraṇyākṣa, who in his pride rolled the Mother Earth like a mat and plunged into the ocean with her. He remained there enjoying the destruction of everything on Earth. Goddess Mother Earth prayed to Lord Vishnu who took the form of the Boar (Varāha), dived into the ocean, killed the demon Hiraṇyākṣa and lifted Mother Earth on His horns and rested her in her original place.

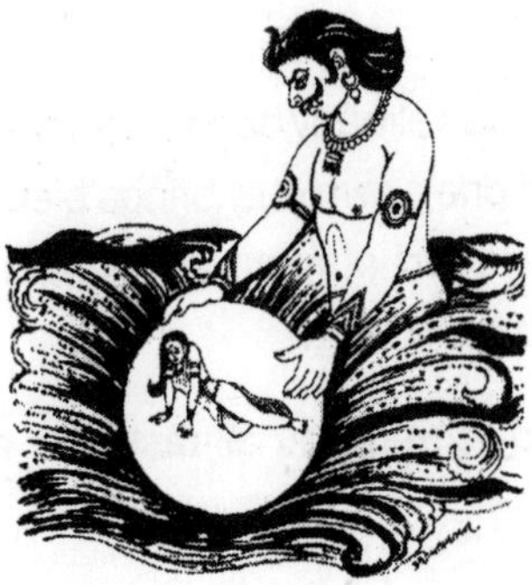

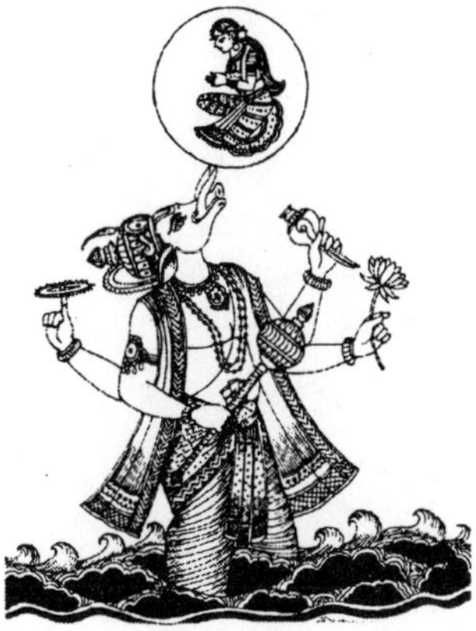

The Mother Earth represents the *sāttvic* and divine qualities such as devotion, faith, love, patience and friendliness. Though we have these qualities of divinity in us as *sādhakas,* the vanity, pride or lust which are demonic qualities may roll and crush all the divine ones and plunge us in the ocean of delusion, infatuation and enamouration.

The Lord residing in each of us saves us, lifts us to evolve intelligently and to reach the highest and the ultimate freedom, which is freedom from sorrow, provided we practise devotedly. This elation is attainable by practising *āsana* and *prāṇāyāma* with reverential attention as a devotee.

Let me remind you before closing, of what Lord Krishna said in the *Bhagavad Gītā.*

Yā niśā sarva bhūtanāṁ tasyām jāgarti saṁyamī /
yasyāṁ jāgrati bhūtāni sā niśā paśyato muneḥ //

(*B.G.,* II.69)

What is night to the evolutes of nature *(prakṛti),* is day for the Self *(puruṣa),* and what is night for the Self is the day for nature.

This is the true essence of what I spoke of, with the interpenetration and internalisation that are observed and followed in the practice of *āsana* and *prāṇāyāma,* so that you live in the waking state of the Self by allowing the *karmendriya, jñānendriya, manas, buddhi, ahaṁkāra, citta* and *antaḥkaraṇa* to go to sleep.

Similarly, when a path is chosen and accepted in the search of Self-realisation, stick to it with steadfastness. The path which you are following becomes the way of life, a religious duty to hold on to even if someone tries to brainwash you that the path you are treading is not a perfect path.

Lord Krishna reminds us not to fall into such traps,

Śreyān svadharmo viguṇaḥ paradharmāt svanuṣṭhitāt /
svadharme nidhanaṁ śreyaḥ paradharmo bhayāvahaḥ //
(B.G., XVIII.47)

It is better to stick with determination on the path that has already been chosen, accepted and carried out imperfectly. Even death in the performance of one's own duty brings blessedness. Turning your coat, thinking that the path you followed is devoid of merit and jumping on to another new path is fraught with confusion and fear even if well done.

So, with steadfast attentive practice of *aṣṭadaḷa yoga,* may you all taste the elixir, the grace of the Self – *ātma-prasāda.*